# Musculoskeletal Examination
## —— of the ——
# Hip and Knee

**Making the Complex Simple**

D1394168

**MUSCULOSKELETAL EXAMINATION**
**MAKING THE COMPLEX SIMPLE**
*SERIES*

*Editor, Steven B. Cohen, MD*

# Musculoskeletal Examination
## of the
# Hip and Knee
## Making the Complex Simple

*Editors:*

*Anil Ranawat, MD*
Sports Medicine and Joint-Preservation
Hospital for Special Surgery
New York, New York

*Bryan T. Kelly, MD*
Sports Medicine and Shoulder Surgery Service
Hospital for Special Surgery
New York, New York

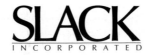

SLACK
INCORPORATED

www.slackbooks.com

# ISBN: 978-1-55642-920-0

Copyright © 2011 by SLACK Incorporated

SLACK Incorporated uses a review process to evaluate submitted material. Prior to publication, educators or clinicians provide important feedback on the content that we publish. We welcome feedback on this work.

Published by:         SLACK Incorporated
                      6900 Grove Road
                      Thorofare, NJ 08086 USA
                      Telephone: 856-848-1000
                      Fax: 856-848-6091
                      www.slackbooks.com

Contact SLACK Incorporated for more information about other books in this field or about the availability of our books from distributors outside the United States.

Library of Congress Cataloging-in-Publication Data

Musculoskeletal examination of the hip and knee : making the complex simple / [ edited by] Anil Ranawat, Bryan T. Kelly.
    p. ; cm.
Includes bibliographical references and index.
ISBN 978-1-55642-920-0 (alk. paper)
1. Hip joint--Examination--Handbooks, manuals, etc. I. Ranawat, Anil S. II. Kelly, Bryan-
[DNLM: 1. Hip Injuries--diagnosis. 2. Diagnostic Techniques and Procedures. 3. Knee Injuries--diagnosis. 4. Musculoskeletal Diseases--diagnosis. WE 855]
  RD772.M87 2011
  617.5'8075--dc22
                              2010030383

Printed in the United States of America.

Last digit is print number: 10  9  8  7  6  5  4  3  2  1

# Contents

Contents    v

# ACKNOWLEDGMENTS

I would like to thank my many mentors who have guided me during my surgical training and career. The list includes many at the Hospital for Special Surgery, University of Pittsburgh, Lennox Hill Hospital, and Schulthess Klinik. However, there are a few individuals who stand out more than the rest. First, my co-editor, Dr. Bryan T. Kelly, has been a friend and mentor. Second, my oldest brother, Dr. Amar Ranawat, has supported, guided, and trained me throughout my entire surgical career. Lastly, I would like to acknowledge my father, Dr. C.S. Ranawat. He has the been the single greatest driving force in my life and career. His advice and example has truly defined the word *mentor*. And of course, I have to thank my wife, Dana, and my 2 children, Cooper and Viviana, who have shown me unwavering love and support. I love you guys and this book is for you.

*Anil Ranawat, MD*

I would first like to acknowledge my co-editor, Dr. Anil Ranawat, who has been the driving force behind this book. His hard work and dedication to further our understanding of the diagnosis and management of injuries to the hip and knee have continuously pushed me to greater heights in my own clinical and research endeavors.

I would also like to acknowledge and thank my primary mentors who have been the foundation of my own knowledge base, surgical and technical tools, and inspiration. Dr. Russell F. Warren has been my constant source of guidance and support from the time that I met him as a medical student in 1995. He has been a role model for the field of sports medicine in general, and for any field that is in the process of active change. His combined efforts in the clinical arena, training room, operating room, and research lab are unsurpassed. Dr. Marc J. Philippon provided me with the opportunity to become an active participant in the field of hip sports injuries and has provided me with the technical tools and clinical skill set that have since formed the primary basis for the majority of my clinical practice. The ever present support of Dr. J. W. Thomas Byrd, Dr. Michael Leunig, and Professor Reinhold Ganz have provided me with a better understanding of the clinical diagnosis and treatment of hip deformity and injury, its challenges, and of all of the opportunity that lies ahead.

Finally, I would like to acknowledge my family, who have provided me with the love, security, and support that has allowed me to pursue my clinical, academic, and research interests. My mother and father have given me all of the opportunity needed to succeed, and my brother, Sean, will always serve as a sounding board and force me to keep life in perspective. My wife, Lois, has selflessly endured the long hours of training, working, and researching, always without complaint and with constant love and support. And my children, Conor, Emma, and Jack, are the 3 people in my life who can always make me smile.

*Bryan T. Kelly, MD*

# ABOUT THE EDITORS

*Anil Ranawat, MD's* research and clinical interest focuses on joint-preserving procedures of both the hip and knee. His interest encompasses nonarthroplasty options of these joint including meniscal, ligament, labral, and capsular surgery with and without concomitant osteotomies. He has a faculty appointment at Weill Medical College of Cornell University in New York, NY and medical staff appointments at Hospital for Special Surgery and New York-Presbyterian Hospital, New York, NY. He refined his area of expertise after his orthopedic residency at the Hospital for Special Surgery by doing 2 years of additional training. He was a sports medicine fellow at the University of Pittsburgh in Pittsburgh, PA, where he focused on knee surgery under Drs. Freddie Fu and Christopher Harner. The following year, he travelled abroad to the Schulthess Klinik in Switzerland where he studied hip surgery under Professor Rheinhold Ganz and Dr. Michael Leunig.

Dr. Ranawat began his academic study at Duke University, Durham, NC, where he attained numerous academic honors. Later, he began his medical training at Weill Medical College and continued his training at Hospital for Special Surgery. Throughout his career, some of the accolades that Dr. Ranawat has received include the T. Campbell Thompson Award for Excellence in Orthopedic Surgery, the Jean C. McDaniel Resident Teaching Award at Hospital for Special Surgery, the Maurice Müller European Traveling Hip Fellowship, and the AAOS Washington Health Policy Fellowship. The latter is evidence of Dr. Ranawat's commitment to providing quality care for all patients, a mission encompassed by his interest in health policy initiatives.

Dr. Ranawat currently serves as the Medical Director of the Physicians Assistants at the Hospital of Special Surgery, Co-Director of Research for Center for Hip Pain and Preservation, Quality Chairman of the Orthopaedic Department of Cornell, and Assistant Team Physician for the New York Mets. Besides his administrative and clinical responsibilities, he has authored over 25 scientific publications, chapters, review articles, and books.

*Bryan T. Kelly, MD* is a specialist in sports medicine injuries and arthroscopic and open surgical management of nonarthritic disorders around the hip. He has faculty appointments at New York Presbyterian's Weill Cornell Medical College as well as the Hospital for Special Surgery (HSS), both in New York, NY. He cares for several sports teams, serving as an associate team physician for the New York Giants and the New York Red Bull's MLS team, as well as team consultant for hip injuries for the New Jersey Nets and several collegiate teams in the tri-state region.

After the completion of his residency at HSS in 2001, Dr. Kelly completed a 2-year fellowship there, specializing in sports medicine and shoulder surgery. Dr. Kelly then completed a fellowship in hip sports injuries and arthroscopy at the University of Pittsburgh Medical Center, Center for Sports Medicine in Pittsburgh, PA under the direction of Dr. Marc J. Philippon. Prior to starting his practice, he also completed an AO International Traveling Fellowship where he spent time with Dr. Herbert Resch at the Landeskliniken Hospital in Salzburg, Austria. He has also spent time with Professor Reinhold Ganz and Dr. Michael Leunig in Bern and Zurich, Switzerland studying advanced techniques in open surgical management of hip injury and deformity through an AO Surgical Preceptorship.

Dr. Kelly currently serves as Co-Director for the Center for Hip Pain and Preservation at HSS, which is designed to provide multi-disciplinary care for patients at all levels with hip injuries. He has a broad range of both clinical and basic science research interests including the development of a clinical outcomes registry; biomechanical studies evaluating conflict patterns in femoroacetabular impingement and techniques in labral refixation; development of synthetic scaffolds for labral reconstruction and cartilage injuries in the hip; and the development of novel surgical techniques for managing soft tissue injuries around the hip joint. He has authored over 75 scientific publications, chapters, review articles, and books.

# CONTRIBUTING AUTHORS

*Olufemi R. Ayeni, MD (Chapter 15)*
Assistant Professor, Orthopedic Surgery
McMaster University
Hamilton, Ontario
Canada

*Martin Beck, MD (Chapter 11)*
Head, Clinic of Orthopaedics
Luzerner Kantonsspital
Lucerne, Switzerland

*Asheesh Bedi, MD (Chapter 7)*
Assistant Professor
Department of Orthopaedic Surgery
University of Michigan
Ann Arbor, Michigan

*James P. Bradley, MD (Chapter 18)*
Clinical Professor, Orthopedic Surgery
Department of Orthopaedic Surgery
University of Pittsburgh School of Medicine
Pittsburgh, Pennsylvania

*Robert L. Buly, MD (Chapter 10)*
Associate Attending Orthopedic Surgeon
Hospital for Special Surgery
Associate Professor
Weill Cornell Medical College
Cornell University
New York, New York

*Sunny Cheung, MD (Chapter 4)*
St. Mary's Specialty Clinic, Orthopedics
Apple Valley, California

*Mark Drakos, MD (Chapter 16)*
Orthopedic Surgery Attending
North Shore—Long Island Jewish Health System
Department of Orthopedics
New Hyde Park, New York

*Freddie H. Fu, MD, DSc(Hon), DPs(Hon) (Chapter 12)*
Distinguished Service Professor
David Silver Professor and Chairman
Department of Orthopaedic Surgery
University of Pittsburgh School of Medicine
Head Team Physician
University of Pittsburgh Athletic Department
Pittsburgh, Pennsylvania

*Reinhold Ganz, MD (Chapter 6)*
Professor Emeritus
Department of Orthopedic Surgery
Inselspital and University of Berne
Bern, Switzerland

*Christopher D. Harner, MD (Chapter 13)*
Blue Cross of Western Pennsylvania Professor, Orthopedic
    Surgery
University of Pittsburgh School of Medicine
Medical Director
UPMC Center for Sports Medicine
Pittsburgh, Pennsylvania

*Victor M. Ilizaliturri Jr, MD (Chapter 9)*
Professor, Hip and Knee Surgery
Universidad Nacional Autónoma de México
Chief, Adult Joint Reconstruction Hip and Knee Service
National Rehabilitation Institute of Mexico
Mexico City, Mexico

*Michael S. H. Kain, MD (Chapter 6)*
Department of Orthopaedic Surgery
Lahey Clinic
Burlington, Massachusetts

*Eric J. Kropf, MD (Chapter 12)*
Assistant Professor, Orthopedic Surgery
Temple University School of Medcine
Division of Sports Medicine
Temple Orthopaedics and Sports Medicine
Philadelphia, Pennsylvania

*Michael Leunig, MD (Chapter 6)*
Head of Orthopedics
Schulthess Clinic and University of Berne
Zürich, Switzerland

*C. Benjamin Ma, MD (Chapter 4)*
Associate Professor
Chief, Sports Medicine and Shoulder Service
University of California, San Francisco
Orthopaedic Insitute
San Francisco, California

*Hal David Martin, DO* (Chapter 1)
Oklahoma Sports Science and Orthopaedics
The Hip Clinic
Oklahoma City, Oklahoma

*RobRoy L. Martin, PhD, PT, CSCS (Chapter 7)*
Associate Professor
Department of Physical Therapy
Duquesne University
Staff Physical Therapist
Center for Sports Medicine
University of Pittsburgh Medical Center
Pittsburgh, Pennsylvania

*Douglas N. Mintz, MD (Chapter 3)*
Radiology Associates of South Florida
Miami, Florida

*Ryan G. Miyamoto, MD (Chapter 8)*
Orthopedic Surgeon
Fair Oaks Orthopaedics
Fairfax, Virginia

*Nicola Mondanelli, MD (Chapter 6)*
Orthopedic Surgeon
Department of Orthopaedics
Azienda Ospedaliero-Universitaria Careggi
Florence, Italy

*Volker Musahl, MD (Chapters 15 and 17)*
Assistant Professor, Orthopedic Surgery
Department of Orthopaedic Surgery
Division of Sports Medicine
University of Pittsburgh Medical Center
Pittsburgh, Pennsylvania

*Michael H. Ngo, MD (Chapter 3)*
Attending Radiologist
Department of Diagnostic Imaging
Kaiser Permanente—Los Angeles Medical Center
Los Angeles, California

*Andrew D. Pearle, MD (Chapter 2)*
Assistant Attending Orthopedic Surgeon
Shoulder and Sports Medicine Division
Hospital for Special Surgery
New York, New York

*Marc J. Philippon, MD (Chapter 8)*
Orthopaedic Surgeon
Steadman Clinic
Vail, Colorado

*Bradley S. Raphael, MD (Chapter 14)*
Sports Medicine Fellow
Kerlan Jobe Orthopaedic Foundation
Los Angeles, California

*Keith R. Reinhardt, MD (Chapter 16)*
Department of Orthopaedic Surgery
Hospital for Special Surgery
New York, New York

*Scott A. Rodeo, MD (Chapter 14)*
Co-chief, Sports Medicine and Shoulder Service
Attending Orthopedic Surgeon
Hospital for Special Surgery
Professor, Orthopedic Surgery
Weill Cornell Medical College
New York, New York

*James R. Romanowski, MD (Chapter 13)*
Director
The Ohio Shoulder Institute
Circleville, Ohio

*Jon K. Sekiya, MD (Chapter 5)*
Associate Professor
MedSport—Department of Orthpaedic Surgery
University of Michigan Medical Center
Ann Arbor, Michigan

*Seth L. Sherman, MD (Chapter 14)*
Orthopedic Sports Medicine Fellow
Rush University
Chicago, Illinois

*Matthew V. Smith, MD (Chapter 5)*
Assistant Professor, Orthopedic Surgery
Sports Medicine
Washington University in St. Louis
Department of Orthopaedic Surgery
St. Louis, Missouri

*Russell F. Warren, MD (Chapter 16)*
Professor, Orthopedics
Weill Cornell Medical College
Surgeon-in-Chief Emeritus
Hospital for Special Surgery
New York, New York

*Thomas L. Wickiewicz, MD (Chapter 17)*
Attending Surgeon
Hospital for Special Surgery
Professor of Clinical Orthopaedic Surgery
Weill Cornell Medical College
Cornell University
New York, New York

*Riley J. Williams III, MD (Chapter 15)*
Associate Attending Orthopedic Surgeon
Hospital for Special Surgery
Associate Professor
Weill Cornell Medical College
Cornell University
New York, New York

*Andrew K. Wong, MD (Chapter 12)*
Resident
University of Southern California
Department of Internal Medicine
Los Angeles, California

# PREFACE

Orthopedic surgery has gone through natural evolutionary progression over the last 100 years. The field was originally a nonoperative specialty focusing on fracture management and bracing for debilitating diseases such as polio and tuberculosis. In the early 1960s, pioneering Swiss and German surgeons were the first to question authority with their revolutionary approach to fracture care championing principles of operative fracture reduction and internal fixation. In the late 1960s and early 1970s, UK and US surgeons as well as innovators around the world began championing arthroplasty of the hip and knee. These procedures eventually proved to be both incredibly successful and durable. They have been shown to decrease both morbidity and mortality associated with debilitating arthritic conditions. In the late 1970s and into the 1980s, less invasive surgical approaches, specifically knee arthroscopy, became much more widespread. These methods, which focused on a younger patient population, explored concepts of maintaining and improving joint function prior to the onset of arthritis. In the late 1990s, nonarthroplasty hip surgery experienced a renaissance with the advent of femoro-acetabular impingement and, more recently, the explosion of hip arthroscopy. In the 2000s, orthopedics has ventured into a biological revolution. Over the last 100 years, many ideas have been proven ineffective (ie, medial inserts) and many others have seen rebirths (osteotomies). The future is still uncertain, but joint preservation and biological arthroplasty appears to be the next great orthopedic revolution.

This book focuses on two fundamental concepts. First, orthopedic procedures will constantly evolve and change, but the principles of anatomy, joint stability, kinematics, and biologic function are more constant. Second, this books attempts to simplify the increasingly complex and emerging field of joint preservation of the hip and knee by making the complex simple.

# FOREWORD

It is indeed an honor for me to provide the Foreword for Drs. Anil Ranawat and Bryan T. Kelly's book on the diagnosis and treatment of hip and knee sports injuries. Actually, I am doubly honored since I was asked to contribute a chapter for the book on the anterior cruciate ligament.

In 2003, Bryan joined our department here at Pitt for a hip arthroscopy fellowship, and Anil was my sports medicine fellow in 2006. I worked closely with both of them here in Pittsburgh, and now they are leaders in the subspecialty of sports medicine and teaching their fellows about how to diagnose and treat sports injuries.

This book is one in a series of 5 books edited by Dr. Steven B. Cohen. Steve also was my sports medicine fellow here at Pitt.

In *Musculoskeletal Examination of the Hip and Knee: Making the Complex Simple*, Drs. Ranawat and Kelly and their contributing authors are, as the title states, trying to make the complex simple by providing the reader with a simplified approach to complicated hip and knee pathologies.

*Freddie H. Fu, MD, DSc(Hon), DPs(Hon)*
Distinguished Service Professor
David Silver Professor and Chairman
Department of Orthopaedic Surgery
University of Pittsburgh School of Medicine
Head Team Physician
University of Pittsburgh Athletic Department
Pittsburgh, Pennsylvania

# Introduction

The diagnosis and treatment of nonarthritic hip and knee disease can be challenging. As weight-bearing joints, dysfunction in the hip and knee can significantly affect one's ability to perform both activities of daily living and sports. Although total hip and knee replacement have proven to be highly successful operations to eliminate pain and improve quality of life, recent advancement in joint preservation have revolutionized the diagnosis, prevention, and treatment of non-arthritic hip and knee pathologies.

This book will cover various topics starting from the basics of the physical exam of hip and knee to the most advanced imaging techniques such as modern MRI cartilage mapping. The focus of this book is to provide a simple approach for the diagnosis and treatment of common pathologies of the hip and knee. These topics include basic meniscal, labral, and cartilage injuries as well as more complex entities such as collateral knee injuries, femoroacetabular impingement, and hip instability. A further aim of this book is to emphasize simple pearls of procedures such as ACL reconstruction, high tibial osteotomy, hip abductor tears, and open hip osteotomies.

The authors of each chapter are highly knowledgeable hip and knee surgeons with vast experience in each topic. Each chapter focuses on common pathologies and outlines the basics and guiding principles of physical exam, diagnosis, and treatment. Each section aims to provide simple algorithms and pearls in the treatment of each of these hip and knee topics while maintaining a comprehensive approach. We hope that this book will be widely used by medical students, residents, fellows, attendings, physical therapists, and other health care providers.

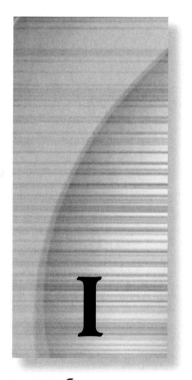

# I

# Physical Examination

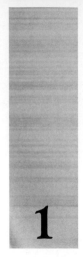

**1**

# PHYSICAL
# EXAMINATION OF
# THE HIP
## *THE BASICS AND SPECIFIC TESTS*

*Hal David Martin, DO*

## INTRODUCTION

The clinical examination of the hip continues to evolve as our understanding advances with newer surgical techniques. Recognition of current hip conditions are a reflection of the contributions by many generations of physicians and surgeons. The utilization of a battery of tests will aid in the early recognition of the hip as the underlying source of pain. A consistent method of performing the history and clinical examination of the hip is important to this objective. The goal of this chapter is to describe how to perform a detailed and comprehensive clinical examination of the hip and to explain why these tests are important.

Ranawat A, Kelly BT. *Musculoskeletal Examination of the Hip and Knee: Making the Complex Simple* (pp. 2-41).
© 2011 SLACK Incorporated

# HISTORY AND PHYSICAL EXAMINATION

## History

Prior to the physical examination of the hip, the patient history is noted. The first factor for consideration of treatment is the age of the patient and the presence or absence of trauma.[1] An account of the present condition is noted, including the date of onset, the presence or absence of trauma, mechanisms of injury, pain location, and factors that increase or decrease the pain. Prior treatments such as rest, physical therapy, ice, heat, nonsteroidal anti-inflammatory drugs, surgery, injections, orthotics, or the use of support aids must be clearly defined. Functional status and current limitations of the patient are recorded, which include getting in or out of a bathtub or car, activities of daily living, jogging, walking, and/or climbing stairs. Related symptoms of the back, abdomen, lower extremities, or neurological system must also be recorded. The presence of associated complaints such as abdominal or back pain, numbness, weakness, sit pain, length of time sitting, and cough or sneeze exacerbation helps to rule out thoracolumbar issues, which is occasionally confused with the hip as a portion or dominant cause of complaint pain.

The location of the presenting pain and the presence or absence of popping will aid in the determination of intra-articular versus extra-articular etiology. Potential sources of disruption to the vascular supply of the femoral head are screened, including metabolic disorders, such as abnormality of lipids, thyroid, homocysteine, and clotting function. The presence or use of tobacco, alcohol, steroids, or altitude issues can also affect the blood supply to the femoral head and are routinely recognized through a review of the patient's social history. Participation in sports and other activities is documented, which can help determine the type of injury because rotation sports such as golf, tennis, ballet, and martial arts have been commonly associated with injuries to the intra-articular structures, including the labrum, iliofemoral ligament, and ligamentum teres.

Finally, treatment goals and expectations are reviewed with the patient. Treatment may vary based upon the patient's expectations and postoperative goals. Unrealistic goals should be addressed before any diagnostic testing and treatment recommendations are given. The expected outcome for each option should be explained thoroughly and completely. Clear communication, time, understanding, empathy, and compassion are of paramount importance in working through differences in expectations and can save much undue hardship later.

A gross level of function is quantified with the use of the Modified Harris Hip Score (HHS) or Merle d'Aubigné (MDA). The modified HHS (Table 1-1) is the most documented and standardized functional score to date that is a quantitative score based on pain and function. However, the high-performing athletic population may be best evaluated by the Athletic Hip Score.[2] Other hip scores for use in more specific patient populations include the Non-Arthritic Hip Score (NAHS), Hip Disability and Osteoarthritis Outcome Score (HOOS), Musculoskeletal Function Assessment (MFA), Short Form 36 (SF-36), and the Western Ontario and McMaster University Osteoarthritis Index (WOMAC).[3] The Hip Outcomes Score (HOS), currently under analysis by the Multicenter Arthroscopy of the Hip Outcomes Research Network (MAHORN) Group, will provide an internationally accepted score and will be useful for the athletic population.[4] This test will help to compare the outcomes and provide a consensus for comparison between examiners, as well as between different centers. The use of a verbal analog score is also subjectively useful.

## The Physical Examination of the Hip

A comprehensive examination of the hip is performed quickly and efficiently to screen the hip, back, abdominal, neurovascular, and neurologic systems and to identify any comorbidities that may coexist with complex hip pathology. It is important that the physical examination of the hip be inclusive enough to rule out other joints as a possible cause of pain. Each examination or physical evaluation has a specific way to be performed, although the inter-observer consistency and practice is one of the most important aspects of the evaluation.[5]

**Table 1-1**

# MODIFIED HARRIS HIP SCORE

## Pain

44  None/ignores

40  Slight, occasional, no compromise in activity

30  Mild, no effect on ordinary activity, pain after usual activity, uses aspirin

20  Moderate, tolerable, makes concessions, occasional codeine

10  Marked, serious limitations

0  Totally disabled

## Function: Gait Limp

11  None

8  Slight

5  Moderate

0  Severe

0  Unable to walk

## Support

11  None

7  Cane, long walks

5  Cane, full-time

4  Crutch

2  2 canes

0  2 crutches

0  Unable to walk

## Distance Walked

11  Unlimited

8  6 blocks

5  2 to 3 blocks

2  Indoors only

0  Bed and chair

## Functional Activities

### STAIRS

4  Normally

2  Normally with banister

1  Any method

0  Not able

### SOCKS/SHOES

4  With ease

2  With difficulty

0  Unable

### SITTING

5  Any chair, 1 hour

3  High chair, ½ hour

0  Unable to sit, ½ hour, any chair

### PUBLIC TRANSPORTATION

1  Able to enter public transportation

0  Unable to use public transportation

*Total Points* _____ x 1.1= _____

*(Total Score)*

The Modified HHS is calculated out of 91 points for pain and function, which is multiplied by 1.1 to give a total possible score of 100.

(Reprinted with permission from *Arthroscopy*, 16(6), Byrd JW, Jones KS, Prospective analysis of hip arthroscopy with 2-year follow up. Copyright 2004 Elsevier.)

Hip complaints are often complex, requiring a thorough assessment in order to separate the co-morbidities that frequently exist. The technique of physical examination is dependent upon the examiner's experience and efficiency. The sequence of the examination is one that is easy on the patient and the flow for the physician and an assistant, if available. The most efficient method of examination begins with standing tests followed by seated, supine, lateral, and ending with prone tests (Table 1-2).[6,7] It is important to schedule a sufficient amount of time with the patient to allow for a comprehensive assessment.[6,7] Most hip examiners have a structured examination that is generally used in all cases and helps to differentiate the specific pathologies upon presentation. The physical examination will be fine-tuned and directed through the review of the history of present illness.

Access for exposure and patient comfort with loose fitting clothes about the waist are helpful. An assistant to record the examination is useful in accuracy and documentation of the examination. A standardized data form aids in the accuracy of the exam record, especially when first starting a comprehensive hip evaluation or when the presentation is complex.

The MAHORN Group identified common trends among hip specialists in the physical examination of the hip. Common standing tests included gait analysis, single leg stance phase test, and laxity. Common supine tests included range of motion (ROM) of hip flexion, internal and external hip ROM, impingement testing, palpation, flexion/abduction/external rotation (FABER), straight leg raise against resistance, muscular strength, passive supine rotation, and the posterior rim impingement test. Common lateral tests included palpation, passive adduction tests, and abductor strength. In the prone position, the femoral anteversion test was commonly performed. The following physical examination of the hip is inclusive of these points.

## INSPECTION

As the patient stands, a general point of pain is noted with one finger and can usually help to direct the examination. The groin region directs a suspicion of intra-articular problems,

**Table 1-2**

## PHYSICAL EXAMINATION OF THE HIP INTAKE FORM

**PHYSICAL EXAMINATION:** HT: _____ WT: _____ T: _____ R: _____
P: _____ BP: _____

### GAIT/POSTURE:

- Shoulder height:    equal        not equal
- Iliac crest height:    equal        not equal
- Active Forward Bend:    _____ degrees
- Spine:    straight
  Scoliosis:    structural        non-structural
- Recurvatum: thumb test elbows        knees        >5 degrees
- Lordosis: normal        increased        paravertebral muscle spasms
- Gait:        normal                antalgic                    pelvic wink
              arm swing            short stride length        short stance phase
              abductor deficient (Trendelenburg)
  Foot progression angle:        external        neutral        hyperpronation
- Single leg stance phase test (Trendelenburg test):        R _____ L _____

### SEATED EXAMINATION:

- Neurologic findings:
  Motor:        _____
  Sensory:        _____
  DTR:        Achilles _____        Patella _____
- Circulation:  DP _____        PT _____
- Skin inspection:   _____
- Lymphatic: lymphedema        no lymphedema        pitting edema: 1+  2+
- Straight leg raise:    R _____    L _____
- Range of motion:   Internal rotation:                External rotation:
                            R _____    L _____            R _____    L _____

### SUPINE EXAMINATION:

- Leg lengths:    R _____ cm        L _____ cm        equal/not equal
- ROM:        Right leg                        Left leg
  Flexion:        80  100  110  120  130  140        80  100  110  120  130  140
  Abduction:  10  20    30    45    50    10        20  30    45    50
  Adduction:  0    10    20    30                        0    10    20    30

(continued)

**Table 1-2 (continued)**

## PHYSICAL EXAMINATION OF THE HIP INTAKE FORM

- Hip flexion contracture test (Thomas test):    R + -   L + -
  FADDIR:    R + -   L + -
- DIRI:    R + -   L + -
- DEXRIT:    R + -   L + -
  Posterior rim impingement test:    R + -   L + -
  Apprehension sign:    R + -   L + -
- Abdomen:    tender   non-tender
- Adductor tubercle:    tender   non-tender
- Palpation pubic symphysis/adductor    tender   non-tender
- Tinels—femoral nerve    R + -   L + -
- FABER (Patrick test):    R + -   L + -
- Straight leg raise against resistance
  (Stitchfield test):    R + -   L + -
- Passive supine rotation test (log roll test):    R + -   L + -
- Heel strike:    R + -   L + -

**LATERAL EXAMINATION:**

- Palpation:
  SI joint    tender   non-tender
  Ischium    tender   non-tender
  Greater trochanter    tender   non-tender
  ASIS    tender   non-tender
  Piriformis    tender   non-tender
  Tinels—sciatic nerve
  G. Max insertion into ITB    tender   non-tender
  Sciatic nerve    tender   non-tender
  Gluteus medius    tender   non-tender
  Abductor strength:
  　　Straight leg _____ Gluteus max_____ Gluteus medius _____
- Tensor fascia lata contracture test:    Grade (1-3)____
- Gluteus medius contracture test:    Grade (1-3)____
- Gluteus maximus contracture test:    Grade (1-3)____
- Lateral rim impingement test:    R + -   L + -
- FADDIR test:    R + -   L + -

*(continued)*

**Table 1-2 (continued)**

## PHYSICAL EXAMINATION OF THE HIP INTAKE FORM

**PRONE EXAMINATION:**

- Rectus contracture test (Ely's test):     R + -   L + -
- Femoral anteversion test (Craig's test): _____ degrees anteversion
- Palpation:
  Spinous processes    +         -
  SI joints              R + -  L + -
  Bursae ischium

**SPECIFIC TESTS:**

Philippon internal rotation test
McCarthy's sign
Scours
Foveal distraction
Leunig bicycle test
Fulcrum
Seated piriformis stretch test
Pace sign
ABDEER
Sampson dynamic trendelenberg

and lateral-based pain is primarily associated with both intra- or extra-articular aspects. A characteristic sign of patients with hip pain is the "C Sign."[5] The patient will hold his or her hand in the shape of a C and place it above the greater trochanter with the thumb positioned posterior to the trochanter and fingers extending into the groin.[5] This can be misinterpreted as lateral soft tissue pathology, such as trochanteric bursitis or the iliotibial band; however, the patient is often describing deep interior hip pain.[5] Posterior-superior pain requires a thorough evaluation in differentiating hip and back pain. Back issues are many times noted concomitantly with musculotendonous hip pathology.

General body habitus is assessed, and issues of ligamentous laxity are determined by the thumb test or hyperextension of the elbows or knees (Figures 1-1C and D). With the patient in the standing position, shoulder height and iliac crest heights are noted to evaluate leg length discrepancies (Figure 1-1A). Incremental wooden blocks placed under the short side heel aid in orthotic considerations. Leg lengths are also assessed with the patient in the supine position (Figure 1-2A). Structural versus nonstructural scoliosis is differentiated by forward bending, and the degree of spinal motion is recorded (Figure 1-1B).

Gait abnormalities often help to detect hip pathology due to the hip's role in supporting body weight (Table 1-3). Joint stability, preservation of the labrum and articular cartilage, and proper functioning of the hip joint involve 3 biomechanical planes of the femur and acetabulum. These relationships are important for the transfer of dynamic and static load to the ligamentous and osseous structures.[8] The ligamentous capsule must maintain the stability of the hip while the musculature of the lower limbs produce the forces required during ambulation and play a part in hip stability.[8] This is especially important with connective tissue disorders and improper osseous alignment, emphasizing the importance of adequate rehabilitation.

The patient is taken into the hallway so that a full gait of 6 to 8 stride lengths can be observed (Figures 1-1E and F). Key points of gait evaluation include foot rotation (internal/external progression angle), pelvic rotation in the X and Y axes, stance phase, and stride length. Gait viewed from the foot progression angle will detect the possibility of osseous or static rotatory malalignment as exists with increased or decreased femoral anteversion versus capsular or musculotendonous issues. The knee and thigh are observed simultaneously to assess any rotatory parameters. The knee may want to be held in either the internal or external rotation to allow proper patellofemoral joint alignment, but may produce a secondary abnormal hip rotation. This abnormal motion is usually present in cases of severe increased femoral anteversion precipitating a battle between the hip and knee for a comfortable position that will affect the gait. In cases of a painful gait, note the anatomical location of pain and at what point within the gait phase pain presents.

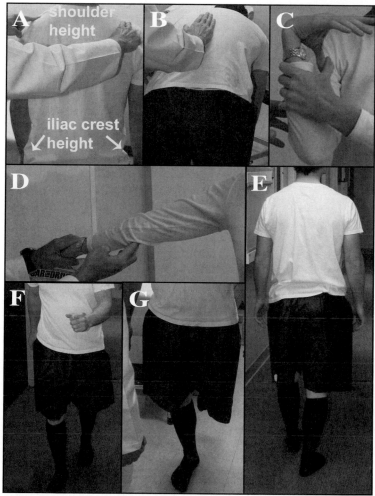

**Figure 1-1.** Standing tests. (A) Shoulder and iliac crest heights are examined with the patient with dynamic loading of the hip joint in the standing position. (B) As the patient bends forward at the trunk, spinal alignment is palpated. The degree of trunkal flexion is noted in full flexion. (C) Laxity of the thumb. (D) Recurvatum of the elbow. (E, F) The patient is taken into the hallway so that 6 to 8 stride lengths can be observed from behind and in front of the patient. Gait evaluation includes foot rotation, stance phase, stride length, pelvic rotation, pelvic shift, and terminal hip extension. (G) The single leg stance phase test is performed bilaterally and observed from behind and in front of the patient. The patients hold this position for 6 seconds. A pelvic shift of greater than 2 cm is positive, indicating abductor weakness or proprioception disruption.

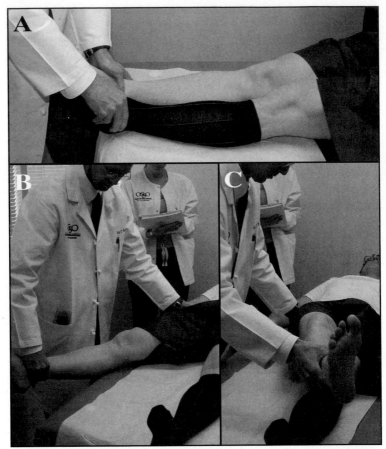

**Figure 1-2.** Supine inspection and range of motion tests. (A) Leg lengths are evaluated in the supine (unloaded) position for comparison to the dynamic (loaded) standing evaluation. The supine position easily allows for (B) passive abduction and (C) adduction range of motion.

Pelvic rotation is assessed by noting iliac crest rotation and terminal hip extension. On average, normal gait requires 8 degrees of hip rotation and 7 degrees of pelvic rotation, equaling a total rotation of 15 degrees.[9] The pelvic wink is demonstrated by an excessive rotation in the axial plane toward the affected hip, thus producing extension and rotation through the lumbar spine to obtain terminal hip extension.

## Table 1-3

### GAIT ASSESSMENT AND INSPECTION SUMMARY

| Examination | Assessment/Association |
| --- | --- |
| Abductor deficient gait | Abductor strength, proprioception mechanism |
| Antalgic | Trauma, fracture, synovial inflammation |
| Pelvic rotational wink | Intra-articular pathology, hip flexion contracture, increased femoral anteversion, anterior capsule laxity |
| Foot progression angle with excessive external rotation | Femoral retroversion, increased acetabular anteversion, torsional abnormalities, effusion, ligamentous injury |
| Foot progression angle with excessive internal rotation | Increased femoral anteversion or acetabular retroversion, torsional abnormalities |
| Short leg limp | Iliotibial band pathology, true/false leg length discrepancy |
| Spinal alignment | Shoulder/iliac crest heights, lordosis, scoliosis, leg length |
| Laxity | Ligamentous laxity in other joints: thumb, elbows, shoulders, or knee |
| Femoral anteversion test (Craig's test) | Detect increased femoral anteversion or retroversion, ligamentous injury, hyperlaxity |

This winking gait can be associated with laxity or hip flexion contractures, especially when combined with increased lumbar lordosis or a forward-stooping posture. Gait changes can affect spinal mechanics and function. Excessive femoral anteversion, or retroversion, can affect a wink on terminal hip extension as the patient will try to create greater anterior coverage with a rotated pelvis. Injury to the anterior capsule can also attribute to a winking gait.

During the stance phase, body weight must be supported by a single leg with the gluteus maximus, gluteus medius, and gluteus minimus providing the majority of support forces. Maximum ground reactive force occurs upon heel strike at 30 degrees of hip flexion.[9] A shortened stance phase can be indicative of neuromuscular abnormalities, trauma, or leg length discrepancies. The abductor deficient gait (common nomenclature: Trendelenburg Gait or abductor lurch) is an unbalanced stance phase attributed to abductor weakness or proprioception disruption. The abductor deficient gait may present in 2 ways: with a shift of the pelvis away from the body (a "dropping out" of the hip on the affected side) or with a shift of the weight over the adducted leg (a shift of the upper body "over the top" of the affected hip). The antalgic gait is characterized by a shortened stance phase on the painful side, limiting the duration of weight bearing (a self-protecting limp caused by pain). A short leg gait is noted by the drop of the shoulder in the direction of the short leg. In abduction gait testing, dysplastic hips will have a reduction in pain, and this observation can aid in the direction of treatment. Excessive external foot progression angle is often associated with decreased femoral anteversion, or retroversion. Decreased foot progression angle, zero or internal, is contrasted in the opposite direction and may be associated with increased femoral anteversion.

The femoral anteversion test (traditionally known as Craig's test) will give the examiner a generalized idea of femoral anteversion/retroversion (Figure 1-3B). With the patient in the prone position, the knee is flexed to 90 degrees, and the examiner manually rotates the leg while palpating the greater trochanter. The examiner positions the greater trochanter so that it protrudes most laterally, thereby placing the femoral head into the center portion of the acetabulum.[10] Femoral anteversion/retroversion is assessed by noting the angle between the axis of the tibia and an imaginary vertical line. Normally, femoral anteversion is between 10 and 20 degrees. This test will help to identify cases of retroversion.

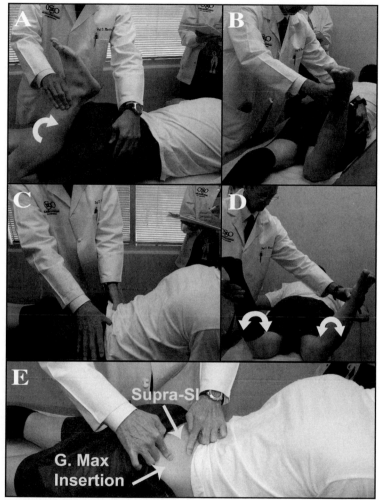

**Figure 1-3.** Prone tests. (A) The rectus contracture test. The lower extremity is flexed toward the gluteus maximus. Any raise of the pelvis or restriction of hip flexion motion is indicative of rectus femoris contracture. (B) The femoral anteversion test. The knee is flexed to 90 degrees, and the examiner manually rotates the leg while palpating the greater trochanter. The examiner positions the greater trochanter so that it protrudes most laterally, noting the angle between the axis of the tibia and an imaginary vertical line. (C) Palpation of the SI joint with lumbar hyperextension. (D) Internal and external rotation in the extended position. Note any side-to-side differences or differences from the seated flexed position. (E) Palpation of the supra-SI and gluteus maximus origin.

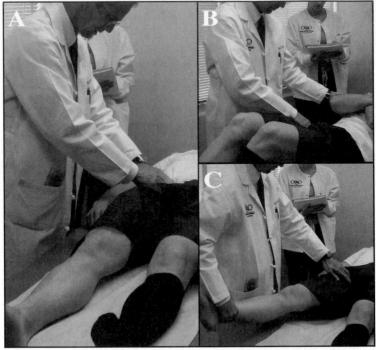

**Figure 1-4.** Supine palpation tests. (A, B) Palpation of the abdomen in the relaxed supine position and with an abdominal contraction. (C) Palpation of the adductor tubercle.

# PALPATION

Palpation of the abdomen is performed with the patient in the supine position, and any abdominal tenderness is appreciated (Figure 1-4A). Abdominal tenderness is differentiated from fascial hernia and/or adductor tendonitis. Resisted torso flexion with palpation of the abdomen will differentiate the fascial hernia from other complaints (Figure 1-4B). Palpation of the adductor tubercle with active testing will detect adductor tendonitis (Figure 1-4C). Common physical exam findings associated with athletic pubalgia include inguinal canal tenderness, pubic crest/tubercle tenderness, adductor origin tenderness, pain with resisted sit-ups or hip flexion, and a tender, dilated superficial ring (Table 1-4).[11]

**Table 1-4**

## SUMMARY OF PALPATION

| Examination | Assessment/Association |
|---|---|
| **SUPINE POSITION** | |
| 1. Abdomen | Fascial hernia, associated gastrointestinal/genitourinary pathology |
| 2. Pubic symphysis | Osteitis pubis, calcification, fracture, trauma |
| 3. Adductor tubercle | Adductor tendonitis |
| **LATERAL POSITION** | |
| 1. Greater trochanter | Greater trochanter bursitis, iliotibial band contracture |
| 2. Sacroiliac joint | Distinguish between hip and back pathology |
| 3. Maximus origin | Gluteus maximus origin tendonitis |
| 4. Ischium | Biceps femoris tendonitis, avulsion fracture, ischial bursitis |
| **PRONE POSITION** | |
| 1. Supra-SI | Mechanical transverse process ilial conflict |
| 2. SI | Sacroilitis |
| 3. Gluteus max insertion | G maximus tendonitis |
| 4. Spine | Detect spinal mechanical pathology |
| 5. With lumbar hyperextension | Rule out spine as a prominent or secondary issue |

The lateral position, with the patient on the contralateral side, allows for palpation of the supra-SI and SI joint, muscles of abduction, and in particular the origin of the gluteus maximus as it inserts along the lateral border of the sacrum, as well as the most posterior aspect of the ilium (Figure 1-5). The next point of palpation is the ischium for detection of avulsions or bursitis (Figure 1-5B). Additionally, the piriformis and sciatic nerve are palpated for any sign of tenderness, along with the abductor musculature, which includes the gluteus maximus, gluteus medius, gluteus minimus, and tensor fascia lata.

The prone position allows for further palpation of 4 distinct areas: the supra-SI, SI, gluteus maximus origin, and spine (facet), identifying the exact area of complaint (see Figures 1-3C and E). Should the pain be identified in the supra-SI joint region in or about the facet, a lumbar hyperextension test can help to identify exact location of suspected pain. If this test is positive, the patient can then be placed into a supine position with knees flexed. If this helps to alleviate the pain, the back should be further evaluated.

## SURFACE ANATOMY

The bony landmarks of the hip are easily recognized in the average individual. In the lateral view of the hip (Figure 1-6), the most prominent landmark is the iliac crest located at the most superior aspect of the pelvis. Distal to the iliac crest is the bony landmark of the greater trochanter as it protrudes laterally from the gluteal region. Two of the gluteal muscles can be identified posterior and superior to the greater trochanter. The largest muscle group in the hip is the gluteus maximus located posterior to the greater trochanter, which arises from the posterior ilium and adjacent sacrum. Superior to the greater trochanter is the gluteus medius, which arises from the superior portion of the iliac wing and inserts on the greater trochanter. The gluteus medius can be felt with hip abduction. Anterior to the gluteus medius is the tensor fascia lata forming the anterior border of the lateral view of the hip. Distal to the greater trochanter, forming the anterior and posterior shape of the thigh, are the vastus lateralis and biceps femoris, respectively. The iliotibial band (ITB) is found bordering the vastus lateralis, which is seen at the distal third of the thigh as it narrows toward its insertion on the tibia.

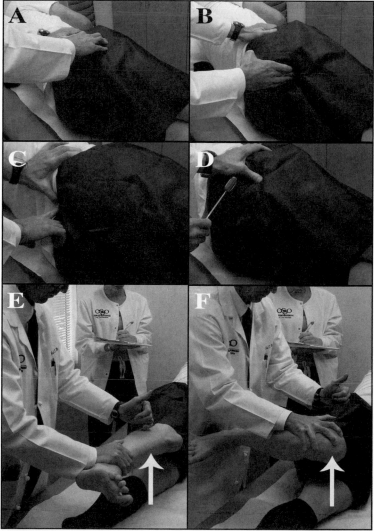

**Figure 1-5.** Lateral palpation and strength assessment. Palpation of the (A) greater trochanter region—gluteus maximus origin, gluteus medius, and bursae; (B) ischium; (C) supra-SI and SI region; and (D) tinels of the sciatic nerve. (E) Gluteus maximus strength is evaluated by active hip abduction with knee extension. (F) Gluteus medius strength is evaluated by having the patient perform active hip abduction with knee flexion.

**Figure 1-6.** Lateral view surface anatomy of the hip. GT, greater trochanter; GMax, gluteus maximus; GMed, gluteus medius; TFL, tensor fascia lata; BF, biceps femoris; VL, vastus lateralis; ITB, iliotibial band.

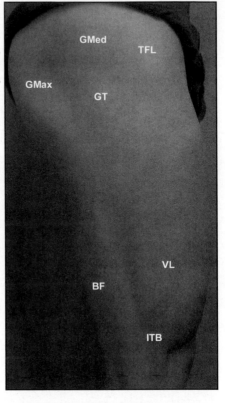

The curve of the iliac crest is the prominent bony landmark of the posterior view of the hip, which curves posteromedially to the posterior superior iliac spine (PSIS). Distal to the PSIS is the sacroiliac joint, which proceeds longitudinally distal from the PSIS. The large gluteus maximus covers much of the posterior landmarks of the hip. The lateral prominence of the greater trochanter can be identified and palpated from the posterior view. The ischial tuberosity is the most inferior portion of the pelvis and is covered by the gluteus maximus. Deep palpation of the inferior portion of the gluteus maximus will allow for locating the ischial tuberosity. Hip flexion will help to identify the ischial tuberosity. Location of the ischial tuberosity is important for evaluation of hip pain as the sciatic nerve lies lateral to this structure and medial to the greater trochanter (Figure 1-7).[12] Medial to the ischial tuberosity lies the pudendal nerve as it enters Alcock's canal.

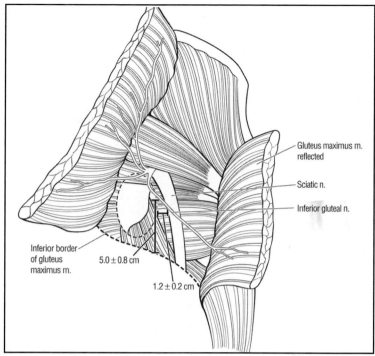

Gluteus maximus m. reflected

Sciatic n.

Inferior gluteal n.

Inferior border of gluteus maximus m.

5.0 ± 0.8 cm

1.2 ± 0.2 cm

**Figure 1-7.** Anatomical locations of the inferior gluteal nerve and sciatic nerve. Posterior, right-sided view. At the lateral border of the ischium, the inferior gluteal nerve is an average of 5.0 ± 0.8 cm from the distal border of the gluteus maximus, and the sciatic nerve is an average of 1.2 ± 0.2 cm from the most lateral aspect of the ischial tuberosity. (Reprinted with permission from Miller SL, Gill J, Webb GR. The proximal origin of the hamstrings and surrounding anatomy encountered during repair. A cadaveric study. *J Bone Joint Surg.* 2007;89(1):44-48.)

# RANGE OF MOTION

The loss of internal rotation is one of the first signs for the possibility of intra-articular disorder; therefore, one of the most important assessments is the internal and external rotation in the seated position (Figures 1-8E and F). The seated position ensures that the ischium is square to the table, thus providing sufficient stability at 90 degrees of hip flexion and a reproducible platform for the accurate rotational measurement. Passive internal and external rotation testing

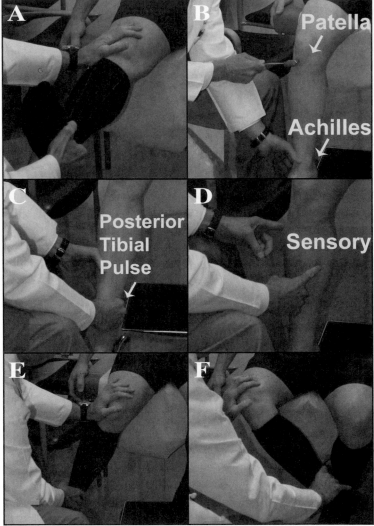

**Figure 1-8.** Seated tests. (A) The patient performs an active straight leg raise, useful for detecting radicular neurological symptoms. (B) Deep tendon reflexes are assessed at the patella and Achilles tendons. (C) Vascular examination of the dorsalis pedis and posterior tibial arteries. (D) Sensory evaluation by lightly touching both sides of the patient's lower leg and asking the patient to compare the sensation with the other leg. (E,F) Passive internal and external rotation testing is compared from side to side. In the seated position, the ischium is square to the table, thus providing sufficient stability at 90 degrees of hip flexion. Internal and external rotation in the seated position offers a reproducible platform for the accurate rotational measurement.

is performed gently and is compared from side to side. Seated rotation ROM is also compared and contrasted to the extended position of the hip (see Figure 1-3D).

Musculotendonous, ligamentous, and osseous control of internal and external rotation is complex; therefore, any differences in seated versus extended positions may raise the question of ligamentous versus osseous abnormality. Sufficient internal rotation is important for proper hip function as there should be at least 10 degrees of internal rotation at the mid-stance phase of normal gait,[9] but less than 20 degrees is abnormal and poorly tolerated for normal activity (Table 1-5). The loss of internal rotation at the hip can be related to diagnoses such as arthritis, effusion, internal derangements, slipped capital femoral epiphysis, and muscular contracture. Pathology related to femoroacetabular impingement or to rotational constraint from increased or decreased femoral acetabular anteversion can result in significant side-to-side differences. An increased internal rotation combined with a decreased external rotation may indicate excessive femoral anteversion, although the hip capsular function will require further assessment, which is correlated with the radiographic and biometric findings.

Passive abduction and adduction ROM is easily assessed in the supine position (see Figures 1-2B and C). Also in the supine position, passive hip flexion ROM is assessed as both knees are brought up to the chest and the degree of flexion is recorded (Figure 1-9A). It is important to note the pelvic position as the hip may stop early in flexion with the end ROM being predominately pelvic rotation. From this position, the hip flexion contracture test (also known as the Thomas test) is performed by having the patient extend and relax one leg down toward the table (Figure 1-9B). Any lack in terminal hip extension, noted by the inability for the thigh to reach the table, demonstrates a hip flexion contracture. Both sides are performed to compare the difference (Table 1-6). An important aspect of the hip flexion contracture test is to obtain the 0 set point for the lumbar spine. Patients with hyperlaxity or connective tissue disorders could result in a false negative. In these patients, the 0 set point can be established with an abdominal contraction. The hip flexion contracture test could also be falsely negative if there is lumbar spine hyperlordosis due to a previous spinal fusion.

**Table 1-5**

## NORMAL RANGE OF MOTION

| Range of Motion Assessment | Normal (degrees) | Abnormal (degrees) |
|---|---|---|
| Seated internal rotation | 20 to 35 | <20 |
| Seated external rotation | 30 to 45 | <30 |
| Extended internal rotation | 20 to 35 | <20 |
| Extended external rotation | 30 to 45 | <30 |
| Supine hip flexion | 100 to 110 | <100 |
| Adduction | 20 to 30 | <20 |
| Abduction | 45 | <45 |

**Table 1-6**

## ADDITIONAL RANGE OF MOTION TESTS

| Examination | Assessment/Association |
|---|---|
| Hip flexion contracture test (Thomas test) | Hip flexor contracture (psoas), femoral neuropathy, intra-articular pathology, abdominal etiology |
| Tensor fascia lata contracture test (Ober's test) | Tensor fascia lata contracture |
| Gluteus medius contracture test (Ober's test) | Gluteus medius contracture/tear (decreased strength with knee flexion, suspect tear) |
| Gluteus maximus contracture test | Gluteus maximus contracture, contribution to iliotibial band |
| Rectus contracture test (Ely's test) | Rectus femoris contracture |

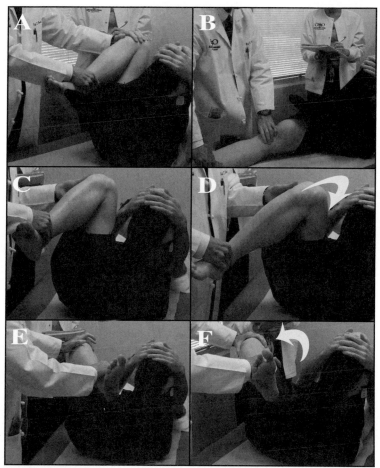

**Figure 1-9.** Supine provocative tests. (A) Zero set point of the pelvis is achieved by having the patient hold the contralateral leg in full flexion, thus establishing neutral pelvic inclination. (B) Hip flexion contracture test. From the start position shown in A, the examined hip is passively extended toward the table. Both hips are examined for side-by-side comparison. If the thigh cannot reach the table (lack of terminal hip extension), this demonstrates a hip flexion contracture. (C, D) DIRI test, dynamic internal rotation test, begins with the hip at 90 degrees flexion or beyond and is passively taken through a wide arc of adduction and internal rotation while decreasing flexion to about 80 degrees. (E, Γ) DEXRIT test, dynamic external rotation test, begins with the hip at 90 degrees flexion or beyond and is dynamically taken through a wide arc of abduction and external rotation.

With the patient in the lateral position, a set of passive adduction tests (most like Ober's test) are performed with the leg in 3 positions (Figures 1-10A through C): extension (tensor fascia lata contracture test), neutral (gluteus medius contracture test), and flexion (gluteus maximus contracture test). Evaluation of gluteus medius tension is achieved by release of the iliotibial band with knee flexion, and the hip should be able to be adducted down toward the table. Any restrictions of these motions are recorded. When performing the gluteus maximus contracture test, the shoulder is rotated toward the side of the table with the hip flexed and knee extended. If adduction cannot occur in this position, the gluteus maximus portion is contracted. The hip should freely be able to come into a full adducted position, and any restriction of the gluteus maximus is recognized. The gluteus maximus is balanced with the tensor fascia lata anteriorly. If the hip does not come beyond the midline in the longitudinal axis of the torso, it is graded as 3+ restriction above torso, 2+ at the midline, and 1+ restriction below. A clear delineation of the exact area of restriction will help to direct physical therapy and peritrochanteric treatment options.

With the patient in the prone position, the rectus contracture test (also known as Ely's test) is performed as the lower extremity is flexed toward the gluteus maximus (see Figure 1-3A). Any raise of the pelvis or restriction of hip flexion motion is indicative of rectus femoris contracture. Internal and external rotation is also assessed in the prone position, and if there is a significant difference of internal rotation in the extended and the seated flexed position, osseous versus ligamentous etiology should be differentiated (see Figure 1-3D).

# STRENGTH TESTING

Manual muscle testing is a basic measure of hip function that is helpful to differentiate muscle strain/injury and hip pain (Table 1-7). Each muscle group is graded in the traditional fashion on a 5-point scale. Abduction strength is assessed with the patient in the lateral position. Gluteus maximus strength testing is performed with the knee extended, while gluteus medius strength testing is performed with the knee flexed (see Figures 1-5E and F) to release the iliotibial band contribution.

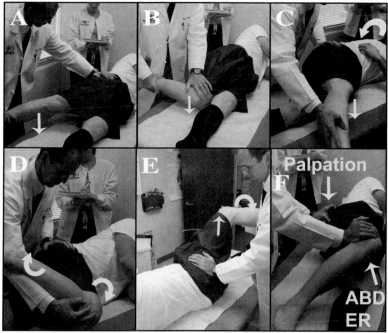

**Figure 1-10.** Lateral tests. (A) The tensor fascia lata contracture test is performed with knee extension. The examiner passively brings the hip into extension and then adduction. (B) The gluteus medius contracture test is performed with knee flexion, thus eliminating contribution of the iliotibial band and zero flexion. The examiner passively adducts the hip toward the exam table. (C) The gluteus maximus contracture test is performed with the ipsilateral shoulder rotated toward the exam table. The examined leg is held in knee extension as the examiner passively brings the hip into flexion then adduction. (D) FADDIR test. In the lateral position, the examiner brings the examined hip into flexion, adduction, and internal rotation, while monitoring the superior aspect of the hip. (E) Rear view of the lateral rim impingement test is performed in the lateral position. The examiner cradles the patient's lower leg with one arm and monitors the hip joint with the opposing hand. The examiner passively brings the affected hip through a wide arc from flexion to extension in continuous abduction while externally rotating the hip. (F) The active piriformis test is performed with the patient in the lateral position as the examiner palpates the piriformis. The patient drives the heel into the examining table, thus initiating external hip rotation as the patient actively abducts and externally rotates against resistance.

**Table 1-7**

## STRENGTH EXAMINATION ASSESSMENT

| Examination | Assessment/Association |
|---|---|
| Single leg stance phase test | Abductor strength, proprioception mechanism |
| Gluteus maximus strength test | Abduction against resistance with the knee extended |
| Gluteus medius strength test | Abduction against resistance with the knee flexed |
| Active piriformis test (Pace's test) | Piriformis syndrome, deep gluteal syndrome |

An active piriformis test is performed by the patient pushing the heel down into the table, abducting and externally rotating the leg against resistance, while the examiner monitors the piriformis (see Figure 1-10F). The active piriformis test is similar to Pace's sign, which is pain and weakness on resisted abduction and external rotation of the thigh in the seated position.[13]

The single leg stance phase test (traditionally known as the Trendelenburg test) is performed during the standing evaluation of the hip. In order to establish a baseline reference for the patient's function, the single leg stance phase test is performed on the uninvolved leg first and then on the involved leg (see Figure 1-1G). During the single leg stance phase test, the examiner stands behind the patient, and the patient should be exposed to the degree that the bony landmarks are easily observed. The patient stands with feet shoulder-width apart, then brings one leg forward by flexing the leg to 45 degrees at the hip and 45 degrees at the knee, thereby simulating the single leg stance phase with load on the examined hip. The single leg stance phase position is held for 6 seconds. As the patient lifts and holds one foot off the ground, the contralateral hip abductor musculature and neural loop of proprioception

**Table 1-8**

---

## SENSORY AND VASCULAR EXAMINATION ASSESSMENT

| Examination | Assessment/Association |
|---|---|
| Neurologic | Sensory nerves originating from the L2-S1 levels, DTR of patella (L2-L4 spinal nerves and femoral nerve) and Achilles (L5-S1 sacral nerves) |
| Straight leg raise | Radicular neurological symptoms |
| Vascular | Pulses of the dorsalis pedis and posterior tibial artery |
| Lymphatics | Skin inspection for swelling, scarring, or side-to-side asymmetry |

---

are being tested. The pelvis will tilt toward or away from the unsupported side if the musculature is weak or if the neural loop of proprioception is disrupted. Normal dynamic mid-stance translocation is 2 cm during a normal gait pattern; a shift in either direction of greater than 2 cm constitutes a positive shift. This test is also performed in a dynamic fashion by some examiners.

# SENSORY TESTING

A thorough neurologic and vascular examination can be performed with the patient in the seated position (see Figure 1-8). The need to check the basics would appear obvious, even in apparently healthy individuals (Table 1-8). Criteria exist for the care of the patient, as well as coding. The posterior tibial pulse is checked first, any swelling of the extremity is noted, and inspection of the skin is performed at this time. A straight leg raise test is then performed by extending the knee into full extension. The straight leg raise test is helpful in detecting radicular neurological symptoms, such as the stretching of an entrapped nerve root. Evaluation of the sensory nerves originating from the L2 through S1 levels are compared (left and right) to assess uniformity. Deep tendon reflexes of the Achilles and patella are also evaluated. Another useful test is Tinels of the femoral nerve. Tinels test is found to be positive with the hip flexion contractures presenting at greater than 25 degrees because of the proximity of the psoas tendon and the femoral nerve.

# PROVOCATIVE TESTS

The importance of multiple examinations is recognized for the detection of intra-articular pathology (Table 1-9). Even in the presence of normal internal and external rotation, there is a need for further delineation as far as the relationships that exist between the musculotendonous, osseous, and ligamentous structure. Tests for impingement can have good specificity and reasonable predictive value for osseous abnormalities; however, no single test is sensitive enough to be used exclusively in the detection of subtle pathology. Furthermore, the ligamentous contribution to ROM varies with flexion and rotation.[14]

## Supine Position

The flexion/abduction/external rotation test (FABER), conventionally known as the Patrick test, is helpful in determining hip versus non-hip complaints (Figure 1-11B). A positive re-creation of pain directed to the hip can be associated with musculotendonous or osseous posterior lateral acetabular incongruence or ligamentous injury. In cases of a coup/contra-coup injury in which the mechanism of injury is initiated posteriorly, pain will be referred to the anterior secondarily.

Tests, which include flexion/adduction/internal rotation test (FADDIR), are used for the detection of impingement or intra-articular pathology.[15] The degree of flexion required in this position of adduction/internal rotation depends upon the degree of impingement and the type and location of impingement. The degree of hip flexion with the amount of pressure of internal rotation is taken on a case-by-case basis depending upon the function required of the patient as well as the patient complaint.

## Table 1-9

# SUMMARY OF PROVOCATIVE TESTS AND ASSESSMENT

| Examination | Assessment/Association |
| --- | --- |
| **SUPINE POSITION** | |
| FADDIR test | Anterior femoroacetabular impingement, torn labrum |
| FABER test (Patrick/Faber) | Distinguish back and hip pathology, specifically sacroiliac joint pathology |
| Dynamic internal rotatory impingement test (similar to McCarthy's test) | Anterior femoroacetabular impingement, torn labrum |
| Dynamic external rotatory impingement test (similar to McCarthy's test) | Superior femoroacetabular impingement, torn labrum |
| Posterior rim impingement test | Posterior femoroacetabular impingement, torn labrum |
| Straight leg raise against resistance test (Stitchfield) | Labral damage, internal derangement |
| Passive supine rotation test (log roll) | Trauma, effusion, synovitis |
| Heel strike test | Trauma, femoral fracture |
| **LATERAL POSITION** | |
| FADDIR test | Anterior femoroacetabular impingement, torn labrum |
| Lateral rim impingement test | Lateral femoroacetabular impingement, torn labrum, instability |

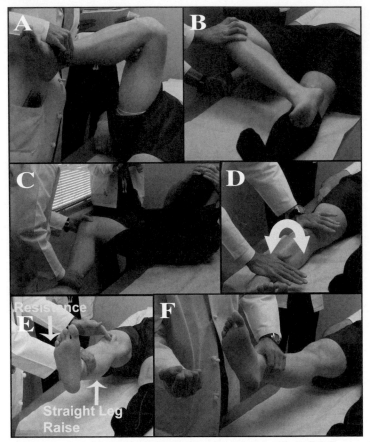

**Figure 1-11.** Additional supine provocative tests. (A) FADDIR test. The examiner brings the examined hip into flexion, adduction, and internal rotation, while monitoring the superior aspect of the hip. (B) FABER test. The examiner brings the leg into 90 degrees of flexion and externally rotates and abducts the leg so that the ipsilateral ankle rests distal to the knee of the contralateral leg. The passive abduction ROM can be measured by "fist widths" and compared side to side. (C) The posterior rim impingement test is performed with the patient at the edge of the examining table. The leg should hang freely at the hip while the patient holds the contralateral leg in full flexion. The examined leg is then brought into full hip extension, abducted, and externally rotated. (D) The passive supine rotation test involves passive internal rotation (shown) and external rotation of the femur, with the leg lying in an extended position. (E) The straight leg raise against resistance test. The patient performs a straight leg raise at 45 degrees of hip flexion as the examiner applies manual resistance. (F) The heel strike is performed by striking the heel abruptly.

Another test is the dynamic internal rotatory impingement test (DIRI). As with the dynamic external impingement maneuver, elimination of lumbar lordosis and a zero pelvic set-point is achieved by the patient holding the non-affected leg in flexion beyond 90 degrees while in the supine position. The examined hip is then brought into 90 degrees flexion or beyond and is passively taken through a wide arc of adduction and internal rotation (see Figures 1-9C and D). A positive result is noted with re-creation of the complaint pain. DIRI can also be performed in the operating theater for direct visualization of femoral neck and acetabular congruence. DIRI is similar to the traditional McCarthy's test, which elicits a pop.[16]

The dynamic external rotatory impingement test (DEXRIT) is conducted with the patient in the supine position. The patient is instructed to hold the non-affected leg in flexion beyond 90 degrees, thus eliminating lumbar lordosis. The examined hip is then brought into 90 degrees of flexion or beyond and is dynamically taken through a wide arc of abduction and external rotation (see Figures 1-9E and F). A positive result is noted with re-creation of the complaint pain. DEXRIT can be performed in the operating theater for direct visualization of femoral neck and acetabular congruence. DEXRIT is similar to the traditional McCarthy's test, which elicits a pop.[16]

The straight leg raise against resistance test (also known as the Stitchfield test) is an assessment of hip flexor/psoas strength and as a sign of inter-articular problems as the psoas places pressure on the labrum. The patient performs an active straight leg raise, with knee extension, to 45 degrees; the examiner's hand is then placed distal to the knee while applying downward force (Figure 1-11E). A positive test is noted with re-creation of the complaint pain or weakness. A heel strike is performed by striking the heel abruptly, which is indicative of some type of trauma and/or stress fracture (Figure 1-11F). The passive supine rotation test (commonly known as the log roll) involves passive internal and external rotation of the femur, with the leg lying in an extended or slightly flexed position (Figure 1-11D). The passive supine rotation test is performed bilaterally, and any side-to-side differences of this maneuver can alert the examiner of the presence of laxity, effusion, or internal derangement.

The posterior rim impingement test can also be performed in the supine position. The patient is positioned at the edge of the examining table so that the examined leg hangs freely at the hip and the patient draws up both legs into the chest, thus eliminating lumbar lordosis. The affected leg is then extended off the table, allowing for full extension of the hip, abducted and externally rotated (Figure 1-11C). The posterior rim impingement test takes the hip into extension, assessing the congruence of the posterior acetabular wall and femoral neck. A variation of this test is the lateral rim impingement test explained in the lateral examination position.

During the course of the supine examination, any pop in this plane can sometimes be related to a snapping iliopsoas tendon. A fan test (the patient circumducts and rotates the hip in rotatory fashion; Figures 1-12E through H) can help delineate the presence of the snapping iliopsoas tendon over the femoral head or the innominate. Many times, this does diminish with an abdominal contraction by decreasing lumbar lordosis, thus affecting the innominate ridge on the anterior wall and eliminating the pop of coxa sultans internus. A hula hoop maneuver (in which the patient stands and twists) or a bicycle test (performed in the lateral position), can help to distinguish the pop internally from the external pop of coxa sultans externus due to the subluxing iliotibial band over the greater trochanter.

## Lateral Position

Passive assessment of FADDIR is performed in a dynamic manner (see Figure 1-10D). The examiner holds the monitoring hand in and about the superior aspect of the hip with the lower leg cradled on the forearm with the knee upon the hand. The hip is then brought into flexion and adduction and is internally rotated. Any reproduction of the patient's complaint and the degree of impingement are noted. FADDIR is commonly performed as part of the supine assessment.[17] The difference is the position of the pelvis. The supine position eliminates lumbar lordosis, whereas the lateral tests the normal dynamic pelvic inclination. Pelvic inclination may affect testing, and both positions are helpful in evaluation.

The lateral rim impingement test is performed with the hip passively abducted and externally rotated (see Figure 1-10E).

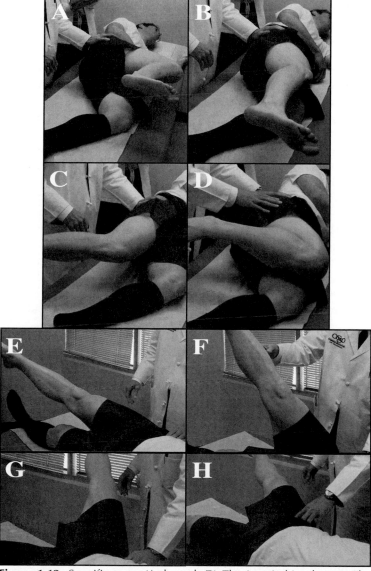

**Figure 1-12.** Specific tests. (A through D) The Leunig bicycle test. The patient mimics the motion of a bicycle pedaling pattern as the examiner monitors the iliotibial band for the detection of coxa sultans externus. (E through H) The fan test. The patient circumducts and rotates the hip in rotatory fashion. This test can help delineate the presence of the snapping iliopsoas tendon over the femoral head or the innominate.

The examiner cradles the patient's lower leg with one arm and monitors the hip joint with the opposing hand. The examiner passively brings the affected hip through a wide arc from flexion to extension in continuous abduction while externally rotating the hip. Reproduction of the patient's pain is scored positive. If the feeling of guarding or the feeling of instability is present, the test is positive for apprehension, which is not to be confused with coup/contracoup. The traditional Patrick test is performed in the supine position and is good for differentiating hip and back pain; however, when performed in the lateral position, the lateral rim impingement test is useful for detection of posterior or lateral impingement issues. Any type of re-creation of a posterior or lateral rim complaint specific to the hip or impingement can be precipitated in this position. The lateral rim impingement, FABER, and posterior rim impingement tests all place the hip into positions of posterior and lateral impingement. The lateral rim impingement test establishes a functional lumbar lordosis with a clear ability to comfortably monitor sites of impingement, which aids in the separation of posterior and lateral points of impingement.

## SPECIFIC TESTS

The McCarthy test is a maneuver associated with a McCarthy sign, a reproducible pop, or a click.[16] The McCarthy test is performed with the contralateral leg held in flexion. The examined hip is brought to 90 degrees flexion, then abducted, externally rotated, and extended. The hip is then brought to 90 degrees flexion, adducted, internally rotated, and extended. A positive McCarthy sign is helpful in detecting anterior femoroacetabular impingement or a torn labrum.

The Scour test is performed in the same manner as DIRI; however, the examiner applies pressure at the knee, thereby increasing pressure at the hip joint, which is helpful in detecting inter-articular congruence.

In the foveal distraction test, inter-articular pressure is alleviated by gently pulling the leg away from the body as the patient is in the supine position. Both the relief of pain or re-creation of pain will help delineate extra- versus intra-articular pathology (Figure 1-13A).

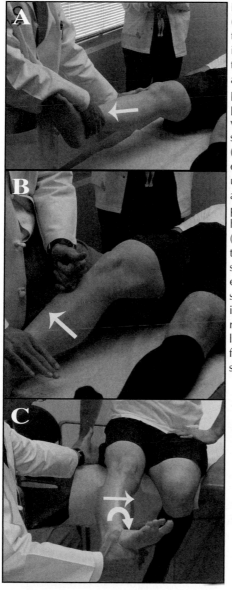

**Figure 1-13.** Specific tests. (A) The foveal distraction test. Inter-articular pressure is alleviated by gently pulling the leg away from the body as the patient is in the supine position. Both the relief of pain or re-creation of pain will help delineate extra- versus intra-articular pathology. (B) The Fulcrum test. The examiner's knee is placed under the patient's knee, acting as a fulcrum, as the patient performs a straight leg test against resistance. (C) Seated piriformis stretch test. The patient is in the seated position with knee extension. The examiner passively moves the flexed hip into adduction with internal rotation while palpating 1 cm lateral to the ischium (middle finger) and proximally at the sciatic notch (index finger).

The Leunig bicycle test is performed with the patient in the lateral position. The patient mimics the motion of a bicycle pedaling pattern as the examiner monitors the iliotibial band for the detection of coxa sultans externus (see Figures 1-12A through D).

During the Fulcrum test, the examiner's knee is placed under the patient's knee, acting as the fulcrum. The patient then performs a straight leg test against resistance (Figure 1-13B). The seated piriformis stretch test is conducted on patients presenting with sit pain and suspected sciatic nerve problems.

The seated piriformis stretch test (Figure 1-13C) is performed in the seated position with the hip at 90 degrees of flexion. The examiner extends the knee and passively moves the flexed hip into adduction with internal rotation, while palpating 1 cm lateral to the ischium (middle finger) and proximally at the sciatic notch (index finger). A positive test is the re-creation of the posterior pain. Freiberg has described sciatic nerve entrapment by the piriformis.[18] The sciatic nerve may be entrapped in other areas, which is best described as deep gluteal syndrome.[19]

The abduction/extension/external rotation test (ABDEER) is performed in the lateral position. The affected leg is passively brought into abduction, extension, and external rotation as forward pressure is applied to the posterior aspect of the hip. Recreation of the patient's complaint pain is a positive test. As with the apprehension test performed on the shoulder, ABDEER is helpful in the detection of any type of anterior capsular laxity or injury. Of note, current research suggests that this position specifically releases the teres ligament.

With the Sampson dynamic trendelenburg test, the patient performs the single leg stance phase test and the examiner applies a slight force or shove to the patient's shoulder. By introducing this dynamic component to single leg standing, the patient must maintain balance through the hip, which may bring out subtle signs of strength or proprioception deficit.

The resisted sit-up test is performed to assess the athletic hernia (sports hernia) or athletic pubalgia. The athletic hernia is described as a condition of a weakened posterior wall of the inguinal canal, which results in chronic pain in the groin that may refer to other surrounding areas and is exacerbated by activity.[11] Although the term *hernia* is associated with a bulge, it is common that no true hernia is present following laparoscopic repair. The majority of patients are involved in sports such as soccer, ice hockey, badminton, squash, rugby, football, golf, and other sports that involve sharp, rapid changes in direction. Diagnosis of the athletic hernia may be difficult because the pain may mimic pain associated with hip labral tears or other hip pathologies. The typical athletic hernia symptoms consist of dull pain in the area of the groin that may radiate to the perineum and inner thigh or across the midline.[11] Common physical exam findings include inguinal canal tenderness, pubic crest/tubercle tenderness, adductor origin tenderness, pain with resisted sit-ups or hip flexion, and a tender, dilated superficial ring.[11]

Using the pudendal nerve block test, 4 clinical features must be present for a diagnosis of pudendal nerve entrapment according to the Nantes criteria.[20] The Nantes criteria includes pain in the area of the urogenital area, pain increased with sitting, pain that does not wake the patient at night, and loss of sensation of the genitalia.[20] If these essential criteria are met, a diagnostic anesthetic pudendal nerve block should be performed, and a relief of symptoms strongly supports these elements of clinical possibilities. This is best performed by a radiologist with experience in this area of complex anatomy.

## Conclusion

The physical examination of the hip encompasses examinations of the hip, back, abdominal, vascular, and neuromuscular systems to lower extremities. In the evaluation of hip pain, it is necessary to also examine joints above and below the hip, record a complete patient history, perform physical examination tests properly and consistently, and be aware of concomitant pathologies that may co-exist with hip pain. The physical examination of the hip will provide a reference grid leading to an accurate diagnosis, a consistent procedure for monitoring the patient during physical therapy and postoperative rehabilitation; and a method of differentiating osseous, ligamentous, and musculotendonous pathology.

As our understanding of hip pathology advances, the physical examination of the hip continues to evolve. A thorough examination of the hip incorporates multiple assessments including palpation, strength, ROM, and provocative maneuvers that are dependent upon patient positioning. Therefore, an efficient physical examination is organized by position, beginning with standing tests and followed by seated, supine, lateral, and prone tests. A consistent physical examination will help identify and distinguish the vast pathologies of the hip in a timely fashion.

## ACKNOWLEDGMENTS

I would like to thank all of the members of the MAHORN Group; Shea A. Shears, RN, BSN, MS; and Ian J. Palmer, PhD for their assistance in the production of this chapter.

## REFERENCES

1. Scopp JM, Moorman CT 3rd. The assessment of athletic hip injury. *Clin Sports Med*. 2001;20:647-659.
2. Philippon M, Schenker M, Briggs K, Kuppersmith D. Femoroacetabular impingement in 45 professional athletes: associated pathologies and return to sport following arthroscopic decompression. *Knee Surg Sports Traumatol Arthrosc*. 2007;15:908-914.
3. Bellamy N, Buchanan WW, Goldsmith CH, Campbell J, Stitt LW. Validation study of WOMAC: a health status instrument for measuring clinically important patient relevant outcomes to antirheumatic drug therapy in patients with osteoarthritis of the hip or knee. *J Rheumatol*. 1988;15:1833-1840.
4. Martin RL, Philippon MJ. Evidence of reliability and responsiveness for the hip outcome score. *Arthroscopy*. 2008;24:676-682.
5. Byrd JWT. Physical examination. In: Byrd JWT, ed. *Operative Hip Arthroscopy*. New York, NY: Springer; 2005:36-50.
6. Braly BA, Beall DP, Martin HD. Clinical examination of the athletic hip. *Clin Sports Med*. 2006;25:199-210, vii.
7. Martin HD. Clinical examination of the hip. *Oper Tech Orthop*. 2005;15: 177-181.
8. Torry MR, Schenker ML, Martin HD, Hogoboom D, Philippon MJ. Neuromuscular hip biomechanics and pathology in the athlete. *Clin Sports Med*. 2006;25:179-197, vii.
9. Perry J. *Gait Analysis: Normal and Pathological Function*. Thorofare, NJ: SLACK Incorporated; 1992.

10. Reider B, Martel J. Pelvis, hip and thigh. In: Reider B, Martel J, eds. *The Orthopedic Physical Examination.* Philadelphia, PA: WB Saunders; 1999:159-199.
11. Swan KG Jr, Wolcott M. The athletic hernia: a systematic review. *Clin Ortho Rel Res.* 2007;455:78-87.
12. Miller SL, Gill J, Webb GR. The proximal origin of the hamstrings and surrounding anatomy encountered during repair. A cadaveric study. *J Bone Joint Surg.* 2007;89(1):44-48.
13. Pace JB, Nagle D. Piriform syndrome. *West J Med.* 1976;124:435-439.
14. Martin HD, Savage A, Braly BA, Palmer IJ, Beall DP, Kelly B. The function of the hip capsular ligaments: a quantitative report. *Arthroscopy.* 2008;24:188-195.
15. Clohisy JC, Knaus ER, Hunt DM, Lesher JM, Harris-Hayes M, Prather H. Clinical presentation of patients with symptomatic anterior hip impingement. *Clin Ortho Rel Res.* 2009;467:638-644.
16. McCarthy JC, Busconi BD, Owens BD. Assessment of the painful hip. In: McCarthy JC, ed. *Early Hip Disorders.* New York, NY: Springer; 2003: 3-6.
17. Klaue K, Durnin CW, Ganz R. The acetabular rim syndrome. A clinical presentation of dysplasia of the hip. *J Bone Joint Surg Br.* 1991;73:423-429.
18. Freiberg A. Sciatic pain and its relief by operations on muscle and fascia. *Arch Surg.* 1937;34:337-350.
19. McCrory P, Bell S. Nerve entrapment syndromes as a cause of pain in the hip, groin and buttock. *Sports Med.* 1999;27:261-274.
20. Labat JJ, Riant T, Robert R, Amarenco G, Lefaucheur JP, Rigaud J. Diagnostic criteria for pudendal neuralgia by pudendal nerve entrapment (Nantes criteria). *Neurourol Urodyn.* 2008;27:306-310.

# 2

# PHYSICAL EXAMINATION OF THE KNEE

## THE BASICS AND SPECIFIC TESTS

*Andrew D. Pearle, MD*

According to the American Academy of Orthopaedic Surgeons (AAOS), in the United States, approximately 10.8 million visits are made to physicians' offices due to a knee problem. It is the most often treated anatomical site by orthopedic surgeons. There are many components to the knee, making it vulnerable for various types of injuries. Its mobility is at the expense of its ultimate stability. Many injuries are successfully treated conservatively, while others require surgery to correct. Given that it is such a common and important site of injury, it stands to reason that a thorough and logical examination technique is the key to correct diagnosis and appropriate management. A detailed examination of the knee is of course preceded by taking the patient's history. This aspect of the

Ranawat A, Kelly BT. *Musculoskeletal Examination of the Hip and Knee: Making the Complex Simple* (pp. 42-68).
© 2011 SLACK Incorporated

clinical approach is vital because it will often be found that a properly taken history will facilitate at least a presumptive diagnosis to be made.

# INSPECTION

## Key Questions

Inspection of the knee joint should begin as soon as the patient enters the examination room. In this way, the knee will be examined while the patient is standing, walking, and lying supine. Comparison with the unaffected side is essential in that it offers a meaningful way to compare form and function that deviates from the norm while bearing in mind those features unique to the patient in question. The knee should be inspected for swelling, bruising, skin color changes, and muscle atrophy.

## Standing

### Lower Limb Alignment

With the patient standing in front of the examiner (with adequate exposure—most commonly barefoot and wearing shorts), alignment can be inspected and subsequently tested. Is there evidence of genu varum (deviation toward the midline distal to the knee; convergence) or valgum (deviation away from the midline distal to the knee; divergence)? An objective measurement may be taken by measuring the distance between the medial femoral condyles (with the medial malleoli touching) for genu varum and the distance between the medial malleoli in the case of genu valgum.[1-3] In a pediatric population, such assessment of lower limb alignment is particularly pertinent, given the opportunity to identify and address malalignment early on before chronic sequelae evolve.[4] For assessment of genu valgum in the 10- to 16-year-old age group, less than 8 cm between the medial malleoli in girls and less than 4 cm in boys is regarded as normal. For assessment of genu varus in the 10- to 16-year-old age group, less than 4 cm in girls between the medial femoral condyles and less than 5 cm in boys is regarded as normal. In those children with genu valgum, rickets should be considered, particularly in those children who exhibit other signs or a background history suspicious for malnourishment. In an adult population, genu valgum is most often associated with rheumatoid arthritis.

### Muscle Atrophy

With the patient standing up straight, particular attention is paid to the quadriceps muscle group. Slight wasting and loss of bulk are normally appreciable upon inspection, particularly when the affected side is compared to the contralateral quadriceps. The vastus medialis in particular is often a useful gauge of quadricep atrophy.[5-7]

Assuming that the contralateral side is normal, substantial wasting may be confirmed by measuring the circumference of the thigh at the same predefined point above the knee on both sides. This objective test may be valuable for repeat assessments to assess progression of disease or assess stage of recovery. Atrophy occurs most commonly due to disuse, generally from joint pain or instability or from infection or rheumatoid arthritis.

## Walking

Watching the patient walk can reveal many features that may guide the physician toward the diagnosis. Are there signs of an antalgic gait? Is the patient favoring one side over the other? Does the patient have a discernible limp?

Key features include the following:
- *Toeing angle*: This is the angle between the long axis of the foot and the direction in which the patient is walking. The foot will normally be seen to make a lateral angle of 10 degrees to 15 degrees with the direction of motion. This angle should be the same on both sides.
- *Tilting of the knee with single-leg stance*: This is manifest when unicompartment wear has occurred due to osteoarthritis (OA). This is a very gradual process in contrast to joint malalignment secondary to ligamentous injury. Medial compartment OA may cause a varus tilt when the knee is close to full extension. This is best appreciated from behind the patient in contrast to lateral compartment OA, which may cause a valgus tilt and is best

appreciated from in front of the patient. Genu recurvatum (knee joint hyperextension) on the other hand is a rare congenital disorder sometimes linked to Osgood-Schlatter disease or Chapple syndrome.[8,9]

# Supine

It is important when assessing a patient in the supine position to pay close attention to 2 features in particular: swelling and flexion deformity.

## Swelling

Small effusions are detected most easily by visible inspection. The first signs are bulging at the sides of the patellar ligaments and obliteration of the hollows at the medial and lateral edges of the patella. With greater effusion into the knee, the suprapatellar pouch may become distended. Effusion is indicative of synovial irritation from trauma or inflammation.

It is important to clarify whether this swelling is confined to the limits of the synovial cavity and suprapatellar pouch (joint effusion, hemarthrosis, pyarthrosis, space-occupying lesion) or beyond the limits of the joint cavity (infection [joint, femur, or tibia], tumor). Is there evidence of prepatellar bursitis (housemaid's knee) or infrapatellar bursitis (clergyman's knee)?

## Flexion Deformity

With the patient supine and relaxed, the examiner grasps both heels and supports them at a height of 10 cm above the examination table, observing whether there is a difference in the flexion angles of each knee joint. This straightforward method does not, however, lend itself to an objective measurement of the deformity. When assessing flexion deformity in the supine position, it is important to establish if such a deformity was present with the patient in the standing position. If a deformity that is manifested upon standing may be reduced in the supine position, it suggests that the deformity is articular in origin.

An alternative method of flexion deformity may be performed with the patient in a prone position on a firm examination table with the knee supported on the surface but the lower limb protruding beyond the table's edge. The heel on the affected side should be seen to be higher than the contralateral heel. This difference in height may be measured.

One caveat when determining if a fixed flexion deformity exists is to establish that the contralateral "normal" side does not have features of genu recurvatum, which could exaggerate a flexion deformity on the affected side or give the impression of a deformity when one does not exist.

## Skin Appearance

Pay attention to the existence and pattern of any peri-articular bruising, which is suggestive of trauma to the superficial tissues or knee ligaments. Is the skin erythematous and thus inflamed? Are there any scars present indicative of prior trauma, surgery, and/or infection (sinus scars)? Is there a distinctive pattern to any abnormal skin appearance, such as in psoriasis?

# PALPATION

## Temperature

Upon first manual contact with the skin, the sensation of heat or cold should be noted and compared with the contralateral limb. Greater heat around the affected knee may suggest inflammation or infection. Heat may also manifest as part of the body's response to injury or in the case of rapidly growing tumors. Meanwhile, a warm knee in combination with a cold foot is suggestive of compromise to the lower limb vasculature. It is always prudent to note whether the patient has just removed a thick bandage or brace. The peripheral pulses should be palpated and recorded.

## Effusion

### Patellar Tap Test

To assess for an effusion, the examiner's hands should be placed on either side of the patella with thumb and middle-to-little fingers "milking" any fluid toward the patella. Meanwhile, the index finger is free to elicit a patellar tap if one exists. The patella is depressed and thus submerged beneath any fluid that may be present, such that it strikes the trochlea producing the "tap." As downward pressure is removed, the patella may "bob" up, given a sufficient effusion. An alternative method sees one hand placed above and across the quadriceps from a point approximately 15 cm proximal to the knee joint. Applying firm pressure, this hand slides toward the upper border of the patella and "milks" any fluid that may be present in the suprapatellar pouch. The tips of the thumb and 3 fingers of the free hand are placed squarely on the patella, and a swift downward pressure is applied to cause the patellar "tap." It is important to remember that the patellar tap test will be negative if there is only a minor effusion present or if the effusion is large enough so that the joint is tense.

### Fluid Displacement Test

The supra-patellar pouch is emptied of fluid as per the patellar tap test. A stroking motion from posterior to anterior applied to the medial aspect of the knee shifts any fluid to the lateral compartment. Next, the lateral compartment is massaged in a similar fashion with attention focused on the medial side to detect any visual evidence of fluid displacement with consequent distention of the medial side.

With a hemarthrosis, the joint may have a "doughy" feel in the suprapatellar region, whereas in the setting of pyarthrosis, there will be associated widespread tenderness.

## Tenderness

When beginning to assess knee joint tenderness, it is best to orientate oneself by palpating the joint lines. Flex the knee while looking for the sulci, which appear at either side of the patellar ligament. Next, apply pressure to these areas to feel the soft hollow of the joint with the bony prominence of the distal femur above and the proximal tibia below. Palpate carefully from alongside the patellar tendon back to the collateral ligaments on either side, noting any tenderness along the joint line or associated with the medial or lateral collateral ligament (MCL/LCL). Localized tenderness at these points at either the medial or lateral joint sulcus is suggestive of meniscus, collateral, and/or fat pad injury. Tenderness in injuries of the MCL is most common at the femoral attachment and in the medial joint line. The LCL can be examined with the heel of the affected side resting on the contralateral proximal tibial crest with the hip abducted (figure-of-4). This serves to render the LCL taut and readily palpable.

Next, palpate the tibial tubercle, which may be tender in a child or adolescent suffering from Osgood-Schlatter's disease and post-avulsion injuries of the patellar ligament and its tibial attachment.

## SURFACE ANATOMY

Surface anatomy is discussed in Table 2-1.

## RANGE OF MOTION

Range of motion should be performed by the patient initially (active) and then by the physician (passive). It is important to establish if there is a great difference between the active and passive ranges observed. The active range may be limited due to pain, and thus passive manipulation should be undertaken with care and sensitivity to the patient's symptoms. Normally, the femur and tibia should form a continuous line when the leg is in full extension, and thus the normal angle of full knee extension is zero. Genu recurvatum is present when the knee extends beyond 0 degrees (ie, hyperextension). When full extension is not possible, this is usually recorded with reference to the 0-degree position (ie, the knee lacks "X" degrees of extension). There are typically 2 types of block to full extension. A springy, soft block is suggestive of meniscal damage with a sliver of cartilage interrupting the joint's full range. A rigid, bony block is often present in severe osteoarthrosis.

The range of flexion should be measured using a goniometer and should be compared to the contralateral knee. Loss of flexion is common after local trauma, effusion, and arthritic conditions. An alternative means of measuring limitation in flexion is to measure the distance from the posterior aspect of the heel to the buttocks.

## STRENGTH TESTING

### Muscle Strength/Power Grading

In the case of known or suspected subnormal knee strength, the following grading system may be applied so as to offer a

**Table 2-1**

# RELEVANT SURFACE ANATOMY

## Anterior Aspect

Supra-articular
- Vastus lateralis muscle
- Vastus medialis muscle
- Lateral femoral condyle
- Medial femoral condyle

Patella

Infra-articular
- Lateral tibial condyle
- Patellar ligament
- Tibialis anterior muscle
- Medial tibial condyle
- Tibial tuberosity
- Head of fibula (lateral)

## Posterior Aspect

Supra-articular
- Semi-tendinosus muscle/tendon and semi-membranosus muscle
- Biceps femoris muscle

Popliteal fossa

Infra-articular
- Medial and lateral head of gastrocnemius

## Osseous Landmarks

Tibial tubercle and patellar tendon

Medial tibial plateau and tibial condyle

Lateral tibial tubercle

Lateral femoral epicondyle

Inferior surface of the patella

Adductor tubercle and medial epicondyle

Medial femoral condyle

Patella

Lateral femoral condyle

Head of the fibula

Trochlear groove

## Soft Tissue Landmarks

Muscular structures

Quadriceps

Vastus lateralis          Rectus femoris

Vastus medialis

Biceps femoris (tendon can be palpated just prior to its insertion into the lateral condyle of the tibia below the joint line)

Iliotibial band

Semi-tendinosus, gracilis, sartorius, pes anserine bursa

Ligamentous structures

Lateral collateral ligament     Medial collateral ligament

meaningful assessment of the patient's strength through the knee joint[10]:

- *Grade 1 (M1)*: Only a trace or flicker of movement is seen or felt in the muscle, or fasciculations are observed in the muscle.
- *Grade 2 (M2)*: Muscle can move only if the resistance of gravity is removed.
- *Grade 3 (M3)*: Muscle strength is further reduced such that the knee joint can be moved only against gravity with the examiner's resistance completely removed.
- *Grade 4 (M4)*: Muscle strength is reduced, but muscle contraction can still move knee joint against resistance.
- *Grade 5 (M5)*: Muscle contracts normally against full resistance.

Knee strength testing is best performed using an isokinetic machine so as to isolate the motion being examined insofar as is possible. Thus, a leg extension machine and a leg flexion machine may be employed effectively. It is important that the knee's axis of rotation is aligned correctly with the weight machine. It is also important when comparing the affected knee to its contralateral counterpart that the resistance pad is placed at an equivalent point on both sides and that the permitted range of motion is also consistent for testing of both sides. Strength outcomes can be expressed as the maximum weight that can be moved for one repetition or as the maximum weight for which a low number of repetitions can be successfully complete (eg, 4 reps).

# SENSORY TESTING

## Sensory Grading

For sensory testing, a similar grading system may be applied as per strength testing above:

- *Grade 0 (SO)*: Absence of all modalities of sensation.
- *Grade 1 (S1)*: Recovery of deep pain sensation.
- *Grade 2 (S2)*: Recovery of protective sensation (skin touch, pain, and thermal sensation).
- *Grade 3 (S3)*: Recovery of protective sensation with accurate localization. Cold sensitivity (and hypersensitivity).

- *Grade 3+ (S3+):* Recovery of ability to recognize objects and texture. Minimal cold sensitivity and hypersensitivity.
- *Grade 4 (S4):* Normal sensation.

When spinal nerve problems are suspected (as opposed to peripheral nerves), examination will be focused upon the relevant myotomes and dermatomes for the knee (Table 2-2).

# SPECIFIC TESTS

Depending on the area of injury and the interest elicited from the general survey that is performed initially, more specific tests may be performed to further assess or localize the injury or abnormality being examined. The following specific tests are arranged with respect to the area of the knee joint being assessed.

## Extensor Apparatus

The extensor apparatus is best assessed with the patient sitting upright with his or her legs over the edge of the examination table. As the patient extends his or her leg, the quadriceps should be palpated to confirm contraction with active extension.

If extension is not possible or is deficient, the extensor apparatus should be examined to rule out a quadriceps tendon rupture.[11] The special test employed in this scenario is the Dreyer test. The patient, in a supine position, is asked to raise his or her fully extended leg. If he or she is unable to do it without stabilization of the quadriceps tendon by the examiner, this is a positive Dreyer test. Other injuries that could produce a positive Dreyer test include patella fracture, patellar ligament rupture, avulsion of the tibial tubercle, and variants of jumper's knee.

## Tibial Tubercle

This bony prominence should be inspected and palpated to ascertain if it is abnormally prominent, enlarged, and/or tender. These features are typically present with Osgood-Schlatter disease or apophysitis.

**Table 2-2**

## *MYOTOMES*

Knee extension: L3, L4

Knee flexion: L5, S1

Dermatomes

Anterior knee: L3

Posterior knee: S2

Peripheral nerves

Femoral nerve (L2, 3, 4)

  Motor distribution (below the inguinal ligament)
  - Quadriceps
  - Sartorius
  - Pectineus

  Sensory distribution (below the inguinal ligament)
  - Anterior thigh (femoral cutaneous branches)

  Testing
  - Inspection: Quadriceps wasting
  - Palpation: Knee extension against resistance (knee-jerk reflex)
  - Sensation: Pin-prick testing in distribution of femoral nerve

Sciatic nerve (L4, 5, S1, 2, 3)

  Motor distribution
  - Hamstrings

Sensory distribution

  Posterior thigh (posterior cutaneous nerve)

  Testing
  - Inspection: Hamstrings wasting
  - Palpation: Knee flexion against resistance
  - Sensation: Pin-prick testing in distribution of sciatic nerve

Lateral cutaneous nerve of thigh (L2, 3)

  Sensory distribution
  - Lateral aspect of thigh

# Patella

The position of the patella should be noted upon inspection. A laterally or highly placed patella (patella alta) may predispose the patient to lateral patellar dislocation and to the development of chondromalacia patellae (CMP). Coexisting genu valgum should be factored into patellar testing given that this malalignment leads to an increase in the quadriceps angle and thus increases the likelihood of patellar dislocation, anterior knee pain, and CMP.

A systematic and thorough patellar palpation should be performed with attention to each aspect of the patella (Figure 2-1). The anterior surface should be checked for the presence of a tender, bipartite ridge. The apex should be examined to rule out the tenderness associated with inflammation of the distal pole of the patella present, which may occur in adolescents as part of Sinding-Larsen-Johansson disease. The medial facet may be tender to palpation as part of an anterior knee pain syndrome, while the lateral facet may be accentuated with pushing of the patella in a lateral direction. Patellofemoral dysplasia will produce lateral impingement, pain, and tenderness along the lateral patellar border. To facilitate palpation of its underlying articular surface, the patella should be pushed medially. Tenderness here is found with CMP.

The patella should also be moved proximally and distally while applying downward pressure such that its articular surface makes firm contact with the femoral condyles. Tenderness elicited from this movement is consistent with CMP and retropatellar OA.

Special tests include the following:
- *Patellar tilt*: The patella is held by the edges between the thumb and index finger, thereby establishing the axis of the patella, which should differ only slightly (10 degree lateral tilt) from the horizontal plane of the knee as seen head-on. The patella may be said to "squint" (convergent or divergent). In general, a convergent squint tends to be associated with anterior knee pain syndrome, and a divergent squint tends to be linked to recurrent patellar dislocation.
- *Patellar apprehension test*: While the patella is pushed firmly in a lateral direction, the knee is flexed from

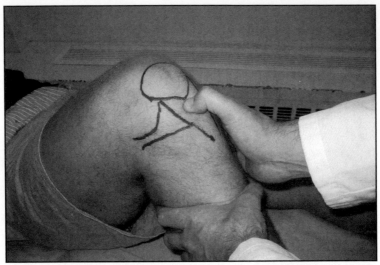

**Figure 2-1.** Care should be taken to palpate around the patella to identify regions of tenderness.

the fully extended position. A patient who suffers from recurrent patellar dislocation will stop the examiner from applying pressure on the patella while the knee is flexed, given his or her apprehension over imminent dislocation. Between 0 and 30 degrees of flexion, the patella is at its highest point with respect to the trochlea, and thus is most vulnerable to dislocation when pressure from the medial side pushes the patella laterally.

- *McConnell test*: This test attempts to provoke patellofemoral pain with isometric contraction of the quadriceps.[12] This is performed with the knee at various degrees of flexion (0, 30, 60, and 120 degrees). In each position, the examiner immobilizes the patient's lower leg while requesting that the patient extend the leg against the examiner's resistance (ie, isometric contraction). If the patient reports pain or a sense of constriction, the examiner medially displaces the patella. In a positive McConnell test, this medial displacement reduces the pain for the patient. This is consistent with the presence of retropatellar pain.

- *Patellar grind test*: The examiner's hand is placed on the front of the knee while the patient performs a full flexion-extension arc. Crepitus may be felt and even patellar catching.

### Assessment of Patellar Stability

The examiner should attempt to displace the patella both medially and laterally. The normal patella excursion is between 25% and 50% of the width of the patella, and greater displacements represent loose patellar restraints (Figure 2-2).

## Mediopatellar Plica

The plica is felt as a cord that rolls under a palpating finger on the medial femoral condyle. It sweeps along the condyle during flexion and may give rise to painful symptoms.

## Menisci

Meniscal testing is broadly based on the fact that stressing an injured medial or lateral meniscus will cause pain. Thus, the specific meniscal tests are designed to accentuate the problems caused by damaged cartilage so that, in eliciting pain, the examiner confirms the injury.[13] The joint line is palpated (Figure 2-3). The most frequently encountered sites of tenderness are overlying or behind the medial collateral ligament. Less frequently, the tender point is found more anteriorly. This is suggestive of a bucket-handle tear of the medial meniscus or injury to the anterior horn of the lateral meniscus. The lateral meniscal tender point may be any of a number of points along the joint line.

Special tests include the following:

- *Posterior meniscal lesions*: The posterior meniscus will be compressed in hyperflexion, and adding tibial rotation serves to add to the diagnostic accuracy compared to a simple flexion-extension maneuver. Sweeping the heel around in a U-shaped arc can elicit clicks accompanied by pain in patients with posterior meniscal lesions.

- *Anterior meniscal lesions*: Firm palpation of the medial and lateral joint lines while extending the joint may be accompanied by a click and pain in the setting of anterior meniscal injuries.

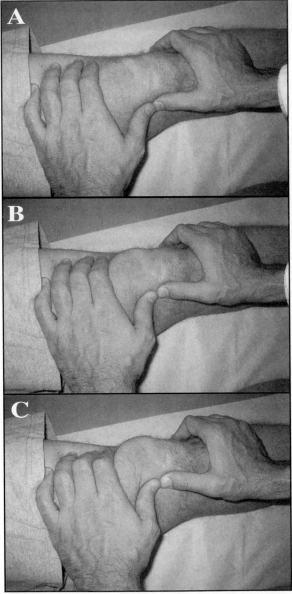

**Figure 2-2.** Assessment of patellar displacement (Sage sign). The examiner's thumbs are used to displace the patella medially or laterally. Excursion of greater than 50% of the width of the patella is found with loose or disrupted patellar restraints.

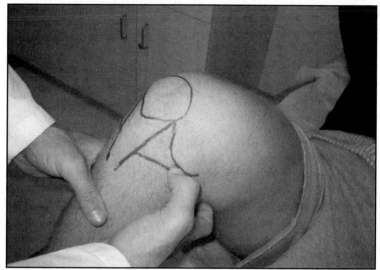

**Figure 2-3.** Tenderness along the medial or lateral joint line is consistent with meniscus pathology.

- McMurray's test:
  - ⅄ *Medial meniscus*: While palpating the medial joint line, the leg is fully flexed; then, the foot is externally rotated and the lower leg is abducted. While maintaining the leg abduction, the joint is extended. A palpable click in the medial joint accompanied by pain suggests a medial meniscus tear.[14]
  - ⅄ *Lateral meniscus*: The test is repeated in a similar fashion to that for the medial meniscus; however, the foot is internally rotated and an adduction pressure is applied while the leg is extended (Figure 2-4).
- *Apley grind tests*: For these tests, the patient is positioned prone with his or her knee flexed.[13] The foot is initially externally rotated, and the knee is flexed fully (Figure 2-5). Next, the foot is internally rotated, and the knee is extended. Then, these motions are repeated with a compression force applied onto the sole of the foot by the examiner. Severe sharp pain is indicative of a meniscus tear.

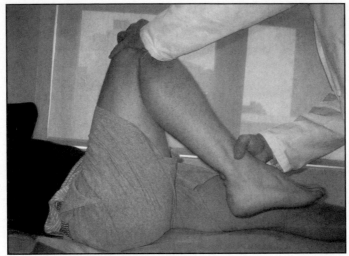

**Figure 2-4.** McMurray's test. To assess the lateral meniscus, palpate the lateral joint, internally rotate the lower leg, and extend the knee from a flexed position. Pain or clicking in the knee during this maneuver represents a positive finding. The medial meniscus is assessed by palpating the medial joint line and externally rotating the lower leg while extending the knee.

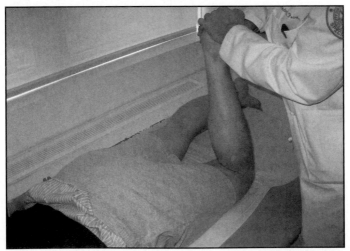

**Figure 2-5.** Apley grind test. The patient is placed in a prone position and downward pressure is applied to the externally rotated tibia to load the knee joint and meniscus. Pain with this examination is likely due to meniscal pathology.

The presence of any meniscal cysts should also be assessed.[15] Cysts of the lateral meniscus may be seen in extension and disappear in flexion. They are by far the most common meniscal cyst. Meanwhile, cystic swellings on the medial side are sometimes due to pes anserinus (insertion of sartorius, gracilis, and semitendinosus) ganglions.

## Knee Stability

Instability of the knee joint can be divided into linear and rotational components, and a systematic physical examination should aim to determine whether the joint displays features of one or both of these forms of instability (see Table 2-3 for instability and associated injury patterns). Linear instability may be assessed in the following ways:

- *Valgus stress test (valgus instability):* With the leg in full extension, grasp the heel with one hand while the other hand is placed against the lateral aspect of the knee. A brisk and brief valgus stress is applied via lower leg abduction. Medial instability is demonstrated if the medial joint line opens up.

  If no instability has been demonstrated with the leg in full extension, the exam is repeated with the leg in 30 degrees of flexion and with the foot internally rotated (Figure 2-6). Some opening of the joint is normal, and thus comparison with the contralateral side is important. An abnormal amount of opening is suggestive of a less extensive injury to the medial structures than that elicited in full extension.

- *Varus stress test (varus instability):* This test is performed in a similar fashion to the valgus stress test but with a varus stress applied in full extension and at 30 degrees (Figure 2-7). Abnormal lateral joint opening in full extension is suggestive of injury to the lateral ligament complex and possibly also the PCL.

- *Anterior drawer test:* With the patient in a supine position, the affected knee is flexed to 90 degrees with the foot flat on the examination table and fixed by the examiner sitting on it or close to it.[16] The examiner's thumbs are placed on the medial and lateral joint sulci so as to receive tactile feedback of any anterior translation produced (Figure 2-8). The test is then repeated at 70 degrees.

**Table 2-3**

## FORMS OF INSTABILITY AND ASSOCIATED INJURY PATTERNS

### Linear Instability

- Valgus instability: Medial collateral ligament tear and, if severe, posterior cruciate ligament (PCL) injury
- Varus instability: Lateral collateral ligament ± PCL injury
- Tibial displacement anteriorly: Anterior cruciate ligament (ACL) injury
- Tibial displacement posteriorly: PCL injury

### Rotational Instability

- Medial tibial condyle anterior subluxation (anteromedial instability): Damage to ACL and medial structures
- Lateral femoral condyle anterior subluxation (anterolateral instability): Damage to ACL and lateral structures
- Lateral tibial condyle posterior subluxation (posterolateral instability)
- Medial tibial condyle posterior subluxation (posteromedial instability)

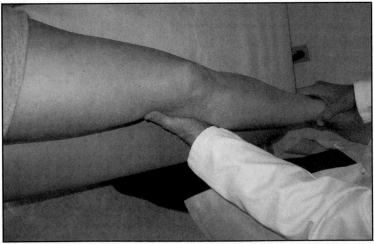

**Figure 2-6.** The valgus stress test is performed at 0 degrees and 30 degrees. Laxity at 30 degrees suggests isolated MCL injury while laxity at full extension suggests combined MCL, cruciate, and capsular injury.

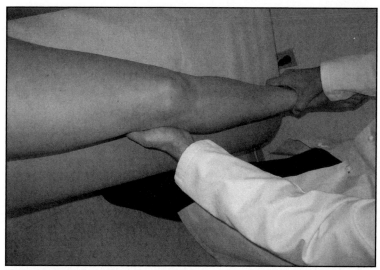

**Figure 2-7.** The varus stress test is done to evaluate for lateral ligament laxity. The test is first performed in 30 degrees of flexion, where the cruciates are in their most relaxed state. Laxity at 30 degrees suggests injury to the LCL. The test is repeated at full extension, where the cruciate ligaments are tauter. Varus laxity at full extension suggests combined cruciate and collateral ligament injury.

It is also repeated at 90 degrees in 15 degrees of external rotation and 30 degrees of internal rotation. Anterior subluxation in either of these positions suggests antero-medial and anterolateral instability, respectively. It is important to be mindful of a pre-existing PCL injury, which would give the affected knee a certain degree of posterior sag, thus potentially demonstrating a false-positive anterior drawer test. This caveat applies to the Lachman test also.

- *Lachman test:* This test is also used to detect ACL disruption. In the manipulative Lachman test, one hand stabilizes the femur while the other attempts to lift the tibia forward.[17] The test is positive if there is a soft endpoint and anterior tibial movement that is 5 to 10 mm greater than the contralateral side (Figure 2-9). In the active Lachman test, the patient's knee is supported at 30 degrees, and the patient is asked to extend it.

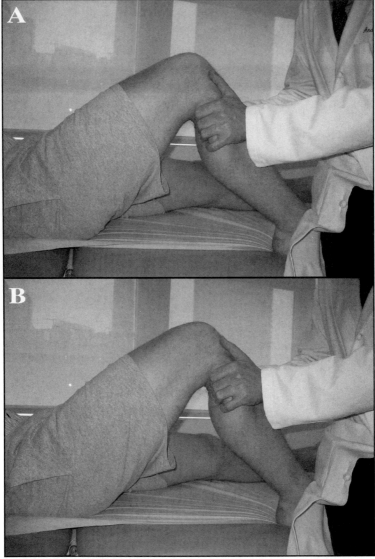

**Figure 2-8.** The anterior drawer test is performed to assess for anterior cruciate ligament injury. The examiner should feel for the amount of translation as well as the endpoint. Translations greater than 5 to 10 mm compared to the contralateral side as well as a soft endpoint are associated with ACL ruptures.

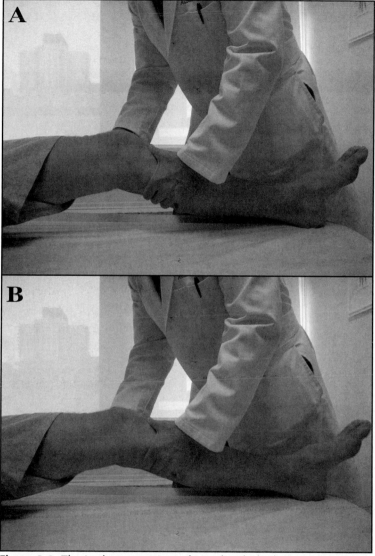

**Figure 2-9.** The Lachman test is performed with the knee in 30 degrees of flexion. An anteriorly directed force is applied to the tibia—a soft endpoint and increased tibial translation compared to the uninjured leg is noted with ACL deficiency.

The test is positive if there is anterior subluxation of the lateral tibial plateau as the quadriceps contracts and posterior subluxation when the muscle relaxes.

- *Posterior cruciate ligament testing:* The knee should be flexed to 20 degrees with a sandbag or similar support placed under the thigh. The patient is instructed to lift his or her heel off of the examination table. Any posterior subluxation should correct.

- *Posterior drawer test:* If the PCL is lax or torn but posterior subluxation has not yet occurred, then anterior pressure on the tibia may cause posterior translation of the tibia relative to the femur.

## Rotational Instability

- *McIntosh pivot shift test:* With the leg in full extension, internally rotated, and with a valgus stress applied, if any anterolateral instability of the tibia exists, the lateral tibial plateau is likely to be subluxed (Figure 2-10).[18-21] Thus, as the knee is flexed, the lateral tibial plateau is reduced. Depending on the severity of the injury, this shift may feel like a glide (Grade 1) or a clunk (Grade 2) to the examiner or a reduction of a frank subluxation (Grade 3).

- *Losee pivot shift:* A valgus force is applied to the knee while the fibular head is pushed anteriorly.[20] The knee should be partly flexed. The knee is then extended with the result that, as full extension is neared, a dramatic clunk may occur as the lateral tibial condyle subluxes forward.

- *Posterolateral instability tests:* First, a posterior drawer test is performed with the patient's foot in external rotation with focus on the lateral side in an attempt to appreciate any excessive motion in this area. Next, an external rotation recurvatum test is performed. With the patient in a supine position, the examiner stands at the base of the examination table and lifts the legs by the big toes. The test is positive if the knee falls into external rotation, varus, and recurvatum. Finally, a dial test is performed. This test is often performed in the prone position and is done at both 30 and 90 degrees (Figure 2-11).

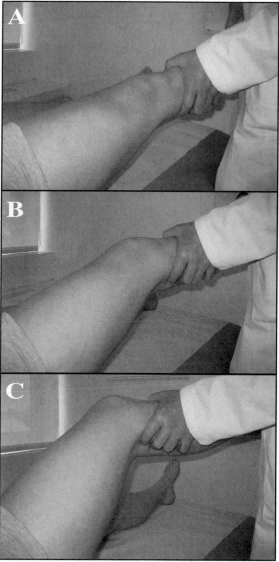

**Figure 2-10.** The pivot shift test recapitulates the functional instability patients experience with ACL deficiency. The test is a subtle maneuver that involves gentle axial load to the foot, a valgus load to the knee, and flexion. External rotation of the foot exaggerates the pivot shift; however, a positive pivot shift with internal rotation of the foot is more specific for ACL deficiency.

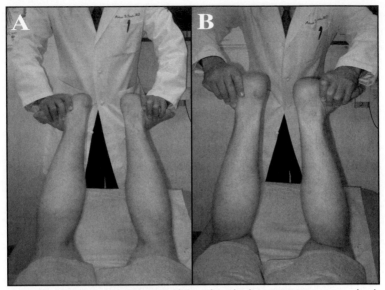

**Figure 2-11.** The dial test is performed with the patient prone at both 30 and 90 degrees. External rotation is applied to the knee by rotating the tibia through the ankle joints. A side-to-side comparison is done with maximal external rotation applied. With an isolated PLC injury, increased external rotation is found at 30 degrees, but symmetric rotation is re-established at 90 degrees of flexion. With a combined PLC and PCL injury, increased external rotation is found at both 30 degrees and 90 degrees.

External rotation is applied to the ankle of both legs at each flexion angle. When external rotation is increased by more than 10 degrees compared to the contralateral side, severe injury to the posterolateral corner of the knee is suspected when the test is performed at 30 degrees. If the PCL is intact, this exaggerated external rotation will disappear at 90 degrees. Increased external rotation at both 30 and 90 degrees is suggestive of a combined PLC and PCL injury.

- *Jakob's reverse pivot shift test:* This test may be employed as a further check for posterolateral instability. The knee is flexed to 90 degrees; the foot is rotated externally, a valgus is applied, and the joint is extended. The test is positive if the posteriorly subluxed lateral plateau suddenly reduces, usually at approximately 20 degrees.[20]

# CONCLUSION

Physical examination of the knee is extremely important given the incidence of knee injury. A thorough assessment should begin as soon as the patient enters the room vis-à-vis inspection of gait and stance. It is very important to examine above and below the knee along with taking a complete history. Performance of the various physical examination tests should be conducted in a consistent manner and with special focus and additional tests when indicated. A complete, accurate, and well-documented knee examination will aid diagnosis, target management effectively, and permit subsequent assessment of rehabilitation and recovery.

# REFERENCES

1. Salenius P, Vankka E. The development of the tibiofemoral angle in children. *J Bone Joint Surg Am.* 1975;57(2):259-261.
2. Shopfner CE, Coin CG. Genu varus and valgus in children. *Radiology.* 1969;92(4):723-732.
3. Wenger DR, Mickelson M, Maynard JA. The evolution and histopathology of adolescent tibia vara. *J Pediatr Orthop.* 1984;4(1):78-88.
4. Heath CH, Staheli LT. Normal limits of knee angle in white children—genu varum and genu valgum. *J Pediatr Orthop.* 1993;13(2):259-262.
5. Jan MH, Lin DH, Lin JJ, et al. Differences in sonographic characteristics of the vastus medialis obliquus between patients with patellofemoral pain syndrome and healthy adults. *Am J Sports Med.* 2009;37(9):1743-1749.
6. Suetta C, Hvid LG, Justesen L, et al. Effects of ageing on human skeletal muscle after immobilization and re-training. *J Appl Physiol.* 2009;107(4):1172-1180.
7. Tsakoniti AE, Stoupis CA, Athanasopoulos SI. Quadriceps cross-sectional area changes in young healthy men with different magnitude of Q angle. *J Appl Physiol.* 2008;105(3):800-804.
8. Bellicini C, Khoury JG. Correction of genu recurvatum secondary to Osgood-Schlatter disease: a case report. *Iowa Orthop J.* 2006;26:130-133.
9. Saito N, Tensyo K, Horiuchi H, et al. Brothers with genu recurvatum. *Knee.* 2007;14(6):500-501.
10. Florence JM, Pandya S, King WM, et al. Intrarater reliability of manual muscle test (Medical Research Council scale) grades in Duchenne's muscular dystrophy. *Phys Ther.* 1992;72(2):115-122; discussion 122-126.
11. Crossley KM, Cowan SM, Bennell KL, et al. Knee flexion during stair ambulation is altered in individuals with patellofemoral pain. *J Orthop Res.* 2004;22(2):267-274.

12. Watson CJ, Propps M, Galt W, et al. Reliability of McConnell's classification of patellar orientation in symptomatic and asymptomatic subjects. *J Orthop Sports Phys Ther.* 1999;29(7):378-385; discussion 386-393.

13. Fowler PJ, Lubliner JA. The predictive value of five clinical signs in the evaluation of meniscal pathology. *Arthroscopy.* 1989;5(3):184-186.

14. Kim SJ, Min BH, Han DY. Paradoxical phenomena of the McMurray test. An arthroscopic investigation. *Am J Sports Med.* 1996;24(1):83-87.

15. Mountney J, Thomas NP. When is a meniscal cyst not a meniscal cyst? *Knee.* 2004;11(2):133-136.

16. Weatherwax RJ. Anterior drawer sign. *Clin Orthop Relat Res.* 1981;154:318-319.

17. Johnson RJ. The anterior cruciate ligament problem. *Clin Orthop Relat Res.* 1983;172:14-18.

18. Lane CG, Warren R, Pearle AD. The pivot shift. *J Am Acad Orthop Surg.* 2008;16(12):679-688.

19. Lane CG, Warren RF, Stanford FC, et al. In vivo analysis of the pivot shift phenomenon during computer navigated ACL reconstruction. *Knee Surg Sports Tramatol Arthrosc.* 2008;16(5):487-492.

20. Leitze Z, Losee RE, Jokl P, et al. Implications of the pivot shift in the ACL-deficient knee. *Clin Orthop Relat Res.* 2005;436:229-236.

21. Pearle AD, Kendoff D, Musahl V, et al. The pivot-shift phenomenon during computer-assisted anterior cruciate ligament reconstruction. *J Bone Joint Surg Am.* 2009;91(suppl 1):115-118.

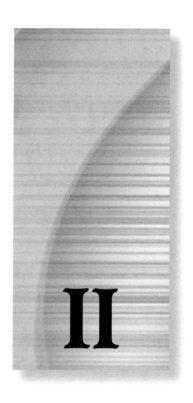

# II

# General Imaging

# 3

# GENERAL IMAGING
# OF THE HIP

*Michael H. Ngo, MD and Douglas N. Mintz, MD*

## INTRODUCTION

This chapter introduces imaging of hip pathologies and familiarizes the reader with the imaging of normal anatomy and common pathologies. It is important to realize that imaging studies must be correlated with the patient's history and physical exam to reach an appropriate diagnosis and treatment plan. This is particularly true in the hip where findings on imaging studies do not necessarily cause patient symptoms. Imaging has become so sensitive that most patients have multiple abnormalities on magnetic resonance imaging (MRI). Knowing the particular patient's presentation will determine which of these abnormalities is clinically relevant.

Ranawat A, Kelly BT. *Musculoskeletal Examination of the Hip and Knee: Making the Complex Simple* (pp. 70-109).
© 2011 SLACK Incorporated

There are currently many ways to image. One should usually start with the most inexpensive and easiest study that will answer the clinical question. For example, if looking for a pelvic fracture, an x-ray, if it demonstrates a fracture, may be the only imaging required and should be obtained before deciding to get a computed tomography (CT) scan.

# TYPES OF IMAGING

There are basically 5 modalities for imaging the hip: radiography (x-ray), CT, MRI, ultrasound, and nuclear medicine imaging (comprising techniques such as bone scan, single positron emission computed tomography [SPECT], and positron emission tomography [PET]). A summary of these modalities is in Table 3-1.

## Radiography

X-rays, first used for imaging in 1895, require ionizing radiation from a source to pass through the body and expose a film. Today, many centers use digital formats rather than the older photographic films. X-rays do not display subtle differences in soft tissues but do provide excellent resolution and detail of bone. Therefore, x-ray is effective for detecting subtle fractures and should be used for the initial evaluation of suspected fractures. Always follow the cortex of bone on x-rays to detect subtle fractures.

One of the disadvantages of radiography is that it projects a 3-dimensional object (the body) into 2 dimensions on the x-ray film. One of the ways to get more information from an x-ray is to change the position of the body or the x-ray beam to create a different view. For the pelvis and the hip, many specialized views have been developed (see "Osseous Trauma" section on p. 80). Normal anatomy on x-ray is determined in part by the relationship among structures. These relationships have been defined so that radiographic measurements and angles become a quantitative way of assessing radiographs of the hip (see discussion on femoroacetabular impingement (FAI) on p. 98 and in Chapter 6).

On radiography, it is the relative ability of tissues to block the x-rays from exposing the film that produce the image,

**Table 3-1**

## Summary of Radiographic Imaging Techniques

| Modality | Utility | Terminology | Advantages | Disadvantages |
|---|---|---|---|---|
| X-ray | Good screening<br>Bone abnormalities | Density/lucency | Inexpensive<br>Available<br>Sensitive for fracture | Not good for soft tissue<br>Insensitive for much pathology<br>Can be difficult to interpret |
| Ultrasound | Superficial structures (muscle/tendon)<br>Guiding injections | Echodense/echogenic<br>echolucent | Excellent resolution<br>Accurate<br>Relatively inexpensive | Not readily available in the United States<br>Operator dependent<br>Cannot see into joint |
| Bone scan | Radiographically occult fractures<br>Multiplicity of lesions<br>To see if a lesion is active | Uptake, activity | Sensitive<br>Images whole body | Not specific |
| CT | People who cannot have MRI<br>Assess fractures | Density/lucency | Excellent bony detail<br>Can get images in one plane and reformat/make models | Ionizing radiation<br>Not very good soft tissue contrast (made better by arthrography) |
| MRI | Most musculoskeletal pathologies | Signal intensity (high/low signal) | Superb anatomic detail<br>Sensitive and specific | Expensive |

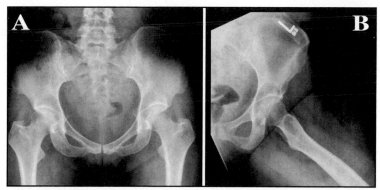

**Figure 3-1.** Normal radiographs of the pelvis and hips. (A) AP and (B) frog-leg lateral views. (Courtesy of Hospital for Special Surgery, New York, NY.)

so images on x-ray are described as (radio)opaque (dense) or radio(lucent). Metal is very dense (blocks all of the x-rays). Bone is less so. Fat is even less so. Air is lucent (blocks none of the x-rays). Soft tissues, such as muscle, are less dense than metal or bone but denser than fat or air, so x-ray is used primarily to look at bony abnormalities (Figure 3-1).

## Computed Tomography

CT or computer assisted tomography (CAT) scanning was invented in the 1970s by the British music company Electric and Musical Industries (EMI). Having been improved and refined since its creation, it is now a mainstay of imaging. Like x-ray, CT uses ionizing radiation, but instead of having a single stationary x-ray source, the source moves around in a circle. The patient lies on a table that slides through the center of that rotating source, like a finger going through a donut hole. The information obtained using this technique allows production of an x-ray slice of the body. Adjacent slices can be stacked to create a 3-dimensional view. Current software allows rapid creation of models that can be manipulated and viewed in any plane (Figure 3-2).

CT has some of the limitations of radiography in that the soft tissue contrast is not ideal. It is best for evaluating bone and calcifications, but muscles, tendons, and fat can also easily be demonstrated. Intra-articular contrast can be used to make

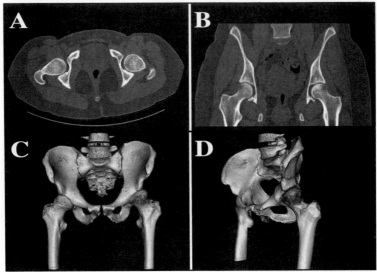

**Figure 3-2.** CT scan. (A) Axial image of the pelvis at the level of the acetabulum. (B) Coronal reformatted image obtained from thin-section axial images. Three-dimensional CT volumetric rendering of the pelvis and hips. (C, D) Thin-section axial images obtained by multi-detector CT scanning can be used to generate 3-dimensional anatomic representations. (Courtesy of Hospital for Special Surgery, New York, NY.)

a CT a CT arthrogram to access articular cartilage defects and labral tears. CT is very valuable in looking for fractures and planning their treatment. It is also excellent for looking at the bony anatomy of patients with dysplasia and FAI and for planning osteotomies. Surgeries can be planned from plastic models created from CT data.

Like x-ray, structures on CT are termed *dense* or *lucent*. Godfrey Hounsfield, a British engineer, created a scale to quantify CT density, using Hounsfield units (HU) ranging from air (-1000 HU) to water (0 HU) to dense bone or metal (+1000 HU).

## Magnetic Resonance Imaging

MRI was initially used for imaging in the early 1980s. Unlike conventional radiography and CT, MRI does not rely on ionizing radiation to produce images of the body. Instead, MRI generates images by using a powerful magnetic field

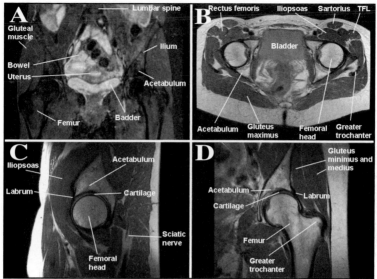

**Figure 3-3.** Normal hip MRI. (A) Body coil IR (inversion recovery) coronal image of the pelvis and hips. (B) Body coil protein density fast spin echo (PD FSE) axial image of the pelvis. Surface coil PD FSE images of the hip of interest in the (C) sagittal and (D) coronal planes are ideal for assessing articular cartilage and labrum. TFL = tensor fascia lata. (Courtesy of Hospital for Special Surgery, New York, NY.)

(up to 7 Tesla) to align the body's protons (hydrogen ions) and then perturb them using radiofrequency pulses. The energy given off by hydrogen nuclei excitation is a radiofrequency signal that can be detected by the scanner to produce an image (Figure 3-3).

MRI imaging has greatly enhanced our ability to diagnose musculoskeletal disorders due to its ability to demonstrate soft tissue and bone abnormalities with exquisite anatomic detail. It is much more sensitive than x-ray, for example, for identifying fractures. As with CT, MRI examinations can be performed with intravenous or intra-articular contrast. Intravenous contrast enhances visualization of certain lesions, while contrast administered directly into a joint, termed *MR arthrography*, can help assess intra-articular abnormalities. MRI also has the ability to produce angiographic images with or without the use of an intravenous contrast agent.

An MRI examination comprises many sequences that image the area of interest. These sequences accentuate different characteristics of the tissues based on behavior of the molecular constituents of the tissues in the magnetic field when subjected to radiofrequency pulses seen as the time that it takes the ions to return to their prestimulation state (relaxation times). T1- and T2-weighted, proton density (PD), inversion recovery (IR), and gradient recalled echo (GRE) are the most common sequences. Chemical suppression of fat can be superimposed on any of them, except inversion recovery (which is already a fat suppression technique).

The imaging characteristics of tissues differ on the different pulse sequences that can be used to differentiate among fluid, fat, blood, muscle, tendon, bone, and cartilage. Fat (ie, bone marrow, subcutaneous fat) is low in signal intensity on fat-suppressed sequences, including a type of inversion recovery sequence termed STIR (short tau inversion recovery; *tau* is also called *inversion time*), while fluid (ie, urinary bladder, bowel, joint synovial fluid) is high-signal intensity. Protein density techniques can be used to evaluate soft tissue (ie, muscle, tendons, intrapelvic structures) and bone. GRE sequences allow for acquisition of images of thin slices but are sensitive to magnetic field heterogeneities (useful for detecting chronic hemorrhage and foreign bodies). Technique is important in producing MRIs and can be quite complex. MRI protocols are not currently standardized, in part accounting for differences in image quality from different imaging centers. High-resolution, thin-sectioned, small field-of-view images will best evaluate anatomy and pathology.

MRI is the most common way to evaluate articular cartilage, labral tears, and avascular necrosis of the hip. It is also the ideal way to assess muscle injury and radiographically occult fractures as well as surrounding soft tissue structures. Indeed, MRI is an excellent tool for evaluating all structures of the hip. Its disadvantage is that it is the most expensive of the techniques described in this chapter. Because MRI uses radiofrequency waves to create the image, the term *signal* describes findings on MRI. Descriptive terminology for *signal* on MRI include high-signal intensity, intermediate signal intensity, and low-signal intensity (or signal void).

The primary disadvantages of MRI include safety issues for patients with implantable medical devices such as pacemakers, high cost, and limited availability. Ferromagnetic instrumentation alters the magnetic field and causes artifact but does not prevent the utility of the examination.

## Ultrasound

Diagnostic ultrasonography uses the same principle as sound navigation and ranging (SONAR). A high-frequency sound-generating probe (which also functions as the receiver) is put on the skin, and the sound waves bounce off structures at various depths to varying degrees to produce images in real time. With the addition of Doppler technique, vascularity can be characterized in detail with high spatial resolution. Ultrasound is extensively used as a diagnostic tool in the fields of obstetrics and gynecology, as well as in abdominal and vascular imaging. The role of ultrasonography in musculoskeletal imaging has been rapidly evolving and expanding due to the continual development and improvement in technology.

Ultrasonography is ideally suited for evaluating superficial structures—shoulder, elbow, wrist, finger, ankle tendons and ligaments, as well as the tendons of the large joints, muscles, and soft tissue masses. Unlike radiography and CT, there is no concern for the harmful effects of ionizing radiation. Unfortunately, it is less commonly used and less available in the United States than in Europe and Australia. One of its advantages is that it can image in real-time, so it can be used to guide injections into the hip joint, iliopsoas, and trochanteric bursae. It is useful to evaluate for tendinosis, tendon tears, and coxa saltans (snapping hip; Figure 3-4). One of its disadvantages is that there has to be an acoustic window, a corridor of soft tissue that the sound waves can pass to get to the area of interest. This fact limits its utility in evaluating intra-articular structures because bone bounces back all of the sound waves.

Because ultrasound images are created by sound reflections, substances on ultrasound are termed *echogenic/echodense* (bone, metal) or *echolucent* (water). Structures can be described as hyper-, iso-, hypo-, or anechoic. Structures that are echogenic can cause an acoustic shadow below them because all of the sound beams are reflected back to the probe.

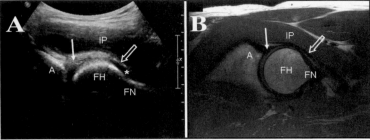

**Figure 3-4.** Normal hip ultrasound. (A) Longitudinal (sagittal) grey scale ultrasound image of the hip. The femoral head (FH), femoral neck (FN), acetabulum (A), labrum (solid arrow), anterior joint capsule (open arrow), iliopsoas muscle (IP), and joint fluid (*) can be identified. (B) MRI sagittal PD image oriented for correlation with the ultrasound image. (Courtesy of Hospital for Special Surgery, New York, NY.)

## Nuclear Medicine Imaging

Nuclear medicine imaging is a type of imaging that is more functional than anatomic. Bioactive radioactive substances are intravenously administered to a patient, and a gamma camera is used to image their distribution. In orthopedics, the most common nuclear medicine test is the bone scan. In a bone scan, a radioactive bone substrate goes to all bones, but more go to metabolically active bones, allowing the radiologist to identify areas of increased turnover secondary to fracture, infection, or tumor. SPECT and PET scanning give 3-dimensional information and can be coupled with CT studies.

The bone scan employs the radiotracer Tc-99m MDP (Tc-99m ligated chemically to the compound methylene-diphosphonate [MDP]), which is absorbed into bone after intravenous injection. Delayed images taken 2 to 4 hours after the injection of Tc-99m MDP can be combined with information regarding blood flow (during injection) and blood pooling just after injection. These are the 3 phases of a 3-phase bone scan. Images of the entire body are obtained as well as specific regions of interest (Figure 3-5). Because bone scan findings are not specific, they should be correlated with other imaging modalities such as radiographs or CT for anatomic correlation and to narrow the differential diagnosis of what is causing the radiotracer uptake. Other nuclear medicine techniques can be used to look for infection and tumors (radioactivity-labeled white blood cell studies and PET, respectively).

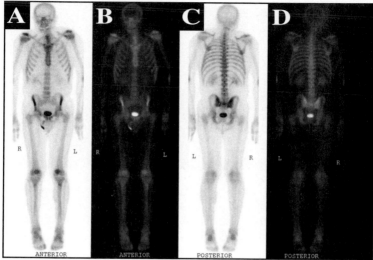

**Figure 3-5.** Normal nuclear medicine bone scan. Planar whole body bone scan in the (A, B) anterior and (C, D) posterior projections. Images are obtained after 3 hours of intravenous administration of the radiotracer Tc-99m MDP. The color scale can be inverted (eg, A versus B) to improve the radiologist's detection of abnormal radiotracer activity. (Courtesy of Hospital for Special Surgery, New York, NY.)

Bone scans are often used to look for metastatic disease, stress or occult fractures, and osteonecrosis. It can also be used as a screening test of the skeletal system—if a lesion is present on a radiograph, one can look for other lesions by bone scanning instead of taking x-rays of the entire body.

Nuclear medicine scans are based on the body incorporating the radionuclide that is seen by the gamma camera. Variations in the amount of absorption cause areas termed *increased/high uptake* or *decreased/low uptake* (photopenic).

## Intervention

Interventional radiology is a subspecialty of radiology in which minimally invasive procedures are performed with image-guidance. Fluoroscopy, CT, ultrasound, and MRI can be used to guide these procedures. Interventional procedures fall under 2 broad categories: either primarily for diagnostic or primarily for therapeutic purposes.

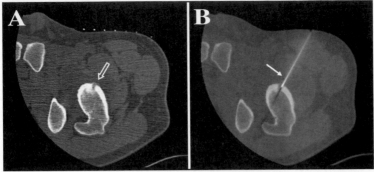

**Figure 3-6.** Osteoid osteoma radiofrequency ablation. CT scan through the left hip during (A) pre-procedural localization and (B) intra-procedural ablation with percutaneous radiofrequency probe (solid arrow) in the osteoid osteoma (open arrow). (Courtesy of Hospital for Special Surgery, New York, NY.)

In the musculoskeletal system, image-guided diagnostic procedures include percutaneous core needle biopsy of soft tissue and bone, joint fluid and extra-articular cyst aspiration, and arthrography.

Therapeutic interventional procedures include osteoid osteoma radiofrequency ablation and therapeutic anesthetic and steroid injections of joints, bursae, interdigital (Morton) neuromas, and tendon sheaths, as well as around nerves (Figures 3-6 and 3-7).

Interventional procedures are usually performed on an outpatient basis, incur minimal risks, and can often delay or even preclude surgery. Patients who are not surgical candidates may undergo an interventional diagnostic study to guide appropriate medical treatment or an interventional therapeutic procedure to alleviate clinical symptoms.

# IMAGING EVALUATION OF HIP PATHOLOGIES

## Osseous Trauma

Evaluation of pelvic and hip fractures typically begins with conventional radiographs. The radiographic views to obtain depend on what pathology is suspected. The views required depend upon whether the examination is for hip fracture,

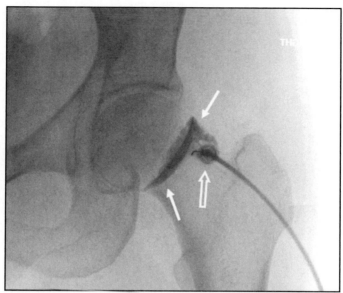

**Figure 3-7.** Fluoroscopic-guided therapeutic hip joint injection. An intra-procedural fluoroscopic image after contrast injection demonstrates characteristic opacification of the hip joint (solid arrows), confirming intra-articular position of the needle (open arrow). After documenting correct needle position, a combination of anesthetic and cortisone is injected through the same needle. (Courtesy of Hospital for Special Surgery, New York, NY.)

pelvic fracture, or acetabular fracture. CT may be useful when plain films are negative in the setting of a high index of suspicion for fracture. CT can be used for preoperative planning to delineate anatomic detail of complex fractures and to identify intra-articular fragments. Radiographs can miss up to 30% of pelvic fractures, up to 40% of intra-articular fragments, and 50% of femoral head fractures identified by CT.[1]

### Hip Fracture

Fractures around the hip most commonly occur at the proximal femur. Fractures can be the result of low-impact falls in people who are elderly or who have osteoporosis. They are best evaluated with 2 views of the proximal femur, usually an AP view of the pelvis and a frog-lateral view of the affected hip (Figure 3-8). These fractures are traditionally categorized

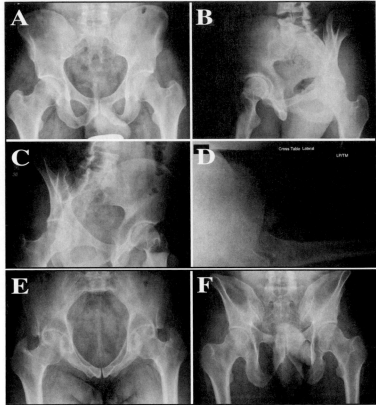

**Figure 3-8.** Trauma series. (A) AP; (B) obturator (internal) oblique left hip; (C) iliac (external) oblique left hip; (D) cross-table lateral (detailed evaluation of bony structures is usually limited due to x-ray beam attenuation by soft tissues). (E) Inlet and (F) outlet views of the pelvis. (Courtesy of Hospital for Special Surgery, New York, NY.)

as either intracapsular fractures (femoral head or neck) or extracapsular fractures (trochanters). Intracapsular fractures are further classified as capital, subcapital, transcervical, and basicervical, depending on their location (in the femoral head, just below the femoral head, across the middle of the femoral neck, or at the base of the femoral neck). These fractures can be difficult to see on radiograph if they are not displaced. A classification system for femoral neck fractures was proposed by Garden[2] (Figure 3-9 and Table 3-2). Extracapsular fractures are further classified as intertrochanteric and subtrochanteric.

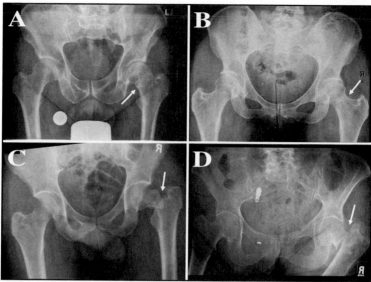

**Figure 3-9.** Garden classification of femoral neck fractures. (A) Garden I. Note cortical discontinuity in the medial left femoral neck and sclerosis representing impaction (arrow). (B) Garden II. (C) Garden III. (D) Garden IV. (Courtesy of Hospital for Special Surgery, New York, NY.)

**Table 3-2**

## GARDEN CLASSIFICATION OF SUBCAPITAL FEMORAL FRACTURES

I.   Incomplete fracture
II.  Complete fracture without displacement
III. Complete fracture with partial displacement
IV.  Complete fracture with full displacement

Osteonecrosis of the femoral head is the most common complication of intracapsular fractures, occurring in up to 15% to 35% of patients due to the tenuous blood supply to the proximal femur. Its presence can be evaluated with MRI or bone scan. Nonunion is also a common complication of post-traumatic femoral neck fractures, occurring in 10% to 44% of patients.

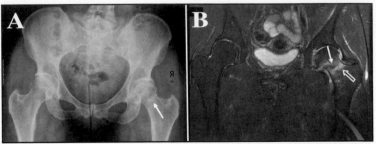

**Figure 3-10.** Subcapital femoral neck insufficiency fracture. (A) AP radiograph of the pelvis demonstrates a sclerotic band (solid arrow) traversing the subcapital femoral neck. (B) MRI coronal STIR image reveals high-signal bone marrow edema (open arrow) surrounding a low signal intensity fracture line (solid arrow), confirming the presence of a stress fracture. (Courtesy of Hospital for Special Surgery, New York, NY.)

Although difficult to see on radiographs, subtle subchondral fractures are a cause of hip pain. These fractures may be related to transient osteoporosis, although it is uncertain if the osteoporosis is cause or effect.

To detect a subtle fracture, the entire femoral cortex should be scrutinized for discontinuity or irregularity. Intramedullary and impacted fractures may appear as a linear sclerotic density within the medullary cavity. The sclerosis may become more conspicuous with time because, as a fracture starts to heal, it can become more dense. A femoral neck fracture can be difficult to distinguish from an osteophyte that surrounds the capsule (apron osteophyte). Radiographically occult femoral fractures are demonstrated on MRI as linear low signal intensity surrounded by an amorphous region of localized bone marrow edema (Figure 3-10).

For patients who are unable to undergo MRI examination, CT scan or radionuclide bone scan can often identify the fracture. On CT, femoral fracture can appear as a cortical break, lucent fracture line, or intramedullary sclerotic density. On a bone scan, a fracture appears as a focal area of increased radiotracer activity, although this finding is not specific for fracture. It can take up to 3 to 7 days for a bone scan to become positive (Figure 3-11). CT is not as sensitive as MRI to identify subtle nondisplaced fractures because MRI adds the conspicuity of edema on the fat-suppressed sequences.

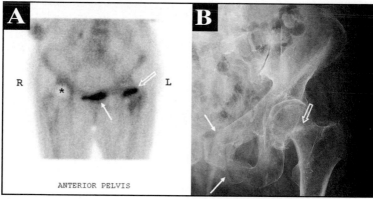

**Figure 3-11.** Subcapital femoral neck fracture. (A) Nuclear medicine bone scan, spot view of the pelvis demonstrates abnormal increased radiotracer activity in the left proximal femur (open arrow) and parasymphyseal pubic bone (solid arrow). Note the "cold" defect in the right proximal femur (*), due to a hip prosthesis. (B) Left hip radiograph confirms fractures of the left subcapital femoral neck (open arrow) and pubis (solid arrows). (Courtesy of Hospital for Special Surgery, New York, NY.)

## Pelvic Fracture

The bony pelvis is considered a nearly rigid ring composed of 3 elements: the sacrum dorsally, joined to 2 innominate bones by the sacroiliac joints. Each innominate bone comprises the ilium, ischium, and pubis; the innominate bones are joined anteriorly by the pubic symphysis (Figure 3-12). Because of the inter-relationship of the individual components within the ring, fractures of the pelvic ring usually occur in pairs. Diastasis of the sacroiliac joints or pubic symphysis can substitute for one of these fractures.

Radiographic evaluation of the pelvic ring should include inlet and outlet views of the pelvis (views taken with the x-ray camera obliqued caudally or cranially, respectively), which are useful for assessing fractures by creating another projection of the bones onto the film. They aid in identifying fractures, improving confidence that they are real, and evaluating their displacement. They also permit evaluation of hemi-pelvis displacement, as well as fractures of the iliac crests, the SI joints, pubic symphysis, and sacrum.

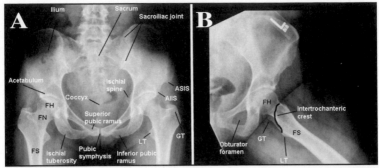

**Figure 3-12.** Normal pelvis and hip radiographs. (A) AP pelvis radiograph. (B) Frog-leg lateral view of the left hip. ASIS = anterior superior iliac spine; AIIS = anterior inferior iliac spine; GT = greater trochanter; LT = lesser trochanter; FH = femoral head; FN = femoral neck; FS = femoral shaft. (Courtesy of Hospital for Special Surgery, New York, NY.)

## Acetabular Fractures

When acetabular fractures are suspected, Judet oblique views (45 degree oblique projections) should be obtained. The obturator oblique view is imaged with the hip of interest rotated toward the film and facilitates inspection of the posterior acetabular rim and the anterior column. The iliac oblique view is imaged with the hip of interest rotated away from the film and facilitates inspection of the anterior acetabular rim and the posterior column (Figure 3-13).

In patients who have sustained pelvic trauma, radiographic evaluation should always include assessment of the following landmarks on the AP view of the pelvis: the iliopectineal line, ilioischial line, anterior rim of the acetabulum, posterior rim of the acetabulum, acetabular roof, "tear drop" (Kohler's), Shenton's arcuate line, and sacral arches (Figure 3-14).

The iliopectineal line is formed by anterior structures of the acetabulum, and disruption of this line represents a fracture of the anterior column. The ilioischial line is formed by posterior structures of the acetabulum, and disruption of this line represents a fracture of the posterior column. The pelvic tear drop represents the anteroinferior aspect of the acetabular fossa at the acetabular notch with contributions from the ischium and superior pubic ramus.[3]

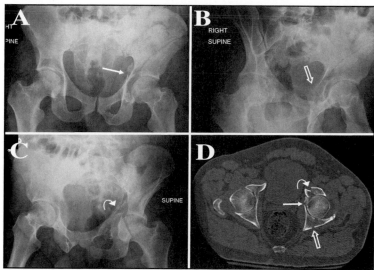

**Figure 3-13.** Acetabular fracture. (A) AP demonstrates a left acetabular fracture (solid arrow). (B) Iliac (external) oblique and (C) obturator (internal) oblique views show disruption of the ilioischial (open arrow) and iliopectineal lines (curved arrow). (D) Axial CT image demonstrates fractures through the medial wall (solid arrow) and anterior (curved arrow) and posterior (open arrow) columns of the left acetabulum. (Courtesy of Hospital for Special Surgery, New York, NY.)

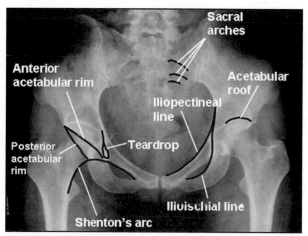

**Figure 3-14.** Radiographic landmarks of the hip and pelvis. These lines should be scrutinized in every patient presenting with pelvis or hip trauma. Disruption of any of these normal radiographic landmarks indicates possible fracture. (Courtesy of Hospital for Special Surgery, New York, NY.)

**Table 3-3**

## CLASSIFICATION OF PELVIC FRACTURES

| Elementary Fractures | Associated Fractures |
| --- | --- |
| 1. Anterior wall fractures | 1. T-shaped fractures |
| 2. Anterior column fractures | 2. Complete 2-column fractures |
| 3. Posterior wall fractures | 3. Transverse and posterior wall fractures |
| 4. Posterior column fractures | |
| 5. Transverse fractures | 4. Posterior column and posterior wall fractures |
| | 5. Anterior column posterior hemitransverse fractures |

Disruption of Shenton's arcuate line, which is drawn from the superior margin of the obturator ring extending laterally to along the medial cortex of the femoral neck, indicates the presence of hip joint subluxation or dislocation.

Acetabular fractures can vary in complexity. The patterns described by Judet and Letournel create a useful classification system. The classification system is divided into 5 simple fracture types and 5 associated fracture types (Table 3-3).[4,5] Four fractures involve both the anterior and posterior column: transverse, T-shaped, anterior column/posterior hemitransverse, and both column-associated fractures. If on radiograph a fracture involves both columns, it will be one of these. The both column-associated fracture is the one that may have the lateral spike described by Judet and Letournel.

With its thin section and multiplanar capabilities, CT is particularly useful for characterizing acetabular fractures and allows accurate classification to facilitate surgical management. Three-dimensional volumetric rendering can be a useful tool for understanding complex fractures for preoperative planning. Trauma centers currently get CT scans for all major trauma cases to assess other injuries. This scan, done with thicker slices, may not provide all of the information, such as the presence of small intra-articular bodies, that the orthopedic surgeon needs to evaluate the fracture (Figure 3-15).

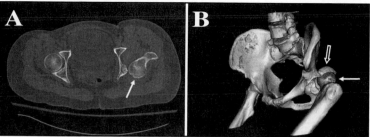

**Figure 3-15.** Hip fracture-dislocation. (A) Axial CT image and (B) 3-D volume rendering demonstrate a right femoral posterior-superior dislocation (solid arrow). A fracture fragment of the posterior acetabulum is also present (open arrow). (Courtesy of Hospital for Special Surgery, New York, NY.)

Even relatively minor trauma (being tackled in a football game) can cause hip dislocation and concomitant fracture of the posterior lip/wall of the acetabulum. This injury can be difficult to see on x-ray. If patient symptoms persist or if x-ray shows no abnormality, further imaging with CT or MRI may be warranted.

### Sacral Fractures

Sacral fractures are common in the elderly. They can occur after minor trauma or even without recognizable trauma. These nondisplaced fractures cause pain but do not require treatment. Discontinuity of the cortical surfaces of the sacral arches can be difficult to appreciate because of the shadows produced by overlying bowel gas, but represents fractures through the sacral foramina. While they may be difficult to see on x-ray, they are readily apparent on CT, MRI, and bone scan.

## Extra-Articular Pathology

### Avulsion Injuries

Injuries to the muscle tendon unit can occur at the muscle tendon junction or the tendinous attachment to bone. Although myotendinous injuries are much more common, avulsions at the muscle attachment frequently occur. In adolescents, these are aphophyseal injuries. Hurdlers, soccer players, and gymnasts are especially prone to avulsion injuries. Common sites for bony avulsions of pelvis include the ischial tuberosity

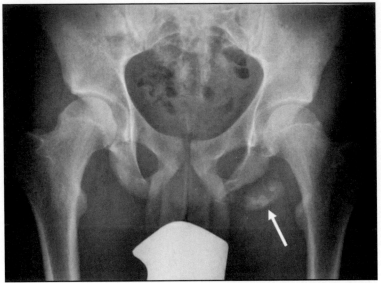

**Figure 3-16.** Left ischial tuberosity avulsion. AP pelvis view shows a large bony fragment (arrow) displaced approximately 1.5 cm from the remainder of the ischial tuberosity, the site of the hamstring origins. (Courtesy of Hospital for Special Surgery, New York, NY.)

(hamstring origin insertion), anterior superior iliac crest (sartorius and tensor fascia lata origins), anterior inferior iliac crest (rectus femoris origin), pubis (adductor origin), and, less commonly, the iliac crest apophysis (abductor musculature/iliotibial band). Avulsion injuries often can be diagnosed on conventional radiograph AP view of the pelvis (Figure 3-16).

## Stress Reaction and Fracture

Runners are prone to stress injuries of the lower extremities, especially of the femur, tibia, and metatarsals. Radionuclide bone scan and MRI are more sensitive than radiographs for the diagnosis of stress fractures (Figure 3-17). Bone marrow edema is demonstrated at the site of injury on MRI. A low signal intensity line represents a fracture. Stress injury to the bone is sometimes visible on MRI before an actual fracture occurs. Stress injuries are also apparent from bony remodeling at tendon insertion sites. Because this stress injury can occur at the gluteus maximus insertion, imaging of hip pain in the athlete should include the proximal femora.

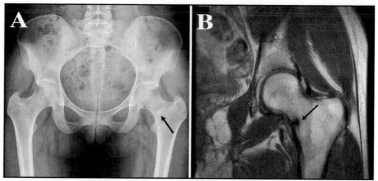

**Figure 3-17.** Stress fracture. (A) AP pelvis radiograph of a marathon runner demonstrates a subtle linear sclerotic density adjacent to the medial cortex of the left femoral neck (arrow). (B) MRI coronal PD FSE of the left hip shows a corresponding low signal intensity focus (arrow) involving only a portion of the medullary cavity, confirming the presence of a stress fracture. (Courtesy of Hospital for Special Surgery, New York, NY.)

## Other Muscle and Tendon Abnormalities

As mentioned previously, injuries to the muscle tendon unit (strain) occur most commonly at the junction of muscle and tendon. Around the pelvis, these injuries occur to the same muscles as described previously with avulsions. Other pathologies include tendon degeneration from chronic overuse and muscle injury from direct trauma.

Tendon degeneration (tendinosis) is more common in older patients and can affect any of the tendons around the hip. Tendinosis commonly affects abductors at their greater trochanter insertion. These tendons may also tear. The iliopsoas also can undergo degeneration but very rarely tear.

Soft tissue injuries are best evaluated with MRI or ultrasound. On MRI, both signal and morphology are important characteristics of muscle and tendon. Low-grade injuries involve only signal abnormalities such as the high signal that may be seen at the normally black (MRI) or white (ultrasound) tendon insertion. Suppressing the fat on a sequence improves the sensitivity of MRI in identifying abnormalities such as with low-grade muscle-tendon junction tear. Morphologic changes that can be seen include tendon thickening and/or tendon discontinuity (Figure 3-18).

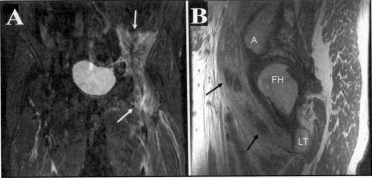

**Figure 3-18.** Iliopsoas tear. (A) MRI coronal STIR of the pelvis shows extensive edema and hemorrhage along the expected course of the iliopsoas muscle (white arrows). (B) Sagittal PD FSE image of the left hip demonstrates complete tear of the iliopsoas tendon (black arrows) with proximal retraction from the lesser trochanter (LT). FH = femoral head; A = acetabulum. (Courtesy of Hospital for Special Surgery, New York, NY.)

Intramuscular hematomas resulting from injury may result in an extra-skeletal non-neoplastic growth of new bone, a process known as heterotopic ossification or myositis ossificans (Figure 3-19). Because of the intense inflammatory reaction in its early stages, myositis ossificans appears aggressive and can be mistaken for a neoplasm. The characteristic zonal appearance of ossification from the periphery to the center differentiates this lesion from neoplasm. Also, myositis ossificans changes more rapidly than tumor; therefore, a radiograph repeated in 1 or 2 weeks will yield a change in early myositis ossificans, but not in tumor.

### Bursitis

Excessive rubbing and friction of one or several of the bursae about the hip or pelvis may lead to painful bursal inflammation. Pelvic and hip bursitis commonly involves the trochanteric, ischial, and iliopsoas bursae. On MRI, bursitis appears as a focal fluid signal intensity lesion in the expected location of a bursa. A bursa around the iliopsoas tendon may be seen either from primary bursitis or from effusion decompressing from the hip joint. Ultrasonography is also a useful modality for the evaluation of suspected bursitis because of

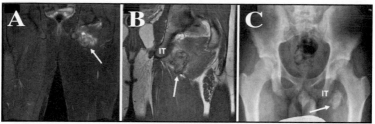

**Figure 3-19.** Myositis ossificans/heterotopic ossification. (A) MRI body coil coronal STIR and (B) surface coil coronal PD FSE of the left hip demonstrates an intermediate signal intensity lesion with low signal intensity irregular margins (white arrow) and adjacent soft tissue edema inferolateral to the left ischial tuberosity (IT). (C) AP pelvis radiograph shows a corresponding focus of heterotopic bone formation (white arrow) in this patient who had sustained a prior hamstring origin avulsion injury. (Courtesy of Hospital for Special Surgery, New York, NY.)

the relative superficial location of bursae. Bursitis on ultrasound appears as a predominantly anechoic fluid collection, although it may also contain echogenic debris and thickened synovium (Figure 3-20). The ultrasonographer can reproduce the patient's symptoms by scanning over an affected bursa with slight pressure, thereby establishing the source of the patient's pain.

## Snapping Iliopsoas Tendon

Ultrasonography is the noninvasive modality of choice for diagnosing iliopsoas tendon subluxation as a cause of hip pain. In this condition, also known as coxa sultans, the iliopsoas tendon slips over a bony prominence such as the anterior inferior iliac spine (AIIS), iliopectineal eminence, or lesser trochanter, producing a painful audible snapping sensation during certain movements of the hip joint. A dynamic ultrasound exam demonstrates iliopsoas tendon subluxation with hip motion in real time and can also identify any associated bursitis. Ultrasound can also identify extra-articular snapping hip syndrome caused by subluxation of the iliotibial band or the gluteus maximus over the greater trochanter.[6]

## Pubalgia/Sports Hernia

A unique consideration in athletes with pain about the pubic symphysis or groin is the condition of athletic pubalgia.

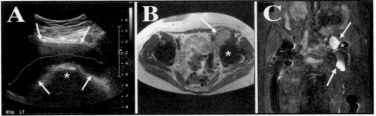

**Figure 3-20.** Iliopsoas bursitis. (A) Ultrasound image of the left hip demonstrates a large anechoic fluid collection (demarcated by arrows and dotted line), superficial to an echogenic structure with posterior acoustic shadowing, in this patient with a left total hip prosthesis (*). (B) Axial PD FSE and (C) coronal STIR confirms the presence of a large iliopsoas bursitis (arrows) adjacent to susceptibility artifact from the joint prosthesis (*). The iliopsoas (IP) is displaced laterally. A right hip prosthesis is also present. (Courtesy of Hospital for Special Surgery, New York, NY.)

Pubalgia is an umbrella term used to describe several causes (or a multifactorial process) of groin pain. The particular cause in a given patient can be difficult to discern. MRI may be helpful in identifying a specific abnormality of regional musculoskeletal structures. These include the lower frontal abdominal musculature, symphysis pubis and pubic rami, and adductor/obturator compartment, as well as the pelvic viscera and inguinal canal. Pubic degeneration and adductor tendinosis or tear are the most readily diagnosable causes of this pain (Figure 3-21).

The sportsman's hernia is another term that has been applied to this condition, but it is a misnomer because a hernia is usually absent. Some believe that the pain is related to rectus abdominus/adductor aponeurosis avulsion from the pubis.[7,8] Others believe that the problem starts with a lack of hip motion, putting more stress on the pubis and causing an overuse injury.

## Intra-Articular Pathology

### Degenerative Joint Disease

Degenerative joint disease is often used synonymously with osteoarthritis or just arthritis. Arthritis, arthrosis, and arthropathy can be used interchangeably, although they have slightly different meanings. It is the loss of cartilage in a

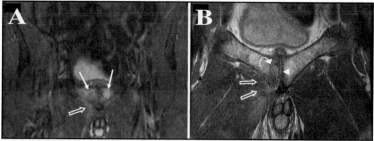

**Figure 3-21.** Pubalgia. (A) MRI coronal STIR and (B) coronal PD images demonstrate degeneration of the pubic symphysis with reactive bone marrow edema (solid arrows), cartilage loss (arrowhead), and subchondral cyst formation (curved arrow). There is also abnormal signal in the right adductor origin (open arrows), representing a partial tear in this triathlete presenting with right groin pain. (Courtesy of Hospital for Special Surgery, New York, NY.)

joint, preventing the normal gliding of one surface over the other, which can cause pain. Osteoarthritis (as opposed to inflammatory arthritis) becomes common with age. It can be primary (idiopathic, degenerative) or secondary. Causes of secondary osteoarthritis of any joint include trauma, infection, osteonecrosis, and underlying inflammatory arthropathies such as rheumatoid arthritis. Conditions predisposing to osteoarthritis specific to the hip are slipped capital femoral epiphysis and developmental dysplasia of the hip (DDH). FAI, discussed on p. 98, has recently been heralded as a cause.

Arthritis can be appreciated on radiographs as joint space narrowing, osteophyte formation, subchondral sclerosis, and subchondral cyst formation. The joint space narrowing is a secondary sign of cartilage loss and is usually more evident in only part of the hip—most commonly superolaterally (Figure 3-22).

Early arthritis, or the loss of some of the articular cartilage of the hip joint, may be difficult or impossible to detect on x-ray. Focal articular cartilage abnormalities—defects or flaps—are radiographically occult. MRI is more sensitive and may be necessary to detect them because it can evaluate the primary abnormality, the cartilage abnormality itself (see Figure 3-22).

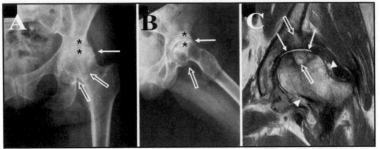

**Figure 3-22.** Left hip osteoarthrosis. (A) AP and (B) frog leg lateral views of the left hip show superior joint space narrowing (solid arrows), subchondral sclerosis and cysts (*), as well as femoral head osteophytes (open arrows). (C) MRI coronal PD FSE image of the left hip demonstrates areas of full-thickness cartilage loss with exposed bone over the acetabular dome and femoral head (white arrows) and large subchondral cysts (open arrows). MRI also reveals a small reactive synovitis (arrowheads). (Courtesy of Hospital for Special Surgery, New York, NY.)

## Inflammatory Arthropathy

Inflammatory arthropathies include seropositive arthopathies (rheumatoid arthritis), seronegative arthropathies (ankylosing spondylitis, psoriatic arthritis, and reactive arthritis [formerly Reiter syndrome]), and infection. The key to diagnosing a noninfectious inflammatory arthritis is often the patient's history. The patient may already know about the disease. Many joints will be affected. Radiographs should show symmetric and concentric joint space loss—both sides and all parts of each side (Figure 3-23). The sacroiliac joints can give a clue as to the type of inflammatory arthritis because they will often be fused in patients with ankylosing spondylitis.

An inflammatory-appearing arthritis that affects only one side may be infectious and should be evaluated with joint aspiration.

### Labral Tear

The acetabular labrum is fibrocartilagenous tissue that surrounds the bony acetabulum, much like the shoulder labrum.[9] Unlike the shoulder, its function in the normal hip has probably less to do with stability and more to do with creating smooth hip dynamics. Athletes engaging in sports-related activities that involve hip hyperextension and external femoral

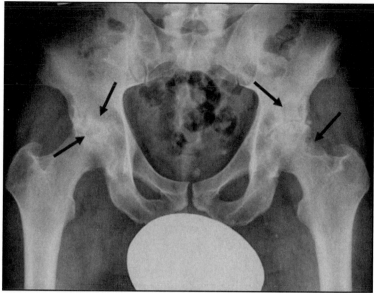

**Figure 3-23.** Rheumatoid arthritis. AP radiograph of the pelvis demonstrates marked central hip joint space narrowing, more severe on the right. Subchondral erosions (arrows) are present bilaterally. Large erosions can be seen in the left femoral head and neck laterally. (Courtesy of Hospital for Special Surgery, New York, NY.)

rotation are susceptible to acetabular labral injuries. Shear injury secondary to contact of the femoral head against the anterior labrum predisposes patients to anterior labral tears.[10] Dysplastic hips usually have a hypertrophic labrum that is susceptible to tear. Most labral tears are of the anterior labrum.

Recognition of labral tears as the etiology of mechanical hip pain in the younger patient is crucial because surgical treatment often provides symptomatic relief. Additionally, labral injury may be one of the precursors to degenerative joint disease.

Although asymptomatic labral tears are common, MRI can confirm the presence of a clinically suspected labral tear. Intra-articular injection of anesthetic can confirm that suspected pain comes from the joint. Pain relief after anesthetic injection indicates that the pain likely comes from the joint rather than the surrounding tissues such as tendons. Whereas MR arthrography is often used to detect labral tears, noncontrast

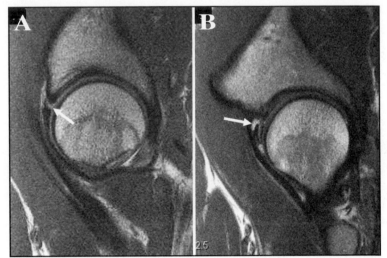

**Figure 3-24.** Labral tear. MRI sagittal MRI PD FSE images demonstrate high signal intensity through the anterior labrum, representing a tear. The normal labrum should be a triangular-shaped homogeneous low signal intensity structure. (Courtesy of Hospital for Special Surgery, New York, NY.)

MRI has been shown to be just as effective.[11] Findings indicative of labral tear are linear high signal intensity through the labrum or identification of joint fluid or contrast imbibition within the labrum (Figure 3-24) . Tears of the labrum can give rise to paralabral cysts, which can themselves cause pain.

## Femoroacetabular Impingement

FAI is a recently described clinical syndrome caused by abnormal contact between the femur and acetabulum, leading to labral tear and cartilage damage.[12] FAI is implicated as a major cause of premature osteoarthritis, especially in young, active patients.[13] The etiology of FAI can be broadly classified as either cam type, which represents abnormal femur morphology, and pincer type, which represents abnormality involving the acetabulum. Asphericity of the anterior femoral head-neck junction (cam type) or overcoverage of the femoral head by the acetabulum (pincer type) results in pathologic contact between the proximal femur and acetabulum during hip joint motion and eventual damage to the labrum and cartilage. In reality, most patients have a combination of cam- and pincer-type impingement.

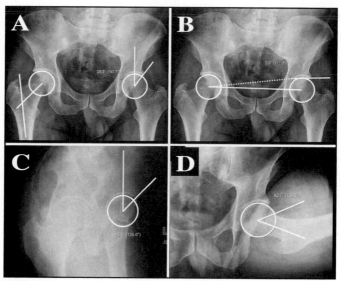

**Figure 3-25.** Standardized hip measurements. (A) AP pelvis radiograph. The femoral neck-shaft angle is formed by a line parallel to the femoral neck axis through the center of the femoral head and a line through the axis of the femoral shaft. The lateral center edge angle is formed by a vertical line through the center of the femoral head and a line to the superolateral most point of the sclerotic sourcil. (B) AP pelvis radiograph. The acetabular index or Tönnis angle is measured by a line connecting the inferior most and superolateral most point of the sclerotic sourcil and a line through the center of the femoral heads. (C) False profile view. The anterior center edge angle is formed by a vertical line through the center of the femoral head and a line to the anterior most point of the sclerotic sourcil. (D) Elongated femoral neck view. The alpha angle is formed by a line through the center of the femoral head and femoral neck axis and a line to the point of the beginning of the femoral head asphericity. Best fit circles are drawn around the femoral head to identify the femoral head center (continued). (Courtesy of Hospital for Special Surgery, New York, NY.)

Patients suspected of having FAI should undergo initial evaluation with radiographs, which includes an AP pelvis view as well as lateral (frog-lateral or false profile) and axial (elongated femoral neck) views of the hip of interest to evaluate for osseous abnormalities (Figure 3-25). Table 3-4 summarizes characteristic findings of FAI and how they are assessed on plain film.

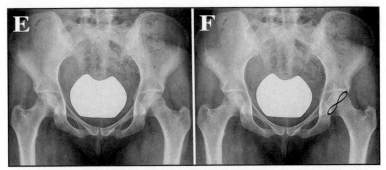

**Figure 3-25 (continued).** Standardized hip measurements. (E, F) Cross-over sign. AP radiographs of the pelvis demonstrate the cross-over sign in the left acetabulum indicating acetabular retroversion, which is a risk factor for femoroacetabular impingement. The cross-over sign is also seen in the contralateral acetabulum. (Courtesy of Hospital for Special Surgery, New York, NY.)

If surgery is contemplated for FAI, the patient should undergo an MRI examination, which includes high-resolution surface coil images of the hip joint as part of an optimized protocol, to assess the status of labrum and articular cartilage. MRI can identify anterosuperior labral degeneration and tears, with or without paralabral cysts. Damage to articular cartilage over the hip joint can manifest as partial or full-thickness defects, fibrillation, or flap formation, usually in the antero-superior acetabulum in cam-type FAI (Figure 3-26). Patients with pincer-type FAI may also develop chondral injury along the posteroinferior acetabulum. The addition of an oblique axial sequence, prescribed as an oblique plane paralleling the femoral neck, or a radial sequence is useful in assessing anterolateral femoral head-neck morphology and lesions, such as herniation pits and osteophytes. The oblique axial or radial plane is also used to assess asphericity and abnormal offset between the femoral head and neck, which can be obvious with significant deformities. More subtle deformities of the femoral head-neck junction can be detected by measuring the alpha angle in the oblique axial plane, with abnormal being more than 55 degrees (Figure 3-27).

**Table 3-4**

## RADIOGRAPHIC EVALUATION OF FEMOROACETABULAR IMPINGEMENT

| Impingement Type | Feature | Assessment |
|---|---|---|
| Cam | Pistol grip deformity | Abnormal femoral head-neck morphology |
| | Coxa vara | Femoral neck-shaft angle <125 degrees |
| | Femoral head-neck junction asphericity | Alpha angle >55 degrees<br>Deficient head-neck junction offset<br>Subcapital osteophytes |
| Pincer | General acetabular overcoverage | Lateral center edge angle >39 degrees<br>Anterior center edge angle >39 degrees<br>Acetabular index angle <0 degrees<br>Coxa profunda<br>Acetabular protrusion |
| | Focal acetabular overcoverage | Acetabular retroversion—crossover sign<br>Prominent acetabular posterior wall—posterior wall sign |
| Secondary findings | Herniation pits | Anterolateral head-neck lucencies |
| | Labral ossification | Os acetabuli |
| | Osteoarthritis | Joint space narrowing, osteophytes, subchondral sclerosis and cysts |

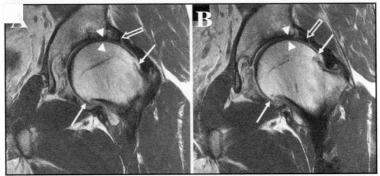

**Figure 3-26.** Osteoarthritis secondary to femoroacetabular impingement. Surface coil coronal PD FSE images of the left hip show a chronically torn and degenerated labrum with intralabral ossification (open arrows) and severe cartilage loss over the acetabular dome and femoral head (arrowheads). Subcapital osteophytes are also present (solid arrows). (Courtesy of Hospital for Special Surgery, New York, NY.)

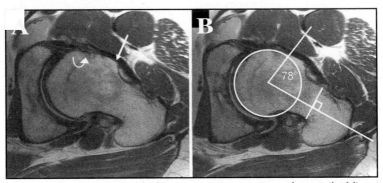

**Figure 3-27.** Femoroacetabular impingement. MRI surface coil oblique axial PD FSE images of the left hip demonstrate an abnormal alpha angle (>55 degrees) caused by femoral head-neck junction bony proliferation (solid arrow). Note the anterior subchondral cysts (curved arrow), which are also associated with FAI. (Courtesy of Hospital for Special Surgery, New York, NY.)

## Avascular Necrosis (Osteonecrosis)

There are many causes of femoral head avascular necrosis (AVN). The most common causes of AVN are steroid use (most common), trauma, sickle cell disease, and vasculitis. AVN can also be idiopathic. The goals of imaging are to diagnose, assess activity, and to determine severity in order to evaluate prognosis. Early stages have a better prognosis than later stages, which may require hip replacement. Radiographs are the first diagnostic imaging modality to assess hip pain but may only show abnormality in the later stages of AVN. Typical findings staged on x-ray are 1) no radiographic abnormality, 2) subchondral linear lucency/sclerosis ("crescent sign"), 3) femoral head collapse, and 4) secondary osteoarthritis.

A bone scan is more sensitive than radiograph at detecting early stages of AVN, usually manifested as decreased uptake in the affected femoral head. MRI is the most sensitive modality for diagnosing AVN. Early identification and intervention may improve a patient's prognosis and prevent collapse of the necrotic segment and subsequent hip arthrosis. MRI is also useful for quantifying the degree of femoral head involvement (predicting outcome) and visualizing early cartilage loss. MRI findings associated with AVN include linear low signal intensity in the femoral head surrounded by bone marrow edema, the "double line" sign representing hypervascular and sclerotic zones, devitalized bone in the necrotic segment, subchondral bone collapse, and joint synovitis (Figure 3-28).

## Synovial Chondromatosis/Osteochondromatosis

Primary synovial chondromatosis or osteochondromatosis is a rare idiopathic monoarticular disease characterized by cartilaginous metaplastic proliferation of the synovial lining. Detachment of these cartilaginous nodules results in multiple intra-articular loose bodies.[14] Primary synovial osteochondromatosis is differentiated from intra-articular loose bodies associated with osteoarthritis, sometimes called secondary synovial osteochondromatosis. These conditions can be distinguished radiographically. Primary synovial osteochondromatosis has multiple calcified or ossified loose bodies of uniform size with preservation of the joint space and possible erosions. In osteoarthritis with loose bodies, the osteoarthritis should be apparent (Figure 3-29). Prior to calcification or ossification of the cartilaginous nodules, synovial osteochondromatosis can present as a nonspecific periarticular soft tissue mass (Figure 3-30).

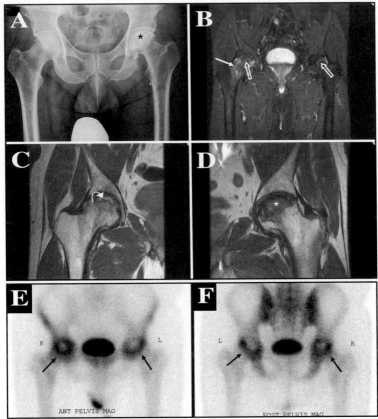

**Figure 3-28.** Bilateral femoral head osteonecrosis. (A) AP pelvis radio-graph demonstrates marked sclerosis in the left femoral head (*) and questionable increased density in the right femoral head. (B) MRI body coil STIR image of the pelvis shows a bone marrow edema pattern in the proximal femur (solid arrow) more pronounced on the right, as well as linear hyperintensity in the femoral heads (open arrows) consistent with bilateral osteonecrosis. (C) Surface coil PD FSE image of the right hip reveals normal bone marrow signal in the femoral head (curved arrow) cir-cumscribed by linear low signal intensity, indicating nondevitalized bone. (D) Surface coil PD FSE image of the left hip shows predominantly low signal (*) corresponding to the sclerosis seen on the radiograph, indicating nearly complete devitalized bone in the necrotic portion of the femoral head. Bilateral femoral head osteonecrosis. (E) Anterior and (F) posterior spot images of the pelvis from a Tc-99m MDP nuclear medicine bone scan of the same patient as A-D demonstrates a ring of abnormal increased radiotracer activity surrounding a focus of relative decreased radiotracer activity in the bilateral femoral heads, characteristic of osteonecrosis. (Courtesy of Hospital for Special Surgery, New York, NY.)

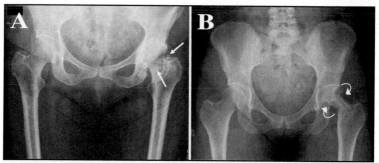

**Figure 3-29.** Synovial chondromatosis. AP view of the pelvis of 2 different patients. (A) AP pelvis radiograph demonstrates multiple ovoid calcified or ossified bodies about the left hip joint (solid arrows). (B) AP pelvis radiograph demonstrates large erosions with scalloping of the left femoral head and neck (curved arrows) without intra-articular calcified or ossified lesions. (Courtesy of Hospital for Special Surgery, New York, NY.)

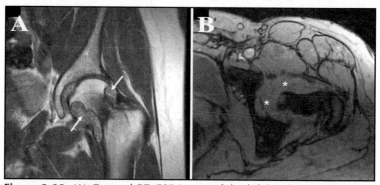

**Figure 3-30.** (A) Coronal PD FSE image of the left hip from patient B in the previous example demonstrates multiple intra-articular intermediate signal intensity lesions of nearly uniform size and shape (solid arrows) associated with large erosions of the femoral head and neck. (B) Axial gradient-recalled echo image of the left hip shows absence of paramagnetic effect (*) indicative of lack of hemosiderin deposition, which makes PVNS unlikely. (Courtesy of Hospital for Special Surgery, New York, NY.)

## Pigmented Villonodular Synovitis

Pigmented villonodular synovitis (PVNS) is a benign synovial hyperplasia that can be focal or diffuse. The hip joint is the second most common site of involvement after the knee.[15] The synovium becomes thick and friable and is prone to bleeding

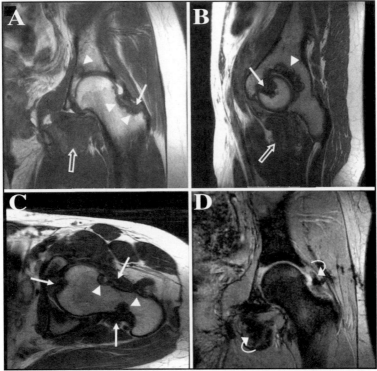

**Figure 3-31.** Pigmented villonodular synovitis. (A) Coronal, (B) sagittal, and (C) oblique axial PD FSE images of the left demonstrate a predominantly intra-articular soft tissue mass (solid arrow) with extracapsular extension (open arrow), associated with erosive changes in the acetabulum and proximal femur (arrowheads). (D) Coronal GRE image shows the "blooming" or dephasing artifact (curved arrows) caused by hemosiderin deposition secondary to chronic hemorrhage within the lesion, a characteristic finding. (Courtesy of Hospital for Special Surgery, New York, NY.)

(hence the *pigmented*). Because PVNS lesions rarely calcify, radiographs may have a normal appearance or demonstrate a nonspecific periarticular soft tissue mass, with bony erosions in more advanced cases. The joint space is usually normal. MRI is the modality of choice for evaluating PVNS where it appears as an intra-articular mass. The hemorrhage can cause areas of low signal (black) that is accentuated by a gradient echo sequence that accentuates the hemosiderin-laden areas and makes them appear larger than they are (termed *blooming artifact*; Figure 3-31).

# Neoplasms

## Osteoid Osteoma

Osteoid osteoma of the hip is a small benign bony tumor that frequently causes pain in young adults. It can occur in any bone, including the cortex of the femoral neck. The diagnosis is often difficult to differentiate clinically from other causes of hip pain, so the diagnosis is often delayed. The typical description of symptoms is pain at night, relieved by aspirin.

In the hip, osteoid osteomas most commonly occur in the proximal femur, manifested as a geographic area of reactive bony sclerosis. The lesion may occasionally be detected on conventional radiographs as a small ovoid lucency in the bone. The radiographic differential diagnosis includes stress fracture and osteomyelitis, especially when periosteal reaction is present. CT is not only the most accurate modality for identifying the lucent center (nidus) but is also used for imaging guidance during radiofrequency ablation of the lesion (Figure 3-32). Percutaneous radiofrequency ablation of osteoid osteomas is a highly effective form of treatment.[16] MRI will detect an associated joint effusion and synovitis if the lesion is intra-articular, but the small lesion itself may be difficult to see because it is often obscured by bone marrow edema. A bone scan is usually positive but not specific.

## Other Tumors

Other bony and soft tissue tumors can occur around the hip and cause symptoms and radiographic abnormalities. Secondary tumors are more common than primary malignancies. Metastases, multiple myeloma, and lymphoma are the most common lesions (Figure 3-33). Other tumors have characteristic imaging findings. The fat in lipomas, for example, can be identified on CT and MRI. Some tumors have typical locations, like the articular surface. Such end-of-bone lesions include giant cell tumor of bone, chondroblastoma, and clear cell chondrosarcoma. Intra-osseous ganglia may have a similar appearance. The shepherd's crook deformity of fibrous dysplasia is characteristic. It is important, first and foremost, to recognize that there is an abnormality. Once something is recognized, referrals and consultation can derive a diagnosis and treatment course.

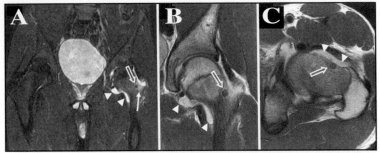

**Figure 3-32.** Osteoid osteoma. (A) Coronal IR image demonstrates a bone marrow edema in the proximal left femur (solid arrow) surrounding an ovoid low signal intensity (open arrow). A high-signal intensity joint effusion is also present, representing a synovitis (arrowheads). (B) Coronal PD FSE also demonstrates the ovoid low-signal intensity (open arrow) focus and joint effusion (arrowhead). The low-signal intensity focus is consistent with calcification or ossification. (C) Axial PD FSE image shows the lesion (open arrow) is in the anterior margin of the femoral neck. (Courtesy of Hospital for Special Surgery, New York, NY.)

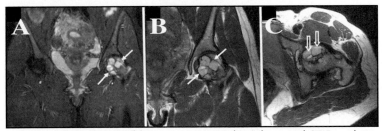

**Figure 3-33.** Aneurysmal bone cyst. (A) Body coil coronal STIR and surface coil PD FSE, (B) coronal, and (C) axial images of the left hip shows a mildly expansile, multilocated high signal intensity lesion in the left femoral head (solid arrows). Subtle fluid-fluid levels (open arrows) are characteristic but not diagnostic and are appreciated on axial images. (Courtesy of Hospital for Special Surgery, New York, NY.)

# CONCLUSION

Hip pathologies are common. Imaging plays an important role in the diagnosis and treatment of these pathologies, so understanding the basics of imaging—available modalities, when to use them, and the appearance of common abnormalities—is an important part of orthopedic training. Images should always be interpreted in clinical context. It is the patient, not the x-ray, that we treat.

This chapter serves as an introduction to the imaging of the hip and the start of understanding a difficult and evolving field.

# REFERENCES

1. Theumann NH, Verdon JP, Mouhsine E, Denys A, Schnyder P, Portier F. Traumatic injuries: imaging of pelvic fractures. *Eur Radiol.* 2002;12(6):1312-1330.
2. Garden RS. Reduction and fixation of subcapital fractures of the femur. *Orthop Clin North Am.* 1974;5:683-712.
3. Bowerman JW, Sena JM, Chang R. The teardrop shadow of the pelvis: anatomy and clinical significance. *Radiology.* 1982;143(3):659-662.
4. Judet R, Judet J, Letournel E. Fractures of the acetabulum: classification and surgical approaches for open reduction. *J Bone Joint Surg Am.* 1964;46:1615-1646.
5. Letournel E. Acetabular fractures: classification and management. *Clin Orthop.* 1980;151:81-106.
6. Pelsser V, Cardinal E, Hobden R, Aubin B, Lafortune M. Extraarticular snapping hip: sonographic findings. *Am J Roetgenol.* 2001;176:67-73.
7. Fon LJ, Spence AJ. Sportsman's hernia. *Br J Surg.* 2000;87:545-552.
8. Zoga AC, Kavanagh EC, Omar IM, et al. Athletic pubalgia and the "sports hernia": MR imaging findings. *Radiology.* 2008;247(3):797-807.
9. McCarthy J, Noble P, Aluisio FV, Schuck M, Wright J, Lee JA. Anatomy, pathologic features, and treatment of acetabular labral tears. *Clin Orthop Relat Res.* 2003;406:38-47.
10. Fitzgerald RH Jr. Acetabular labrum tears: diagnosis and treatment. *Clin Orthop.* 1995;211:60-68.
11. Mintz DN, Hooper T, Connell D, Buly R, Padgett DE, Potter HG. Magnetic resonance imaging of the hip: detection of labral and chondral abnormalities using noncontrast imaging. *Arthroscopy.* 2005;21(4)385-393.
12. Ito K, Minka MA 2nd, Leunig M, Werlen S, Ganz R. Femoroacetabular impingement and the cam-effect. A MRI-based quantitative anatomical study of the femoral head-neck offset. *J Bone Joint Surg Br.* 2001;83:171-176.
13. Beck M, Kalhor M, Leunig M, Ganz R. Hip morphology influences the pattern of damage to the acetabular cartilage: femoroacetabular impingement as a cause of early osteoarthritis of the hip. *J Bone Joint Surg Br.* 2005;7:1012-1018.
14. Crotty JM, Monu JE, Pope TL Jr. Synovial osteochondromatosis. *Radiol Clin North Am.* 1996;34(2):327-342.
15. Dorwart RH, Genant HK, Johnston WH, Morris JM. Pigmented villonodular synovitis of synovial joints: clinical, pathologic, and radiologic features. *Am J Roentgenol.* 1984;143:877-885.
16. Lindner JN, Ozaki T, Roedl R, Gosheger G, Winkelmann W, Wortler K. Percutaneous radiofrequency ablation in osteoid osteoma. *J Bone Joint Surg Br.* 2001;83:391-396.

**4**

# GENERAL IMAGING OF THE KNEE

*C. Benjamin Ma, MD and Sunny Cheung, MD*

As in the hip, imaging studies of the knee should be considered as an adjunct to help the clinician make the appropriate diagnosis. Most of the time, a thorough history and physical exam will lead the clinician to a narrow list of differential diagnoses, and then obtaining a few specific imaging studies is all that is needed to confirm the diagnosis.

## PLAIN RADIOGRAPHY

Plain radiography is the workhorse imaging study for evaluating knee complaints. Images obtained in this fashion not only reveal bony abnormalities, but can also reveal clues about the soft tissue as well. Soft tissue swelling, joint effusions, and

Ranawat A, Kelly BT. *Musculoskeletal Examination of the Hip and Knee: Making the Complex Simple* (pp. 110-134).
© 2011 SLACK Incorporated

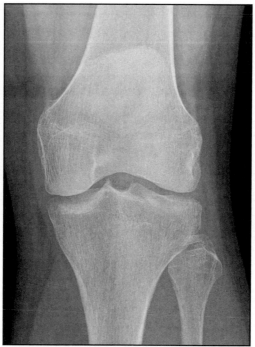

**Figure 4-1.** AP radiograph of a normal left knee.

chondrocalcinosis can all be discerned. The following is a brief guide to the work-up of various pathologies and the typical radiographs that are ordered for the knee.

# Trauma and/or Nonspecific Pain (Younger Patient)

*Typical views:*
- ⊁ *Anterior-Posterior (AP), supine (Figure 4-1)*
- ⊁ *Lateral 30 degrees flexion*

The AP, supine view is good for general evaluation of the knee, mostly to rule out fractures, tumors, and perhaps soft-tissue swelling. Oblique views may also be ordered, mostly to assess fractures of the tibial plateau. One should not forget to carefully examine the patella as well as it is often overlooked due to being overlapped by the distal femur. Bipartite patellas may also be seen on this view (as discussed later).

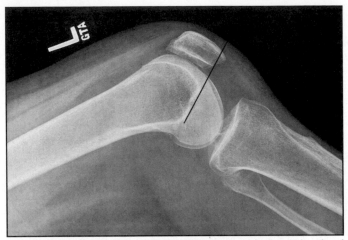

**Figure 4-2.** Lateral 30 degrees flexion radiograph. Note the distal pole of the patella is at the level of Blumensaat's line (black line).

While osteophytes and other bony stigmata of osteoarthritis can be visualized in this view, it is difficult to assess the degree of cartilage wear and joint space narrowing because it is nonweight-bearing (see arthritis section).

The lateral view, 30 degrees flexion, horizontal (Figure 4-2) is excellent for evaluation of transverse patella fractures and distal femur posterior condyle fractures. It is also good for the evaluation of patella height (patella alta or baja), which can be a source of patellofemoral pathology. The Insall-Salvati ratio is most commonly used to check for patella alta. It is the ratio of the length of the patella tendon to the patella length. A patella tendon/patella bone ratio of greater than 1.2 indicates patella alta and can be a contributing cause of patellofemoral subluxation or dislocation. A ratio of less than 0.8 indicates patella baja, which means the patella is abnormally low, and is associated with soft tissue contracture, hypotonia of quadriceps muscle following surgery, or trauma to the knee.[1] This may also indicate arthrofibrosis, leading to restricted range of motion in the knee and chronic pain. Another way to quickly determine patella height is looking at the distal pole of the patella in relation to Blumensaat's line, which represents the roof of the intercondylar notch. In the normal patella, the tip of the distal pole should be just at the level of Blumensaat's line with the knee flexed at 30 degrees (see Figure 4-2).

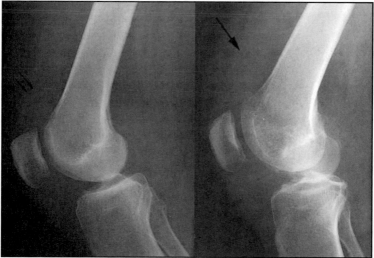

**Figure 4-3.** Joint effusions in the suprapatella pouch on lateral radiographs. (Left) Smaller effusion (black double arrows). (Right) Larger effusion (large black arrow).

Joint effusions can be seen as a radiodensity in the suprapatella pouch (Figure 4-3). Intra-articular fractures may also exhibit a fluid-fat level (fat-blood interface sign) in the pouch, indicating lipohemarthrosis.

## Patellofemoral Pain

*Typical views*
- *Sunrise (115 degrees flexion)*
- *Merchant (45 degrees flexion)*
- *Laurin (20 degrees flexion)*

The sunrise view (115 degrees flexion) is a tangential view of the patella and is more suited for visualizing vertical patella fractures. Because most nonacute sources of patellofemoral pain (such as subluxation) occur in the lower angles of knee flexion, this view is not used very often and is not part of the standard knee radiograph series.

The Merchant view (45 degrees flexion; Figure 4-4) is used to evaluate patellofemoral instability. The patella index can be determined, which is the ratio of the width of the patella to the difference between the lateral and medial facets.

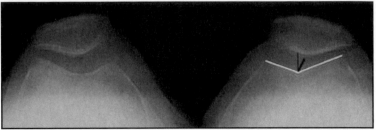

**Figure 4-4.** Merchant view. Sulcus angle (white) is 140 degrees. The congruence angle is formed by the bisector of the sulcus angle (thin black line) and a line from the sulcus to the patella apex (thick black line), which should be medial to the bisector normally. This person has a positive congruence angle and is consistent with patella maltracking or instability.

The medial facet is small in patients with patellofemoral instability.[2] The normal ratio is 15 for male patients and 17 for female patients. The sulcus angle should be less than 138 degrees. A larger angle indicates a shallow groove and lateral trochlear dysplasia.

The congruence angle can be measured on this view. This is determined by bisecting the sulcus angle to give a reference line. Then, a second line is drawn from the sulcus to the patella apex. The angle formed by the second line to the reference line is the congruence angle. The second line should be medial to the reference line and, by convention, is a negative value. The normal congruence angle is -6 degrees. A positive angle (lateral to the bisector) is associated with patellofemoral disorders.

The Laurin view (20 degrees flexion) is probably the easiest view to evaluate patellofemoral disorders. The lateral patellofemoral angle is determined by a line drawn across the top of the medial and lateral femoral condyle and the line across the lateral facet. A normal angle should diverge ("open") laterally. If the lines are parallel or even convergent, then this would indicate patella instability (Figure 4-5).[3] As in the Merchant view, if a plain radiograph indicates a normal sulcus angle (less than 138 degrees), then further radiographic work-up for patellofemoral malalignment would be unlikely to reveal additional useful information. The severity of other features of dysplasia of the extensor mechanism is correlated with increasing sulcus angle.[4]

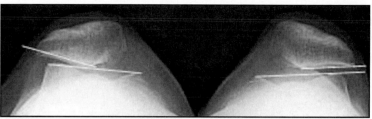

**Figure 4-5.** Another example of patella subluxation. White lines show a parallel patellofemoral angle on the right and a more normal divergent angle on the left.

The tilt of the patella and relative wear of the cartilage can be quantified by the patellofemoral index. This is a ratio of the thickness of the medial patellofemoral joint space (the shortest line from the most lateral edge of the medial facet to the medial femoral condyle) to the lateral patellofemoral joint space (the shortest line between the lateral facet to the lateral femoral condyle). The ratio should be less than or equal to 1.6. Laurin's original study indicated that 93% of patients with patellofemoral chondromalacia had an index greater than 1.6.[3]

# Arthritis or Post-Surgical Evaluation

*Typical views:*
- ⌃ *Posterior-anterior (PA) 30 degree views, weight bearing*
- ⌃ *Rosenberg*
- ⌃ *Notch*

In PA 30 degree views, weight bearing (Figure 4-6), evaluation of the arthritic knee must include the patient in a weight-bearing (standing) mode in order to assess the amount of cartilage wear, as manifested by the remaining "clear space" within the medial and lateral compartments. Because early osteoarthritis usually affects the posterior femoral condyles, a partially flexed view of the knee has been found to be more valuable than the knee in extension.[5] Osteophytes, which are abnormal bony changes due to increased wear, may also be visualized as "squaring" of the condyles. These are also known as *Fairbanks changes*.

The Rosenberg view is similar to the previously described view, except it is taken with weight-bearing PA 45 degrees

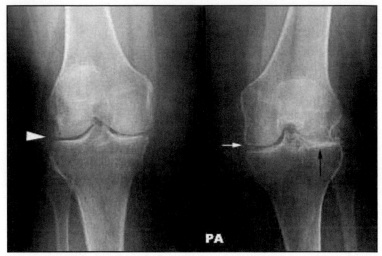

**Figure 4-6.** PA standing view in flexion. Severe bone-on-bone lateral compartment osteoarthritis is shown (black arrow). Fairbanks changes (squaring of the condyles indicating less severe arthritis) are present on the medial compartment (white arrow). Osteophytes are present (white triangle).

flexion instead. This view also effectively demonstrates loss of cartilage due to osteoarthritis.[6]

The notch (tunnel) view (Figure 4-7), as the name implies, shows the intercondylar notch, tibial spines, and tibial plateau. The view is taken in 60 degrees of flexion, supine. It is helpful for evaluation of arthritis (notch osteophytes), loose bodies, and osteochondral lesions in the intercondylar regions.

## COMPUTED TOMOGRAPHY

New advances in multi-detector computed tomography (CT) have reduced imaging time and metallic artifacts, while allowing increased resolution and 3-dimensional reconstructions. Still, this modality is mostly used for evaluating bony tumors and complex fractures of the knee, such as preoperative templating for open reduction internal fixation by orthopedic traumatologists. Occasionally, it may reveal some information on patella tilt.

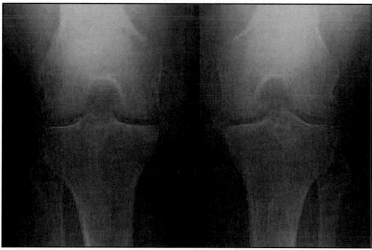

**Figure 4-7.** PA standing notch view of a normal knee.

# MAGNETIC RESONANCE IMAGING

This has become the diagnostic tool of choice for most soft pathologies of the knee, with the exception of arthritis. A detailed explanation of the technical aspects of magnetic resonance imaging (MRI) is beyond the scope of this chapter, but the reader is referred to Chapter 3 for a more detailed explanation of the various MRI sequences. In brief, there are basically 2 modes of imaging (T1- and T2-weighted), plus various modes to suppress the fat signal, which is always bright (hyperintense). Any fluid content is generally bright and solid material is generally dark (Table 4-1 and Figure 4-8). Often, the T2 sequence is modified by a short tau inversion recovery (STIR), which suppresses the bright fatty signal, making the bright fluid signal stand out better (which is usually located at the area of pathology).

The usual thickness of each MRI slice is 3 to 4 mm, allowing the visualization of most soft tissues around the knee. MRI is not without its limits, as metallic objects (plates, joint prostheses, anchors, or bullet shrapnel) can obscure the images with signal artifact. Also, one must be cognizant of the magic angle

**Table 4-1**

## VARIOUS TISSUES AND THEIR CORRESPONDING SIGNAL INTENSITY ON MRI

|  | T1 | T2 | T2 STIR (Fat Suppression) |
|---|---|---|---|
| Fat | Bright | Bright | Dark |
| Muscle | Intermediate (gray) | Intermediate (gray) | Intermediate (gray) |
| Fluid (pus, synovial fluid, edema) | Intermediate | Bright | Bright |
| Hyaline cartilage | Intermediate | Intermediate (but brighter in arthritis) | Intermediate (but brighter in arthritis) |
| Calcium and fibrous tissue (labrum, menisci, tendons) | Dark | Dark | Dark |
| Cancellous bone | Bright | Bright | Dark |
| Cortical bone | Very dark | Very dark | Very dark |
| Stress fracture | Dark | Dark | Dark |

effect that occurs in the T2-weighted images. As collagen fibers (tendons and ligaments) form an angle of 55 degrees with respect to the main magnetic field, the T2 relaxation time becomes longer and therefore generates a hyperintense signal that can be misleading for pathology.

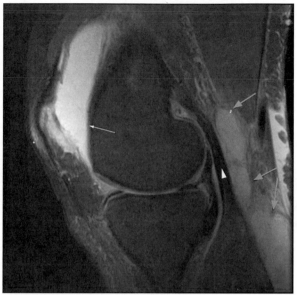

**Figure 4-8.** T2-weighted sagittal image of a knee with a loculated Baker's cyst (gray arrows). A joint effusion is also present (white arrow). Note that fluid is bright on T2-weighted sequences, while bone and tendon (white triangle, gastrocnemius tendon) are dark.

# MAGNETIC RESONANCE ARTHROGRAPHY

The magnetic resonance arthrography (MRA) mode of imaging is essentially an MRI with an intra-articular injection of gadolinium. This increases the accuracy of diagnosing recurrent meniscal tears after previous repair or meniscectomy greater than 25%.[7]

# FUTURE OF MAGNETIC RESONANCE IMAGING

As MRI technology continues to evolve, new modalities and sequences have been developed that provide more information. Quantitative MRI collects information about the tissue rather than just an image, such as the amount of cartilage present on a joint surface. Because data are actually quantified, the results should be independent of the MR machine (assuming the magnetic field strength, pulse sequences, etc, are the same). This allows "standardizing" MRI data into reproducible results, regardless of the MR machine, and pooling of data in multicenter trials. In addition, quantitative MRI is being used increasingly to stage disease and monitor the progress of disease or treatment (ie, ongoing cartilage loss).[8] Another sequence with exciting potential is the T1RHO sequence, otherwise known as Spin-Lock MRI. Early studies have shown it to be highly sensitive to molecular changes in cartilage degeneration, and it may become the modality of choice in evaluating early arthritis.[9]

## ANGIOGRAPHY

This imaging modality is the gold standard to rule out vascular injury from acute traumatic dislocation of the knee. Once a dislocated knee is reduced, the circulation should be assessed. If any of the posterior tibialis or dorsalis pedal pulses are abnormal, or if the ankle brachial index (ABI) is less than 0.9, then immediate angiography should be obtained to look for popliteal artery injury.

## NUCLEAR IMAGING WITH TECHNETIUM-99

This modality may be used to evaluate stress fractures, early degenerate joint disease, or complex regional pain syndrome. Combined with the indium white blood cell labeled scan, it may also be used to distinguish aseptic loosening versus infection in total knee arthroplasties.

## ULTRASOUND

This modality is still somewhat new. Its uses are limited to evaluation of bursae and other fluid collections around the knee, soft tissue masses (such as Baker's cysts), and superficial

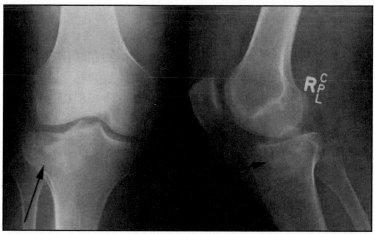

**Figure 4-9.** AP (left) and lateral (right) radiographs of a split depression lateral plateau fracture. A large fragment has been impacted below the joint line (black arrows).

tendon and ligament injuries. It can also be used for detection of arthrofibrosis after total knee arthroplasty. Findings include synovial membrane thickening greater than 3 mm and neovascularity.[10]

# IMAGING EVALUATION OF COMMON KNEE PATHOLOGIES

## Fractures

A standard series of nonweight-bearing views including AP, lateral, and sometimes patella (Laurin or Merchant) views are obtained (Figure 4-9). If there is suspicion of an intra-articular tibial plateau fracture, internal and external oblique views may also be ordered. Low-energy fractures may be subtle and can be missed; if initial radiographs do not reveal any osseous abnormalities, then a CT scan without contrast may be helpful, especially to evaluate fractures involving joint impaction on the tibia or posterior femoral condyle fractures ("Hoffa fracture"). Although frank fractures involving the cortex (including stress fractures) can be seen on T1-weighted

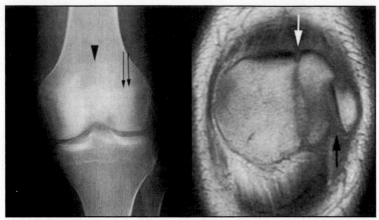

**Figure 4-10.** (Left) AP radiograph in a trauma series of a left knee. This patient suffered a direct blow to his knee causing a vertical fracture (black triangle) and also separation of his bipartite patella (double black arrows). (Right) T1-weighted coronal MRI of the vertical fracture (white arrow) and the bipartite patella piece that has been displaced and flipped 90 degrees (black arrow).

images, subtle injuries to the cancellous bone are best visualized in the T2-weighted images (Figure 4-10). Bony edema due to microfractures in the trabeculae is bright on T2-weighted images (see Figure 4-16D).

Stress fractures can be identified by a simple bone scan with technitium-99. However, MRI is becoming more popular because it provides better resolution and can also track the progress of healing. Stress fractures appear on T1-weighted images as low signal (the "dreaded black line") inside the bright signal of the normal bone. In the tibia, it usually appears on the anterior aspect, perpendicular to the diaphysis. On T2-weighted images, it will appear as a bright signal (due to bony edema), whereas normal bone is dark.

## Osteonecrosis

Osteonecrosis (or avascular necrosis; Figure 4-11) is difficult to visualize on plain radiographs unless it has already progressed to the late stages with subchondral collapse. It can be detected early by MRI. Osteonecrosis may be seen on both T1- and T2-weighted images. It usually has a "geographic" border, and areas of bright signal on T2 indicate the area of

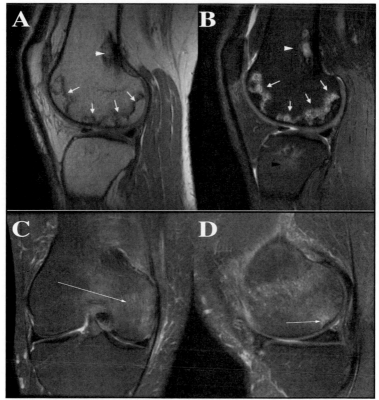

**Figure 4-11.** MRI. (A) T1-weighted sagittal image and (B) T2-weighted sagittal image showing osteonecrosis on the femoral condyle. Note the "geographic" pattern of the lesion (white arrows). Evidence of a previous ACL reconstruction can be seen. (White triangle: femoral tunnel; black triangle: tibial tunnel). (C) T2 coronal and (D) sagittal weighted images showing spontaneous osteonecrosis of the knee (SONK; white arrows). Notice the more diffuse pattern of bony edema in SONK compared to avascular necrosis.

reactive, inflamed bone. Areas of dark signal in the middle of bright cancellous bone on T1 imaging denote necrotic bone. Spontaneous osteonecrosis of the knee (SONK) is a phenomenon diagnosed on MRI that is seen typically in elderly women with osteoporosis. Although the etiology is unclear, it is thought that osteoporotic bone is more vulnerable to microfractures from minor trauma. This sets up a cycle of edema, fluid accumulation, bony ischemia, and ultimately necrosis.

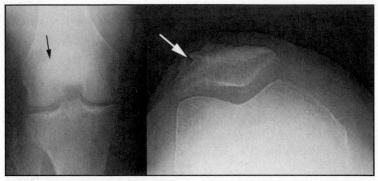

**Figure 4-12.** Plain radiographs of bipartite patella. (Left) AP view and (right) patellofemoral view. The black arrow shows the accessory fragment on the AP view, and the white arrow shows the irregular contour on the patellofemoral view.

## Bipartite Patella

While the bipartite patella is more an anatomic variant rather than disease entity, failure to recognize this may lead to unnecessary further work-up and patient anxiety over a possible fracture. In about 2% of the population, the ossification centers in the patella fail to fuse, and an accessory bone (known as a bipartite patella) can be visualized.[11] The most common location for the accessory bone is in the superior lateral pole of the patella. The other locations include the lateral pole and inferior pole. The presence of a distinct well-defined cortex in the smaller fragment and a smooth, regular, semi-lunar radiolucent defect between the 2 pieces usually alerts the clinician to this typically asymptomatic condition. However, bipartite patellas can be a source of pain due to acute trauma or repetitive microtrauma as motion develops in the fibrocartilage separating the 2 pieces (see Figures 4-1, 4-10, and 4-12).

## Avulsion Injuries

Injuries to the muscle tendon unit can occur at the tendonous attachment to bone. Ligamentous avulsions may also occur. Adolescents are more vulnerable because the tendon and ligaments tend to be stronger relative to the bone, which is still growing and remodeling. Common tendon avulsion

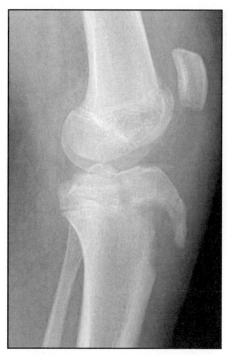

**Figure 4-13.** Lateral radiograph of tibial tuberosity avulsion fracture in a teenager.

injuries include a tibial tuberosity fracture (common in jumpers, such as basketball players, as the patella tendon literally pulls the bone away; Figure 4-13), and the biceps femoris tendon (insertion to the fibula head). Ligamentous injuries commonly include avulsion of the ACL off of the tibial eminence (Figure 4-14) and the PCL off of the posterior tibia. A standard series of nonweight-bearing radiographs can often reveal these lesions.

## Abnormal Calcification

Plain radiographs may reveal areas of abnormal calcification. Common entities include chondrocalcinosis, otherwise known as pseudogout and calcium pyrophosphate deposition disease (CPPD). It is caused by deposits of calcium pyrophosphate crystal in the intra-articular soft tissue including synovium, meniscus, and hyaline cartilage. On plain radiograph AP views, the outlines of the menisci are faintly

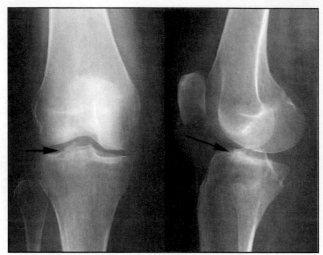

**Figure 4-14.** (Left) AP and (right) lateral radiographs of an avulsion fracture (black arrows) of the tibial eminence by the anterior cruciate ligament.

calcified and visible. Confirmation of this disease includes joint aspiration and analysis for rhomboid crystals that are weakly positive birefringence on polarized light microscopy.

A Pellegrini-Stieda lesion is calcification of the MCL origin off of the femoral condyle. It is not an avulsion injury, but rather abnormal calcification indicating previous MCL tear or injury.

A fabella ("little bean" in Latin) is a sesamoid bone embedded in the tendon of the lateral head of the gastrocnemius muscle (Figure 4-15). It is found in 10% to 30% of the population and can be mistaken for a loose body or fracture.[12] This is best visualized on a lateral view of the knee.

## Ligamentous Injuries

The ACL and PCL can best be seen on MRI sagittal T1 images (Figure 4-16). ACL tears characteristically leave bone contusions that can be seen high signal in the middle femoral condyle and posterior tibial condyle (Figure 4-16D). As the ACL is torn, the tibia slides anterior relative to the femur, and

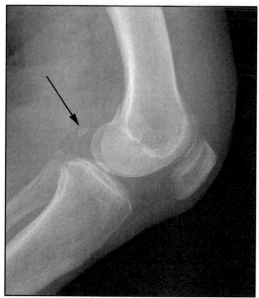

**Figure 4-15.** Lateral radiograph of a normal knee with a fabella (black arrow), which is sesamoid bone embedded in the tendon of the lateral head of the gastrocnemius muscle. This is a normal finding.

the middle portion of the femur collides against the posterior aspect of the tibia. Occasionally, ACL ruptures can be diagnosed on an AP plain radiograph by the "Segond fracture," which is an avulsion fracture of the lateral aspect of the proximal tibia below the articular surface. The mechanism of injury is caused by internal rotation and varus stress, leading to abnormal tension on the central portion of the lateral capsular ligament.

Medial collateral ligament (MCL) injuries can be seen on the T2 coronal plane. Injuries to the posterior lateral corner (PLC), which mainly consists of the popliteofibular ligament, popliteus tendon, and lateral collateral ligament (LCL), are best viewed on the axial T2 image. Injuries to the medial patellofemoral ligament (MPFL) lead to traumatic patella subluxation or dislocation and can be seen on the axial T2 image.

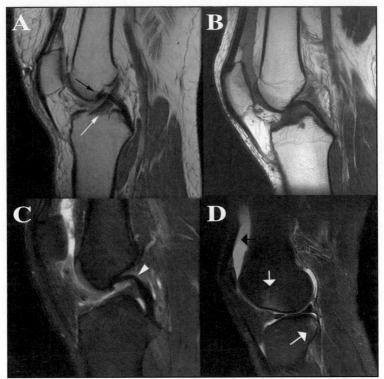

**Figure 4-16.** (A) Sagittal PD image of a normal ACL (thin white arrow) and PCL (thin black arrow). (B) Sagittal PD image of a torn ACL and a normal PCL. Note the "empty wall" sign where the ACL used to insert but is now missing. A small stump of the ACL on the tibial eminence is visible. (C) Sagittal T2 FS image of an acute ACL tear. Although the ligament itself is visible, it has detached off of its origin from the femoral condyle and has "draped" over the PCL (white triangle). (D) Sagittal T2 FS image showing the typical pattern of bony edema following ACL tear (wide white arrows). Note also the joint effusion (wide black arrow).

## Menisci

Meniscal tear patterns can vary depending on age, pre-existing arthritis, and mechanism of injury. MRI is the modality of choice in the evaluation of suspected meniscal injuries. Complex degenerative tears and horizontal flap tears are usually due to arthritis and are not amenable to repair, whereas vertical peripheral tears within the vascularized "red" portion

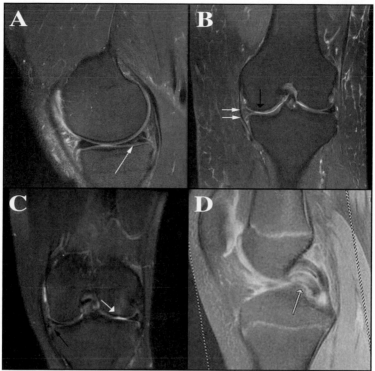

**Figure 4-17.** (A) T2 sagittal FS image of a horizontal flap tear on the undersurface of the posterior medial meniscus (white arrow). (B) T2 coronal FS image of a complex degenerative tear (not repairable) of the medial aspect of the extruded medial meniscus (double white arrow). Also note the chondromalacia on the medial femoral condyle (wide black arrow) and medial osteophytes on the femoral and tibial surface, which likely contributed to the meniscal tear. (C) T2 coronal FS image of a vertical peripheral tear in a teenager, which was later repaired at surgery (black arrow). Also note the cartilage defect on the lateral femoral condyle with associated bony reaction (wide white arrow). (D) T2 sagittal image of the double PCL sign (thin white arrow), in which a bucket-handle tear of the medial meniscus has flipped into the notch underneath the PCL *(continued)*.

of the meniscus can be repaired (Figures 4-17A through C). A classic double PCL sign is pathognomonic for a bucket handle meniscal tear (Figures 4-17D and E). Medial meniscal extrusion greater than 3 mm from the tibial margin is associated with severe meniscal degeneration usually due to osteoarthritis.[10]

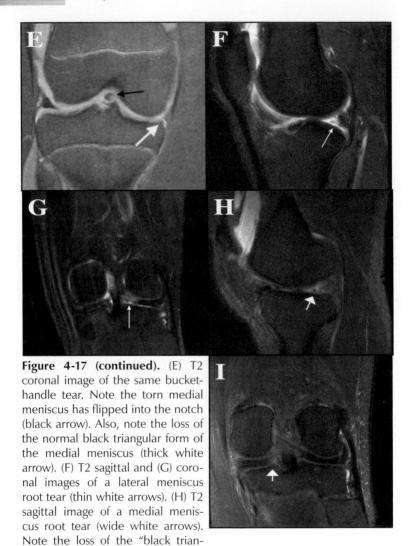

**Figure 4-17 (continued).** (E) T2 coronal image of the same bucket-handle tear. Note the torn medial meniscus has flipped into the notch (black arrow). Also, note the loss of the normal black triangular form of the medial meniscus (thick white arrow). (F) T2 sagittal and (G) coronal images of a lateral meniscus root tear (thin white arrows). (H) T2 sagittal image of a medial meniscus root tear (wide white arrows). Note the loss of the "black triangular wedge" visible on both sagittal views. (I) coronal images of a medial meniscus root tear (wide white arrows). Note the loss of the "black triangular wedge" visible on both sagittal views.

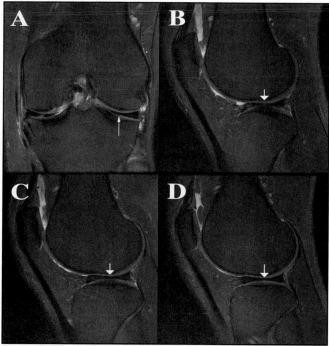

**Figure 4-18.** (A) T2 coronal image of a discoid lateral meniscus (white arrow). A medial meniscus horizontal flap tear with the torn flap flipped into the joint capsule is also present (black arrows). (B through D) T2 consecutive sagittal images (from medial to lateral) of the discoid meniscus. If the black meniscus "bowtie" is visible on 3 consecutive images (wide white arrows), then the meniscus is discoid.

Root tears occur when the posterior horn attachments to the bone are ruptured, leading to an unstable meniscus that can easily "flip" into the joint compartment. This is relatively harder to detect on MRI (Figures 4-17F through I). The presence of a continuous lateral meniscus on 3 consecutive sagittal images usually indicates a discoid lateral meniscus. The prevalence is estimated to be 4% to 5% in the United States but occurs in a higher percentage of Asian patients and can be a cause of painful snapping (Figure 4-18).[13]

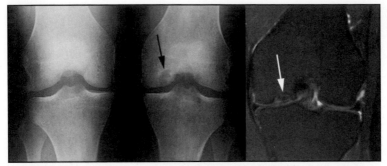

**Figure 4-19.** (Left and center) PA standing radiographs showing an osteochondral defect of the medial femoral condyle (black arrow). (Right) T2 coronal MRI of the same defect (white arrow).

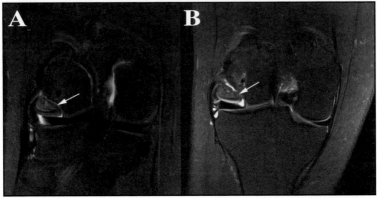

**Figure 4-20.** (A) T2 coronal MRI of a large lateral condyle osteochondral defect (white arrow) in a teenager with open physes that was treated with a bioabsorbable screw. (B) After 3 months postoperatively, the osteochondral defect failed to heal and displaced (white arrow).

## Osteochondral Defects

Osteochondral defects are usually due to traumatic impaction, most often on the medial femoral condyle. They may be subtle findings on plain AP radiographs, but the diagnostic modality of choice remains the MRI (Figure 4-19). Occasionally, very large defects in adolescents with open physes may be amenable to fixation with bioabsorbable screws (Figure 4-20).

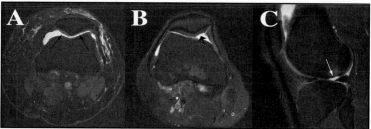

**Figure 4-21.** MRI T2 FS images of cartilage injury. (A) Axial image of an arthritic knee with joint effusion. Notice the irregular contour and thin cartilage over both facets of the patella (thin black arrows). (B) Axial image of a younger patient with isolated cartilage loss over the medial facet (wide black arrow). Note that the normal cartilage on the lateral facet is much thicker. (C) Bright signal on the subchondral surface of the lateral femoral condyle denoting a large grade IV cartilage defect (white arrow). The cartilage has been delaminated off the subchondral bone.

## Cartilage Injuries

Evaluation of cartilage lesions is best on MRI using fat-suppressed, proton density, fast spin-echo (FS PD FSE) or PD FSE images. The sagittal and coronal images can best show any irregular contours in the femoral and tibial cartilage (see Figures 4-17B and C and Figure 4-21C). Axial views can demonstrate cartilage lesions in the patellofemoral joint (Figures 4-21A and B).

## CONCLUSION

Plain radiographs in the weight-bearing mode and patellar views are an excellent initial diagnostic study for evaluation of the knee. However, if soft tissue pathology is suspected, then noncontrast MRI can provide valuable information about the meniscus, ligaments, and the health of the cartilage.

## REFERENCES

1. Grelsamer RP, Meadows S. The modified Insall-Salvati ratio for assessment of patellar height. *Clin Orthop Relat Res.* 1992;282:170-176.

2. Cross MJ, Waldrop J. The patella index as a guide to the understanding and diagnosis of patellofemoral instability. *Clin Orthop Relat Res.* 1975;110:174-176.

3. Laurin CA, Dussault R, Levesque HP. The tangential x-ray investigation of the patellofemoral joint. *Clin Orthop Relat Res.* 1979;144:16-26.

4. Davies AP, Costa ML, Donnell ST, Glasgow MM, Shepstone L. The sulcus angle and malalignment of the extensor mechanism of the knee. *J Bone Joint Surg Br.* 2000;82-B:1162-1166.

5. Davies AP, Calder DA, Marshall T, Glasgow MMS. Plain radiography in the degenerate knee. A case for change. *J Bone Joint Surg Br.* 1999:81(4):632-635.

6. Rosenberg TD, Paulos LE, Parker RD, Coward DB, Scott SM. The forty-five degree posteroanterior flexion weight-bearing radiograph. *J Bone Joint Surg Am.* 1988;70:1479-1483.

7. Stoller DW, Li AE, Anderson LJ, Cannon WD. The knee. In: Stoller DW, ed. *Magnetic Resonance Imaging in Orthopaedics and Sports Medicine.* Baltimore, MD: Lippincott; 2007.

8. Tofts PS. Magnetic resonance: An overview. In: Sharp PF, Perkins AC, eds. *Physics and Engineering in Medicine in the New Millennium.* York, UK: Institute of Physics and Engineering in Medicine Fairmount House; 2000.

9. Lejay H, Holland BA. Technical advances in musculoskeletal imaging. In: Stoller DW, ed. *Magnetic Resonance Imaging in Orthopaedics and Sports Medicine.* Baltimore, MD: Lippincott; 2007.

10. Averion-Maloch T. Imaging. In: Kibler WB, ed. *Orthopaedic Knowledge Update: Sports Medicine 4.* Rosemont, IL: American Academy of Orthopaedic Surgeons; 2009.

11. Lawson JP. Symptomatic radiographic variants in extremities. *Radiology.* 1985;157:625-631.

12. Pritchett JW. The incidence of fabellae in osteoarthrosis of the knee. *J Bone Joint Surg Am.* 1984;66:1379-1380.

13. Jordan MR. Lateral meniscal variants. *Operative Techniques in Orthopaedics.* 2000;10:234-244.

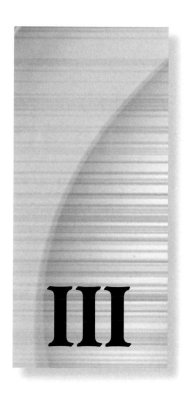

# III

# Common
# Conditions of
# the Hip

# 5

# HIP INSTABILITY

*Matthew V. Smith, MD and Jon K. Sekiya, MD*

## INTRODUCTION

The depth and conformity of the articulation between the femoral head and acetabulum provides a great deal of intrinsic stability to the hip joint. Despite this, hip instability does occur and can be debilitating. There is evidence to support traumatic and atraumatic capsular laxity as a source of hip pain and persistent disability.[1-3] Traumatic hip instability can result from high-energy trauma, like that seen in motor vehicle accidents. It can also result from low-energy injuries seen in athletic competition.[4,5] Proposed causes of atraumatic capsular laxity include generalized ligamentous laxity, collagen disorders like Ehlers-Danlos, and microtrauma from repetitive activities

Ranawat A, Kelly BT. *Musculoskeletal Examination of the Hip and Knee: Making the Complex Simple* (pp. 136-158).
© 2011 SLACK Incorporated

that force the hip into external rotation as seen in golfers, gymnasts, dancers, or throwers.[1-3] Dynamic and transient incongruency can lead to abnormal joint forces which may result in capsular and labral injuries, capsular redundancy, and femoral neck impingement at high flexion angles (secondary impingement). Although diagnosing hip instability can be challenging, identifying the cause of hip instability is important because it can help guide the surgeon toward the most appropriate treatment. The appropriate diagnosis relies upon a combination of clinical suspicion, physical examination, and radiographic findings.

# HISTORY

Traumatic hip dislocation commonly occurs in motor vehicle accidents when the knee impacts the dashboard with the hip in a flexed and adducted position. This position most often results in a posterior dislocation. Less commonly, forced abduction and external rotation can cause an anterior hip dislocation. Low-energy hip subluxations or dislocations can occur in athletic competition from a fall onto a knee with a flexed and adducted hip or from a hit from behind when down on all 4 limbs (Table 5-1).[4] This most commonly happens in sports like football, skiing, gymnastics, rugby, biking, and soccer.[6-8] In most cases, patients with traumatic instability describe a specific event where they feel a sensation of subluxation or sustain a frank dislocation. Patients with acute traumatic subluxation or dislocation will often complain of severe pain in the groin because of a significant soft tissue injury and hemarthrosis.[4] Hip dislocations commonly occur in combination with acetabular posterior wall fractures, especially in high-energy injuries, but they can occur without fractures.

Unlike traumatic instability, patients with instability related to atraumatic capsular laxity may have a more insidious onset of pain, hip snapping, weakness, or mechanical symptoms (see Table 5-1). Often, there is no clear inciting event but rather a gradual onset of symptoms with specific activities like swinging a golf club or throwing a ball. Patients may also complain of pain or snapping during the mid-swing phase of gait.[1]

**Table 5-1**

# HELPFUL HINTS

| Type of Instability | Mechanism/Pathology | Presentation |
|---|---|---|
| **TRAUMATIC** | | |
| Anterior | High-energy injury | Severe pain with motion |
| | Forced external rotation and extension or abduction | Hip held in extension and external rotation |
| Posterior | Often high-energy injury from hip flexion and adduction | Severe pain with motion |
| | Low-energy injuries seen in athletic competition from flexion and adduction or from getting hit while on all 4 limbs | Hip held in flexion and internal rotation |
| | | After reduction, flexion abduction and external rotation improves pain because it maximizes capsular volume |
| | Labral tear, posterior rim fractures, iliofemoral ligament tear, and hemarthrosis common | May have recurrent instability because of resultant capsular laxity |
| **ATRAUMATIC** | | |
| Anterior | Iliofemoral ligament microtrauma from repetitive axial load and external rotation (eg, golf) | Increase external rotation in 0 degrees of hip flexion |
| | | Pain and apprehension with hip extension and external rotation |
| | Generalized ligamentous laxity | Labral tears common |
| | | Coxa saltans (aka, snapping hip) |
| | Collagen disorders (eg, Ehlers-Danlos) | Iliopsoas tendonitis and trochanteric bursitis |

| Imaging | Important Views | Findings |
|---|---|---|
| Plain radiographs | AP pelvis, lateral, Judet (traumatic), traction (atraumatic) | Cam and pincer impingement, acetabular rim fractures (traumatic), vacuum sign (atraumatic) |
| CT scan | Thin cuts with coronal and sagittal reconstructions (traumatic) | Acetabular rim fractures, marginal impaction, intra-articular fragments, femoral head and neck fracture |
| MRI (± arthrogram) | Coronal, sagittal, and axial | Chondral defects, loose bodies, labral tears, hemarthrosis, capsule disruption |

Because the differential diagnosis for patients with these symptoms is broad, it is often difficult to distinguish other causes of hip pain from capsular laxity and instability. It is critical to consider the age and skeletal maturity of the patient when forming a differential diagnosis. It is also important to determine the timing of symptoms, precipitating factors, and the specific location of the pain as this information can narrow the differential diagnosis. The nature of the pain and presence of mechanical symptoms can also narrow the differential diagnosis. For example, coxa saltans (snapping hip syndrome) has been associated with idiopathic hip instability.[1] When the diagnosis is unclear, it is important to consider underlying capsular laxity and subluxation as a contributing factor.

## EXAMINATION

A patient with an acute traumatic hip dislocation will usually have severe pain, especially with attempts at motion. The position of the leg can help determine the direction of dislocation (see Table 5-1). A patient with a posterior hip dislocation will hold the affected leg in a flexed and internally rotated position. A patient with an anterior dislocation will usually hold the affected leg in an extended and externally rotated position. If a patient experiences a subluxation event, even without a frank dislocation, a significant hemarthrosis may develop, causing severe pain and hip irritability.[4] If this happens, the patient will likely hold the leg in a flexed, externally rotated, and abducted position because this maximizes capsular volume. Attempts to move the hip in this situation will cause severe discomfort.

In cases of atraumatic hip instability, a thorough physical examination is critical to differentiate the causes of hip pain (Table 5-2). It is important to watch the patient walk to evaluate gait abnormalities like an abductor lurch or a trendelenburg gait. These may be subtle findings but can provide clues about muscle weakness. A thorough assessment of active and passive hip range of motion (ROM) is critical. In general, active and passive ROM should be similar. If pain is provoked during passive ROM, intra-articular pathology should be suspected.[9]

**Table 5-2**

## METHODS FOR EXAMINING THE HIP FOR PAIN AND INSTABILITY

| Examination | Technique | Illustration | Grading | Significance |
|---|---|---|---|---|
| Range of motion | Active and passive motion<br><br>1. Flexion and extension<br><br>2. Internal and external rotation (0 and 90 degrees flexion)<br><br>3. Abduction | | | Pain with passive motion likely indicates underlying pathology<br><br>↑ external rotation at 0 degrees of flexion indicates anterior capsular laxity |
| Ligamentous laxity | 1. Bilateral (B) thumb-to-forearm | 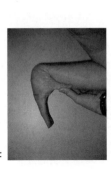1. | Beighton score: 9 points<br><br>0-3 = no laxity<br><br>4-6 = hypermobility<br><br>7-9 = ↑ hypermobility | Positive finding may indicate an increased risk for hip capsular laxity |

*(continued)*

**Table 5-2 (continued)**

## METHODS FOR EXAMINING THE HIP FOR PAIN AND INSTABILITY

| Examination | Technique | Illustration | Grading | Significance |
|---|---|---|---|---|
| Ligamentous laxity (continued) | 2. B elbow hyperextension >10 degrees | 2. 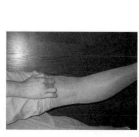 | Beighton score: 9 points<br><br>0-3 = no laxity<br><br>4-6 = hypermobility<br><br>7-9 = ↑ hypermobility | Positive finding may indicate an increased risk for hip capsular laxity |
| | 3. B knee hyperextension >10 degrees | 3. | | |

(continued)

**Table 5-2 (continued)**

## Methods for Examining the Hip for Pain and Instability

| Examination | Technique | Illustration | Grading | Significance |
|---|---|---|---|---|
| Ligamentous laxity (continued) | 4. B 5th MCP hyperextension >90 degrees<br><br>5. Forward flexion of trunk to put hands flat on floor with knees extended | 4. 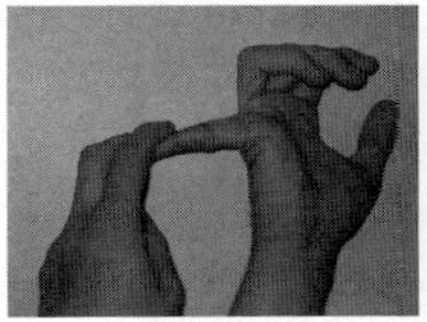   5. 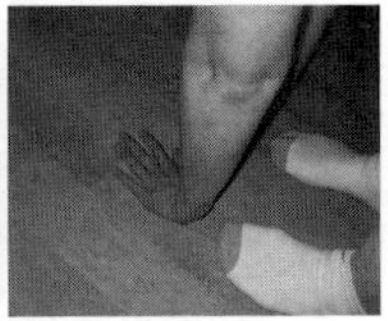 | Beighton score: 9 points<br><br>0-3 = no laxity<br>4-6 = hypermobility<br>7-9 = ↑ hypermobility | Positive finding may indicate an increased risk for hip capsular laxity |
| Palpation | 1. Greater trochanter<br>2. Ischial tuberosity<br>3. Anterior superior/inferior iliac spines<br>4. Pubic symphysis | | | 1. Trochanteric bursitis<br>2. Apophyseal injury (child) or insertional tendonitis<br>3. Apophyseal injury (child) or insertional tendonitis<br>4. Osteitis pubis |

*(continued)*

**Table 5-2 (continued)**

## METHODS FOR EXAMINING THE HIP FOR PAIN AND INSTABILITY

*Specific Tests*

| EXAMINATION | TECHNIQUE | ILLUSTRATION | GRADING | SIGNIFICANCE |
|---|---|---|---|---|
| FAI | 1. Flex hip to 90 degrees then internally rotate<br><br>2. Flexion-abduction-external rotation (FABER) | 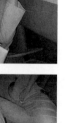 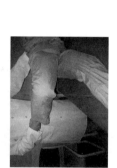 1.   2. | Pain = impingement | 1. May be secondary impingement from capsular laxity<br><br>2. ↑ distance between lateral genicular line and exam table likely anterolateral FAI |
| Ober's test | With the patient lying on the unaffected side, extend the affected hip with the knee flexed to 90 degrees, then ask the patient to allow the knee to adduct. |  | Knee does not adduct to or beyond neutral = IT band is tightness | IT band tightness may be a result of underlying capsule laxity causing chronic contraction of dynamic stabilizers of the hip |

*(continued)*

**Table 5-2 (continued)**

## METHODS FOR EXAMINING THE HIP FOR PAIN AND INSTABILITY

| EXAMINATION | TECHNIQUE | ILLUSTRATION | GRADING | SIGNIFICANCE |
|---|---|---|---|---|
| Hyperextension-external rotation | Hyperextend and externally rotate the affected hip | 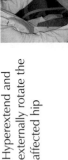 | Pain or a sense of instability | Suspect underlying capsular laxity if this causes pain or a sense of instability |
| Iliopsoas/rectus femoris tendonitis | Ask the patient to flex the affected hip against resistance with the knee:<br>1. Extended<br>2. Flexed | | Pain with knee:<br>1. Extended = rectus tendonitis<br>2. Flexed = iliopsoas tendonitis | Iliopsoas/rectus pain may be a result of underlying capsule laxity causing chronic contraction of dynamic stabilizers of the hip |

*(continued)*

**Table 5-2 (cont nued)**

## *Methods for Examining the Hip for Pain and Instability*

| Examination | Technique | Illustration | Grading | Significance |
|---|---|---|---|---|
| Iliopsoas snapping | Take hip from FABER position to extension, adduction and internal rotation | | Pain or snapping | Snapping likely, iliopsoas snapping over iliopectineal eminence, femoral head, or lesser trochanter |
| IT band snapping | Take hip from flexion to extension and internal rotation/external rotation | 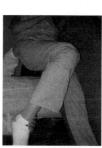 | Pain or snapping | Snapping likely, IT band over the greater trochanter |
| Piriformis | Flex the hip to 60 degrees and adduct the knee across mid-line | | Pain = piriformis tightness | |

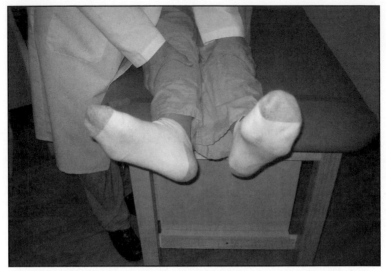

**Figure 5-1.** Physical examination demonstrating increased external rotation of the hip in full extension, suggesting anterior capsular laxity.

It is also important to assess the patient for generalized ligamentous laxity by checking the amount of bilateral elbow hyperextension, bilateral 5th metacarpal-phalangeal joint hyperextension, bilateral thumb-to-forearm apposition, bilateral knee hyperextension, and forward trunk flexion with the knees extended.[10] Anterior hip capsular laxity may be present if there is increased external rotation with the hip in neutral flexion/extension (Figure 5-1). Palpation of the bony prominences around the hip and pelvis can aid in the diagnosis of bursitis, insertional tendonitis, apophyseal injuries, or muscle strains.

There are several tests that can narrow the differential diagnosis for hip pain (see Table 5-2). If hip flexion to 90 degrees with adduction and internal rotation causes pain, femoral acetabular impingement (FAI) should be considered. In addition, pain with flexion, abduction, and external rotation (FABER) may signify anterolateral FAI. External rotation and hip hyperextension can cause pain or apprehension in patients with anterior capsular laxity. Ober's test helps to define iliotibial (IT) band tightness. IT band tightness can aggravate trochanteric bursitis. Ober's test is performed by passively extending the hip with the knee flexed to 90 degrees while the patient is in the lateral decubitus on the contralateral side. If the knee does not adduct past neutral in this position, the IT band is likely tight. To assess for iliopsoas pathology, the patient is asked to flex the hip against resistance with the knee flexed and extended. Pain with the knee extended indicates pain originating from both the rectus femoris and iliopsoas tendons. Pain with the knee flexed points to the iliopsoas as the main source of pain because knee flexion relaxes the rectus femoris. Iliopsoas snapping can also be reproduced, taking the hip from the FABER position to an extended, adducted and internally rotated position. Last, piriformis tightness and associated pain is tested by flexing the hip to 60 degrees and adducting the knee across the body.

## PATHOANATOMY

The hip joint relies upon its osseous anatomy for stability. However, the hip has a ligamentous capsule that helps to provide stability throughout its ROM. It consists of the iliofemoral ligament (Y-ligament of Bigelow) anteriorly, the ischiofemoral ligament and the deep arcuate ligament posteriorly, and the zona orbicularis inferiorly. Each of these ligaments is a discrete structure that has a specific function to resist translation during extremes of motion (Table 5-3). These ligaments also have differing mechanical strengths.[11] The iliofemoral ligament is the strongest ligament in the hip capsule.[11] The iliofemoral ligament helps to resist anterior hip translation during standing, thereby reducing the need for muscle contraction to maintain an erect posture.[12] The ischiofemoral ligament resists internal rotation and adduction when the hip is flexed.[12] The deep femoral arcuate ligament stabilizes the hip in extreme flexion and extension. The zona orbicularis resists inferior distraction forces in the hip.[13]

Traumatic hip dislocation during athletic competition is usually a low-energy event that often results in a pure dislocation or a dislocation with only small acetabular rim fractures. MRI often reveals that there is an acute disruption of the iliofemoral ligament anteriorly, hemarthrosis, and bone contusions in the femoral head and acetabular rim.[4]

**Table 5-3**

## PERTINENT ANATOMY IN HIP INSTABILITY

| Structure | Function | Importance |
|---|---|---|
| Femoral-ace-tabular bone | Deep acetabulum with high degree of femoral-acetabular congruency allows rotation but not much translation | Depth and congruence provides intrinsic stability |
| Labrum | Deepens acetabulum, provides femoral-ace-tabular seal, increases fluid pressure, may resist femoral head translation in extremes of motion | Its seal creates a suction effect with improved hip stability. Increased fluid pressure protects cartilage from consolidation. May provide increased stability |
| Iliofemoral ligament | Located in anterior capsule. Strongest ligament in the hip capsule. Resists hip hyperextension and external rotation | Protects the hip from anterior dislocation in extension and external rotation. Subject to microtrauma with repetitive external rotation |
| Ischiofemoral ligament | Located in posterior capsule. Resists internal rotation and adduction in hip flexion | Protects hip from posterior dislocation in flexion and adduction |
| Deep arcuate ligament | Located in posterior capsule. Stabilizes the hip in extremes of flexion and extension | Reinforces hip stability in extremes of motion |
| Zona obicularis | Located inferior to the femoral head. Resists distraction forces | Keeps femoral head located in the acetabulum |

There have been reports of recurrent hip instability with minimal trauma after an initial traumatic hip dislocation.[5,14] The intraoperative findings in these reports suggested capsular redundancy and labral pathology as the cause of persistent instability. In addition to posterior labral tears, anterior labral tears do occur with a posterior dislocation.[8] Despite the stability imparted by the osseous anatomy of the hip, a traumatic dislocation can cause significant damage to the surrounding supportive soft tissues, leading to persistent pain, instability, and disability.

Atraumatic hip instability may be due to repetitive axial load and external rotation of the hip, resulting in microtrauma to the capsule, gradual stretching of the iliofemoral ligament, and increased capsular volume. Additionally, collagen disorders or generalized ligamentous laxity can cause capsular laxity in the hip. The dynamic stabilizers that cross the hip such as the iliopsoas and the hip abductors work harder to help support the joint during normal motion. It has been reported that capsular laxity contributes to symptomatic iliopsoas and iliotibial (IT) band snapping.[1] Capsular laxity can also exacerbate trochanteric bursitis from excess motion and subsequent tightening of the IT band. Chronic iliopsoas contraction from excess motion can lead to a hip flexion contracture.[8] This can also contribute to low back pain as the pelvis flexes to accommodate the flexion contracture. Additionally, secondary FAI can occur because of increased translation of the femoral head during hip motion due to capsular laxity.[2,3] When patients have a wide spectrum of complaints about the hip, consider capsular laxity and subtle hip instability as a possible underlying cause.

# IMAGING

Imaging is a critical component to evaluating patients with hip instability (see Table 5-1). In the case of an acute traumatic subluxation or dislocation, plain x-rays provide a quick and important assessment of the injured hip. An anterior-posterior (AP) view of the pelvis, a lateral view of the hip, and Judet views are performed to confirm a congruent reduction, to look for associated femoral head or neck fractures, and to assess for associated acetabular fractures. An AP pelvis should always be obtained after reducing a dislocated hip. Widening of the joint space between the femoral head and acetabulum after reduction should raise suspicion of an incarcerated fragment preventing a congruent reduction. In the acute traumatic setting, a post-reduction computed tomography (CT) scan is also helpful to look for subtle acetabular rim fractures, femoral head and neck fractures, or fragments in the joint space.

In the case of atraumatic hip instability, an AP pelvis and a cross-table lateral x-ray of the affected hip is the standard initial evaluation. The AP pelvis gives a good assessment of the presence of acetabular retroversion and the presence of acetabular dysplasia as measured by the center-edge (CE) angle. The "cross-over" sign indicates acetabular retroversion. This is seen when the shadow of the anterior acetabular rim is more inferolateral and crosses the shadow of the posterior acetabular rim (Figure 5-2A). The posterior wall shadow crosses in the center of the femoral head rather than the femoral neck.[15] The presence of a "cross-over" sign suggests pincer impingement. The acetabular version can also be estimated on the cross-table lateral, but a "false profile" view is more of true lateral view.[16] The CE angle is the measured angle between the line drawn from the center of the femoral head to the superolateral rim of the acetabulum and the line drawn perpendicular to the horizontal line connecting the center of both femoral heads (Figure 5-2B). A CE angle of less than 20 degrees is indicative of acetabular dysplasia. A CE angle between 20 and 25 degrees is considered borderline. Abnormalities of the femoral head suggesting cam impingement can be seen on both the AP and cross-table lateral views. Last, a traction view of the affected hip may be helpful to look for abnormal distraction seen as a "vacuum" sign (Figure 5-3).[1]

Magnetic resonance imaging (MRI) has become a useful imaging technique for patients with both traumatic and atraumatic hip instability. In traumatic injuries, an early MRI can help define labral tears, cartilage injuries, loose bodies, and the location and degree of capsular tears. It is also helpful to get an MRI 6 weeks after the injury to assess for early signs of avascular necrosis (AVN).[4] This information can help guide recommendations regarding weight-bearing status and return to play. In patients with atraumatic hip instability,

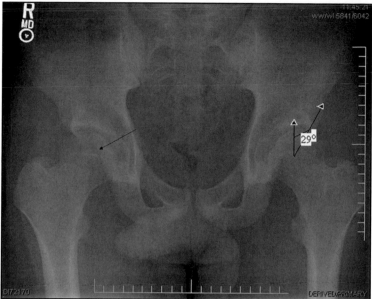

**Figure 5-2.** (Left) AP pelvis view demonstrating a "cross-over" sign where the shadow of the anterior acetabular rim crosses the shadow of the posterior acetabular rim (arrow). (Right) AP pelvis view demonstrating the CE angle measurement. The CE angle in this patient is 29 degrees. This patient has anterior impingement with a "low-normal" CE angle.

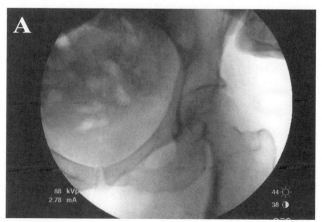

**Figure 5-3.** (A) Fluoroscopic AP view of the left hip without traction *(continued)*.

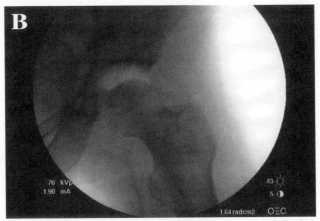

**Figure 5-3 (continued).** (B) Fluoroscopic AP view of the left hip demonstrating a "vacuum" sign with traction applied.

MRI can accurately define intra-articular abnormalities as well as other problems in the bone and surrounding soft tissues that may contribute to pain and dysfunction.[17] MR arthrography has also become a valuable imaging technique to evaluate intra-articular pathology including chondral damage and labral tears. MR arthrography increases the sensitivity for detecting intra-articular pathology at the cost of doubling the false-positive rate.[18] An injection of intra-articular bupivacaine can reliably predict (~90%) the presence of intra-articular pathology as the source of pain.[18,19]

## TREATMENT

In an acute traumatic hip dislocation, it is critical to reduce the hip immediately. After reduction, an incarcerated fragment in the joint requires urgent surgical excision to minimize damage to the articular cartilage. Patients who develop a painful hemarthrosis after an acute dislocation or subluxation should undergo urgent aspiration of the hip for pain control. This also reduces intracapsular pressure that may lower the risk of AVN.[8] Obtaining a MRI acutely after hip reduction can help determine if there is a chondral injury or a loose body that would prompt early operative intervention. Good results

have been reported with microfracture of full-thickness chondral injuries in the hip.[20] It is not clear whether there is any
value in performing a microfracture acutely after hip dislocation before the absence of AVN is confirmed.

Most traumatic hip subluxations or dislocations in athletes can be treated nonoperatively even if there is a small
acetabular rim fracture (<25% to 30%). As long as the hip is
concentrically reduced and there are no loose bodies, active
and passive ROM can start immediately. If the patient sustained a posterior dislocation, do not allow hip flexion beyond
90 degrees or hip internal rotation more than 10 degrees for at
least 6 weeks.[8] For an anterior dislocation, protect the patient
from hip hyperextension and external rotation for the same
period of time. Toe-touch weight-bearing is recommended for
6 weeks. After 6 weeks, a repeat MRI should be done to look
for evidence of AVN and loose bodies.[4,8] Patients who have
no signs of osteonecrosis or loose bodies can safely return to
sports when they are asymptomatic. Patients in whom osteonecrosis is diagnosed at 6 weeks are at risk for collapse and joint
degeneration. These patients should be treated with protected
weight-bearing for another 6 weeks. They should be counseled about ending their sports participation. Patients with
recurrent hip instability have been treated successfully with
operative intervention. There are reports of good outcomes
after open posterior labral repair and capsular plication.[5,14]

Treatment for atraumatic capsular laxity that leads to
hip instability is becoming more common. The challenge in
making the diagnosis and lack of a full understanding of the
clinical implications has made treatment for this problem
a relatively new concept. Open capsular plication has been
described to treat atraumatic hip instability.[1] There have
also been good results using thermal capsular shrinkage to
reduce capsular volume.[3] More recently, arthroscopic capsular plication has become the standard for treating capsular
laxity as it avoids the complications associated with thermal
capsular shrinkage that have been seen in the shoulder.[21]
Arthroscopic capsular plication can be done in the central or
peripheral compartment. Performing this procedure in the
peripheral compartment avoids the need for prolonged traction. In addition, the amount of plication can be estimated
well because it is done under direct visualization (Figure 5-4).

**Figure 5-4.** (A) Arthroscopic image showing an anterior capsular window viewed from the peripheral compartment. (B) Arthroscopic image showing a hooked suture shuttle in a limb of the anterior capsule. (C) Arthroscopic image showing PDS suture that was passed through the suture shuttle and fed into the joint for retrieval *(continued)*.

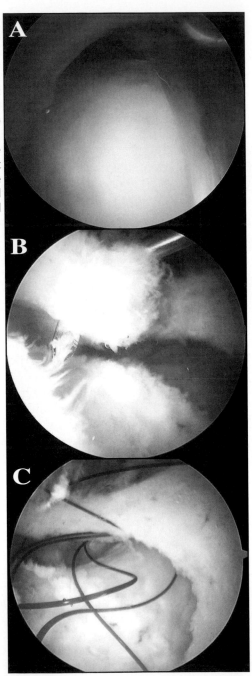

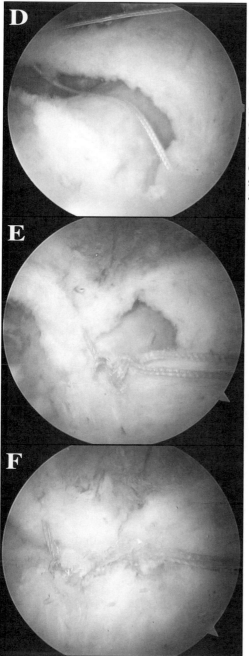

**Figure 5-4 (continued).** (D) Arthroscopic image showing a nonabsorbable braided suture that was pulled through both limbs of the anterior capsule. (E) Arthroscopic image showing the suture tied down to close the capsule. (F) Arthroscopic image showing the final capsular plication after a second suture was passed and tied.

The disadvantages of arthroscopic capsulorrhaphy are that it is technically demanding with current hip arthroscopy equipment, it requires protected motion until the capsule heals, and there is potential for recurrent instability.

Our current algorithm for patients with hip pain and instability is as follows. First, we perform an intra-articular hip injection with 6 cc of 1% lidocaine, 6 cc of 0.25% marcaine, and 80 mg of Kenalog. We ask the patient to record the percentage of pain relief within 2 hours after the injection. This helps us verify that a large part of the pain is related to intra-articular pathology because physical examination is not always reliable in predicting this.[22] If the patient reports a sensation of instability or apprehension with external rotation and hip hyperextension or if he or she demonstrates increased external rotation with the hip in full extension on exam, we consider performing a capsular plication at the time of surgery. If the patient has a labral tear and demonstrates symptoms of FAI without osseous abnormalities consistent with cam or pincer impingement, secondary impingement from capsular laxity may be the cause. We would consider a capsulorrhaphy at the time of surgery, especially if the hip easily distracts with traction. Last, if the patient has generalized ligamentous laxity and an array of hip problems including femoral acetabular impingement, labral tear, coxa saltans, iliopsoas tendonitis, and IT band tendonitis, capsular laxity should be consider as an underlying cause and it should be treated, if clearly present, along with management of concomitant diagnoses.

## CONCLUSION

Traumatic and atraumatic hip instability can be a debilitating problem for patients. Although nonoperative treatment is effective in many cases, surgical intervention can provide relief in those patients who have persistent pain and disability. Soft tissue abnormalities like traumatic or atraumatic capsular laxity may be a pathological factor causing hip instability. Open and arthroscopic techniques have been described to treat capsular laxity in the hip with good success. Arthroscopic capsular plication, although technically challenging, enables the surgeon to clearly visualize the amount of capsular tightening, likely reduces perioperative morbidity, and provides adequate stability until the capsule heals. When evaluating patients with multiple hip complaints, generalized ligamentous laxity, evidence of hip apprehension with provocative maneuvers, coxa saltans, and an easily distractible hip with traction, capsular laxity should be considered as an underlying problem and should be treated.

# REFERENCES

1. Bellabarba C, Sheinkop MB, Kuo KN. Idiopathic hip instability: an unrecognized cause of coxa saltans in the adult. *Clinic Orthop Relat Res.* 1998;355:261-271.
2. Ranawat AS, McClincy M, Sekiya JK. Anterior dislocation of the hip after arthroscopy in a patient with capsular laxity of the hip: a case report. *J Bone Joint Surg Am.* 2009;91(1):192-197.
3. Philippon MJ. The role of arthroscopic thermal capsulorrhaphy in the hip. *Clin Sports Med.* 2001;20(4):817-829.
4. Moorman CT 3rd, Warren RF, Hershman EB, et al. Traumatic posterior hip subluxation in American football. *J Bone Joint Surg Am.* 2003;85-A(7):1190-1196.
5. Liebenberg F, Dommisse GF. Recurrent post-traumatic dislocation of the hip. *J Bone Joint Surg Br.* 1969;51(4):632-637.
6. Giza E, Mithöfer K, Matthews H, Vrahas M. Hip fracture-dislocation in football: a report of two cases and review of the literature. *Br J Sports Med.* 2004;38(4):E17.
7. Mitchell JC, Giannoudis PV, Millner PA, Smith RM. A rare fracture-dislocation of the hip in a gymnast and review of the literature. *Br J Sports Med.* 1999;33(4):283-284.
8. Shindle MK, Ranawat AS, Kelly BT. Diagnosis and management of traumatic and atraumatic hip instability in the athletic patient. *Clin Sports Med.* 2006;25(2):309-326, ix-x.
9. Kelly BT, Williams RJ 3rd, Philippon MJ. Hip arthroscopy: current indications, treatment options, and management issues. *Am J Sports Med.* 2003;31(6):1020-1037. Review.
10. Beighton P, Horan F. Orthopaedic aspects of the Ehlers-Danlos syndrome. *J Bone Joint Surg Br.* 1969;51(3):444-453.
11. Hewitt JD, Glisson RR, Guilak F, Vail TP. The mechanical properties of the human hip capsule ligaments. *J Arthroplasty.* 2002;17(1):82-89.
12. Fuss FK, Bacher A. New aspects of the morphology and function of the human hip joint ligaments. *Am J Anat.* 1991;192(1):1-13.
13. Ito H, Song Y, Lindsey DP, Safran MR, Giori NJ. The proximal hip joint capsule and the zona orbicularis contribute to the hip joint stability in distraction. *J Orthop Res.* 2009;27(8):989-995.
14. Nelson CL. Traumatic recurrent dislocation of the hip. Report of a case. *J Bone Joint Surg Am.* 1970;52(1):128-130.

15. Reynolds D, Lucas J, Klaue K. Retroversion of the acetabulum: a cause of hip pain. *J Bone Joint Surg Br.* 1999;81(2):281-288.
16. Delaunay S, Dussault RG, Kaplan PA, Alford BA. Radiographic measurements of dysplastic adult hips. *Skeletal Radiol.* 1997;26(2):75-81.
17. Mintz DN, Hooper T, Connell D, Buly R, Padgett DE, Potter HG. Magnetic resonance imaging of the hip: detection of labral and chondral abnormalities using noncontrast imaging. *Arthroscopy.* 2005;21(4):385-393.
18. Byrd JW, Jones KS. Diagnostic accuracy of clinical assessment, magnetic resonance imaging, magnetic resonance arthrography, and intra-articular injection in hip arthroscopy patients. *Am J Sports Med.* 2004;32(7):1668-1674.
19. Martin RL, Irrgang JJ, Sekiya JK. The diagnostic accuracy of a clinical examination in determining intra-articular hip pain for potential hip arthroscopy candidates. *Arthroscopy.* 2008;24(9):1013-1018.
20. Crawford K, Philippon MJ, Sekiya JK, Rodkey WG, Steadman JR. Microfracture of the hip in athletes. *Clin Sports Med.* 2006;25(2):327-335.
21. Good CR, Shindle MK, Kelly BT, Wanich T, Warren RF. Glenohumeral chondrolysis after shoulder arthroscopy with thermal capsulorrhaphy. *Arthroscopy.* 2007;23(7):797.e1-797.e5.
22. Martin RL, Sekiya JK. The interrater reliability of 4 clinical tests used to assess individuals with musculoskeletal hip pain. *J Orthop Sports Phys Ther.* 2008;38(2):71-77.

**6**

# FEMOROACETABULAR IMPINGEMENT

*Nicola Mondanelli, MD; Michael S. H. Kain, MD;*
*Reinhold Ganz, MD; and Michael Leunig, MD*

## INTRODUCTION

Femoroacetabular impingement (FAI) is a term used to describe morphologic alterations of the proximal femur, the acetabulum, or both that result in the intra-articular damage and the early onset of secondary osteoarthritis (OA). FAI can be a result of conditions such as slipped capital femoral epiphysis (SCFE), Legg-Calvé-Perthes disease (LCPD), coxa vara, or morphological alterations such as acetabular retroversion or coxa profunda. Regardless of the etiology, the main problem is a mismatch in geometry of the proximal femur and the acetabulum that results in restricted motion and abnormal joint loads. This morphological mismatch of the femur and acetabulum,

Ranawat A, Kelly BT. *Musculoskeletal Examination of the Hip and Knee: Making the Complex Simple* (pp. 159-182).
© 2011 SLACK Incorporated

combined with the forceful activities, can lead to mechanical damage of the hip joint and the early onset of OA, as it has been observed during the open surgical treatment of FAI.[1-4]

# HISTORY

FAI tends to occur in young and active patients with a slow onset of groin pain.[3] The onset of pain can also begin after sustaining a minor trauma, but patients are most likely unable to recall the initial onset.[3,5] Patients commonly complain of sharp groin pain with hip flexion and internal rotation or abduction, and there are common complaints of groin pain after sitting for a prolonged period or while climbing up stairs.[1,5] Other positions may trigger lateral or posterior hip pain; for instance, athletes with FAI may report difficulty with squatting, lateral/cutting movements, and starting/stopping.[5-7]

During the initial stages of the disease, the pain is intermittent and is exacerbated by athletic activities or prolonged walking that causes the hip to be repetitively placed into the position of impingement. Referred gluteal pain can be a sign of posterior FAI, either from abutment of the femoral neck or the greater trochanter impinging posteriorly on the ischium or posterior acetabular wall. Trochanteric pain is also seen in FAI and occurs in as high as 61% of cases and is associated with conditions such as abductor weakness or bursitis.[5] Therefore, a thorough history and physical examination in addition to various imaging modalities are necessary to rule out other possible origins of pain. The differential diagnosis for hip pain should include both local causes (osteonecrosis of the femoral head, stress fracture of the proximal femur, psoas tendinitis, etc) and other pathologies causing referred hip pain (sacroiliitis, vertebral disk disease, fracture of pubic rami, athletic pubalgia, etc).

# EXAMINATION

The physical examination of a FAI hip is similar as for other pathologic conditions of the hip, and it should include evaluating range of motion (ROM), isometric strength, gait analysis, leg length, neurovascular analyses, and provocative tests specific for FAI (Table 6-1). Patients with FAI commonly have decreased flexion and internal rotation, but external rotation and abduction can also be limited.[4] A decrease in hip ROM is often seen but may not be noticed by patients. The "impingement test"[8] is performed with the patient lying supine; the hip is passively brought to 90 degrees of flexion and then forced into maximal internal rotation and adduction. The test is positive if this maneuver reproduces the deep anterior groin pain experienced by the patient. Patients with FAI nearly always have a positive impingement test.[3,5]

Although less commonly positive, a posterior impingement may be assessed by the "posterior impingement test,"[3] placing the hip in extension and external rotation. Pain or decreased motion has been reported in patients with posterior impingement lesions. Pain during the FABER test (flexion, abduction, and external rotation) is not specific to FAI; however, lateral hip pain has been clinically observed to be a frequent complaint in FAI patients during the FABER maneuver.[7] Additionally, an increased vertical distance between the lateral edge of the knee and the examination table has been observed in FAI patients during the FABER examination when compared with the contralateral limb.[5] When the origin of pain is unclear, it may be useful to perform an intra-articular injection of anesthetics under fluoroscopic or ultrasound guidance to determine if the pain is intra-articular in origin.[9]

## PATHOANATOMY

Observations made in the early treatment of FAI through a surgical dislocation approach to the hip joint[10] provided insight into how various FAI morphologies lead to different patterns of joint degeneration.[1] The 2 main types of FAI described are pincer and cam impingement, although a combined form occurs in approximately 70% of our cases (Table 6-2 and Figure 6-1).[1,2] The *pincer type* is characterized by a focal (eg, acetabular retroversion) or global (eg, coxa profunda or protrusio) overcoverage of the acetabulum and leads to linear impact of the acetabular rim against the head-neck junction, trapping the labrum in between.

**Table 6-1**

## METHODS FOR EXAMINING THE HIP FOR FEMOROACETABULAR IMPINGEMENT

| Examination | Technique | Illustration | Grading | Significance |
|---|---|---|---|---|
| Range of motion (ROM) | Examine passive and active and compare to contralateral side | 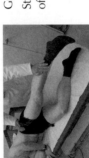 | In degrees | Look for limited ROM in internal/external rotation with hip flexed at 80 to 90 degrees |
| Strength of abductors | Patient lateral on table with affected side up | | Graded 0 to 5 Standard grading of muscle strength | Abductor strength |

*(continued)*

**Table 6-1 (continued)**

*METHODS FOR EXAMINING THE HIP FOR FEMOROACETABULAR IMPINGEMENT*

| Examination | Technique | Illustration | | Grading | Significance |
|---|---|---|---|---|---|
| | | Positive | Negative | | |
| Trendelenburg sign | Patient stands on long leg for minimum of 30 seconds to see if he or she can hold the pelvis level | 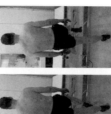 | | Positive/negative | Tests fatigue ability of abductors on side patient is standing on |
| Bicycle test | Patient lateral on table and affected side up performs bicycle motion with leg | | | Positive/negative | Indicates trochanteric bursitis |

*(continued)*

**Table 6-1 (continued)**

## METHODS FOR EXAMINING THE HIP FOR FEMOROACETABULAR IMPINGEMENT

| Examination | Technique | Illustration | Grading | Significance |
|---|---|---|---|---|
| Impingement test (anterior) | Hip is flexed to 80 to 90 degrees, then internally rotated with adduction | 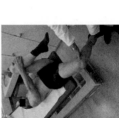 | Positive/negative | A positive test is considered with a reproduction of groin pain |
| Posterior impingement test | Hip is extended and externally rotated with abduction | | Positive/negative | Reproduction of posterior gluteal pain |

(continued)

**Table 6-1 (continued)**

## METHODS FOR EXAMINING THE HIP FOR FEMOROACETABULAR IMPINGEMENT

| Examination | Technique | Illustration | Grading | Significance |
|---|---|---|---|---|
| FABER test | Hip is flexed, abducted, and externally rotated | 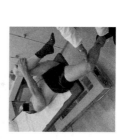 | Positive/negative | To indicate lumbar, sacro-iliac joint, or posterior hip pathology |
| Apprehension test | Hip is in neutral and externally rotated with leg adducted then abducted | | Positive/negative | If patient feels discomfort with adduction, this is a sign of instability |

(continued)

**Table 6-1 (continued)**

## *METHODS FOR EXAMINING THE HIP FOR FEMOROACETABULAR IMPINGEMENT*

*Common Correlations Between Pathology and Location of Impingement*

| | |
|---|---|
| SCFE | Anterolaterally |
| LCPD | Anterolaterally |
| Acetabular retroversion | Anterolaterally |
| Coxa profunda | Generalized |
| Coxa valga | Anteromedially |
| Coxa vara | Anterolaterally |
| Short femoral neck | Extra-articular |

## Table 6-2

# HELPFUL HINTS

## Types of Impingement

|  | HISTORY | RADIOGRAPHIC FINDINGS | LOCATION OF IMPINGEMENT |
|---|---|---|---|
| Cam | Patients are frequently young athletic men; pain during and after activity and while sitting; limited internal rotation | Alpha angle >50 to 55 degrees, flat area at junction of femoral head and neck (no offset) | Anterosuperior |
| Pincer | Patients are usually women; more likely to have a positive posterior impingement sign | Large lateral center edge angle (LCE), coxa profunda, protrusio acetabuli, impingement cysts, labral ossification | Generalized, also countercoup lesion posteroinferiorly |

## Radiology

|  | STUDY | SIGNIFICANCE | FINDINGS |
|---|---|---|---|
| Plain radiographs | AP pelvis; well-centered and avoiding excessive pelvis lordosis | Assess overall pelvis, look at LCE; acetabular version (cross-over sign, posterior wall sign, ischial spine sign), coxa profunda; femoral neck angle (varus or valgus); assess for impingement cysts | Coxa profunda with LCE >35 degrees, acetabular retroversion with positive cross-over sign, posterior wall sign, and ischial spine sign |
|  | Cross-table lateral | Measure alpha angle, assess femoral head-neck junction for flattening and offset and posterior joint space, presence of impingement cysts | Alpha angle >50 degrees |

*(continued)*

## Table 6-2 (continued)

### HELPFUL HINTS

*Radiology*

| | STUDY | SIGNIFICANCE | FINDINGS |
|---|---|---|---|
| MRI and MRA | MRI radial cuts | Assess cartilage and labrum of the entire acetabular rim; measure alpha angle | Coxa profunda with LCE >35 degrees, acetabular retroversion with positive cross-over sign, posterior wall sign, and ischial spine sign |
| | Gadolinium-enhanced MRA | Improved assessment of the articular cartilage and identification of labral tears | Alpha angle >50 degrees |

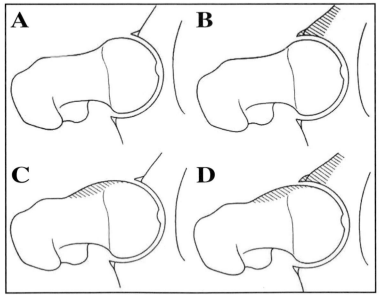

**Figure 6-1.** Femoroacetabular impingement. (A) Normal hip, (B) pincer FAI, (C) cam FAI, (D) combined FAI. (Reprinted with permission from Lavigne M, Parvizi J, Beck M, Siebenrock KA, Ganz R, Leunig M. Anterior femoroacetabular impingement: part I. Techniques of joint preserving surgery. *Clin Orthop Relat Res.* 2004;418:61-66.)

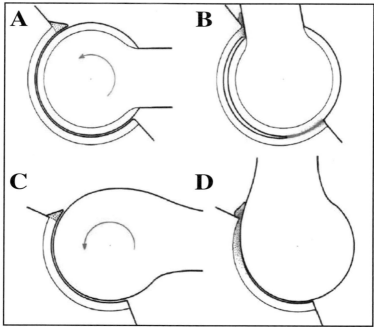

**Figure 6-2.** Mechanism of lesion of FAI. (A, B) pincer type and (C, D) cam type. (Reprinted with permission from Beck M, Leunig M, Parvizi J, Boutier V, Wyss D, Ganz R. Anterior femoroacetabular impingement: part II. Midterm results of surgical treatment. *Clin Orthop Relat Res.* 2004;418:67-73.)

As a result of this repetitive traumatic "squeeze," the labrum is the first structure to degenerate with intra-substance fissuring, ganglion formation, and substance degeneration. Secondarily, the acetabular cartilage adjacent to the involved labrum degenerates. Over time, the impaction area on the femoral neck shows a saddle-like erosion. The femoral head cartilage remains uninvolved over a long period; later on in the process, a cartilage abrasion in the posteroinferior joint, on the head, and/or on the acetabulum (called *countercoup lesion*) can be observed (Figures 6-2A and B).

The *cam-type* impingement is the result of a nonspherical femoral head or lack of head-neck offset. The nonspherical portion of the head impacts into the acetabular rim after superiorly displacing the labrum. Initially, the labrum remains uninvolved while the first structure to fail in pure cam impingement is the acetabular cartilage, which avulses from the labrum and delaminates off of the subchondral bone of the adjacent acetabulum rim. Often, impingement cysts can develop at the head-neck junction.[11] The cartilage of the nonspherical portion of the head (nonweight-bearing area) shows surface damage early in the disease process. Once the defect on the acetabular cartilage is large enough, the femoral head will migrate into it, at which point the cartilage of the spherical portion of the head (weight-bearing area) begins to erode (Figures 6-2C and D).

Although FAI can occur in a variety of locations in the joint, it most commonly occurs in the anterolateral region and is produced by flexion and internal rotation of the femur. Pincer impingement is seen more frequently in active middle-aged women, while cam impingement is more common in young and athletic men. Cam FAI causes more local destruction than pincer FAI, which tends to cause more global involvement of the joint. In the initial stages of pincer impingement, symptoms are often more pronounced than in cam FAI. For instance, women suffering from pincer impingement reported increased pain compared to men with cam FAI.[12] The rationale for this is that the pain begins when the labrum becomes involved because the labrum is known to contain nociceptive fibers.[13]

# IMAGING

A supine anteroposterior (AP) pelvis and a cross-table lateral or Dunn plain x-rays are the first exam to be ordered for a young patient with hip pain (see Table 6-2). Numerous and useful information can be drawn from these views, but care should be taken to maintain neutral pelvic tilt and rotation in AP radiographs as they both affect the interpretation of acetabular version and can either mask or falsely identify pincer lesions.[14] Pincer-type FAI can be detected on AP radiographs by the "crossover" and "posterior wall" signs[15] (Figure 6-3) as well as signs for coxa profunda and protrusio acetabuli or retroversion (eg, global pincer FAI). Lateral-based cam lesions ("pistol grip" deformities) can also be seen on AP pelvis X-rays (Figure 6-4).

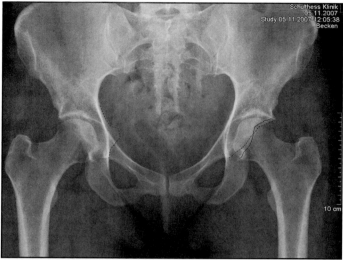

**Figure 6-3.** AP pelvis radiograph with cross-over and posterior wall signs (left hip: dot line = anterior wall; continued line = posterior wall) and projection of ischial spine into the pelvis (right hip).

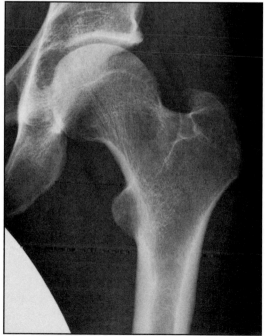

**Figure 6-4.** Pistol grip deformity.

An insufficient anterior femoral head-neck offset has also been reported as a cause of cam FAI and is best viewed with a Dunn or a cross-table lateral with the femur internally rotated.[16] The "alpha angle" is used to describe the point where the femoral head becomes aspherical, and an alpha angle greater than 50 to 55 degrees is considered to be abnormal.[17] The "alpha angle" can be measured either on the lateral plain radiograph (Figure 6-5) or on a modified axial magnetic resonance imaging (MRI) in the plane of the femoral neck.[17] However, even using these sequences might miss femoral head asphericity. As a result, radial sequences were developed to assess the entire anterosuperior quadrant of the hip joint to aid in identifying femoral head asphericity and labral pathology. Gadolinium-enhanced magnetic resonance arthrography (MRA) is also used to evaluate the intra-articular pathology of the labrum and articular cartilage (Figure 6-6), being more effective in detecting labral than chondral lesions.[4,9,18,19] Ultimately, correlating findings from a good physical exam with the findings from properly taken images will enable the physician to make an accurate diagnosis of FAI.

## TREATMENT

### Nonsurgical Treatment

This includes restriction of athletic activities and a course of nonsteroidal anti-inflammatory drugs. Physical therapy to improve passive ROM or stretching is frequently counterproductive and might exacerbate symptoms. Nonsurgical management can be temporarily successful; however, because of the typically high activity level and athletic ambitions of these patients, such treatment usually fails to control the symptoms.[5] Furthermore, the pathomechanism of FAI leads to progressive advancement of labral and chondral lesions, and subsequently to early OA.[1]

### Operative Treatment

The aim is to obtain an impingement-free ROM, to improve symptoms, and to stop (or slow down) the progression of joint damage; it consists of removing any osseous deformity on

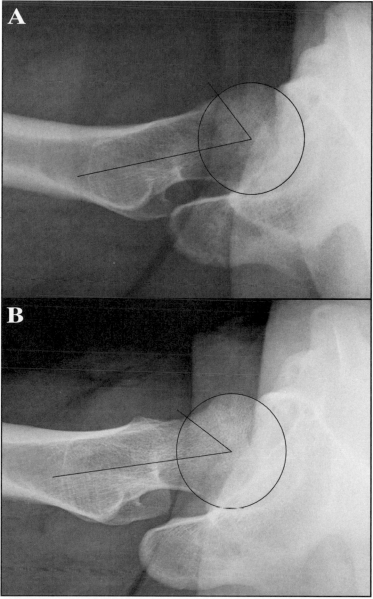

**Figure 6-5.** The "alpha angle" on a Dunn view (A) preoperatively and (B) after arthroscopic osteochondroplasty of the femoral head-neck junction.

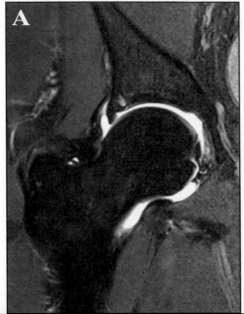

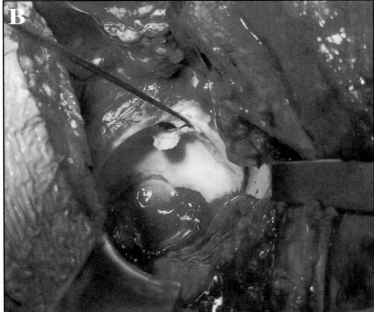

**Figure 6-6.** Labrum and cartilage damage. (A) MRA evaluation and (B) intraoperative picture.

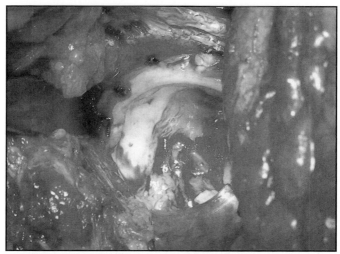

**Figure 6-7.** Surgical dislocation; the labrum has been re-fixed with suture-anchors after acetabular trimming.

either side of the joint and eventually addressing the subsequent labral and chondral lesions secondary to FAI. In pincer FAI, the labrum is taken down (as part of the approach), and the acetabular rim is resected to remove excessive coverage. There is some evidence that labral refixation is beneficial with respect to clinical and radiographic results,[20] so the degenerative labrum is débrided, and the healthy portion is reattached to the acetabular rim with suture anchors at the end of the procedure (Figure 6-7). It is only resected if it is severely damaged. In cam FAI, the primary goal is to excise the prominent bump, which represents the aspherical portion of the femoral head-neck (Figure 6-8). In doing so, attention must be paid to not damage the superolateral epiphyseal vessels (end-branches of the medial femoral circumflex artery) entering the femoral head in the retinacular fold. In the acetabulum, after the rim trimming, cartilage flaps can be débrided and microfractures performed in any remaining bare areas. To perform the required intra-articular procedures, the hip can be approached in various ways including the technique of surgical dislocation, a minimally invasive anterior approach, using the arthroscope or other means to achieve these goals.

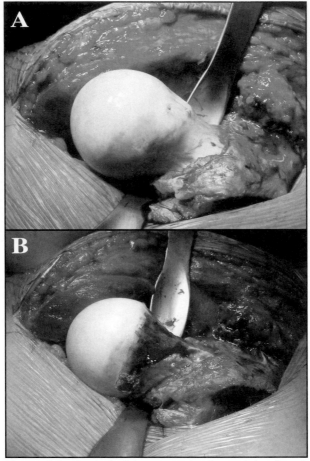

**Figure 6-8.** Surgical dislocation; the femoral head-neck offset (A) before and (B) after osteochondroplasty.

## Surgical Dislocation of the Hip

This technique is considered the gold standard treatment and allows for both sides of the joint to be treated. The use of this exposure has allowed for a better understanding of the patho-anatomy of FAI.[2,20-22] Anatomical studies have clearly demonstrated that vascular supply to the femoral head lies on the deep branch of the medial femoral circumflex artery (MFCA) and its constant anastomosis with the inferior gluteal artery.[23,24]

The surgical dislocation approach as described by Ganz et al was developed to protect this blood supply and allow for the safe dislocation of the hip in order to treat intra-articular pathology of the hip such as FAI.[10,25]

The patient is placed in the lateral decubitus position and the hip is approached through the interval between the gluteus maximus and the tensor fasciae latae. The gluteus maximus is posteriorly retracted, and a trigastric (glutei medius and minimus and vastus lateralis muscles) trochanteric osteotomy is made. The interval between the gluteus minimus and piriformis is then developed, and the minimus is elevated off of the capsule while mobilizing the trochanteric fragment anteriorly to expose the joint capsule. A Z-shaped capsulotomy is made and an anterior dislocation of the hip joint is performed while preserving the attachments of all of the external rotators. Preservation of the external rotators, particularly the obturator externus, allows for the main branch of the MFCA to the femoral head to be protected. This approach allows for visualization and complete access to the femoral head and acetabulum. The intra-articular procedures (acetabular trimming, femoral head-neck osteochondroplasty, labral/chondral procedures) can be performed as necessary. Extra-articular components of FAI and associated deformities can also be treated via this approach at the same time. The capsule should be loosely repaired to prevent tension on the vessels in the retinaculum, and the trochanteric osteotomy is reattached with lag screws.

## Hip Arthroscopy

Recent advances in arthroscopic techniques and the understanding of the pathology have also led to the development of arthroscopic procedures for the treatment of FAI.[26-28] Hip arthroscopy is a valid treatment option for intra-articular disorders without structural abnormality (eg, labral and chondral lesions, loose bodies) and for mild structural abnormality with intra-articular deformity (cam FAI, focal pincer FAI, cam impingement secondary to mild slipped capital femoral epiphysis) in the absence of advanced joint deterioration.[6,29] Our technique uses 2 portals (anterolateral and mid-anterior), with the patient in the supine position. The hip is placed in traction to distract the joint to allow access to the central

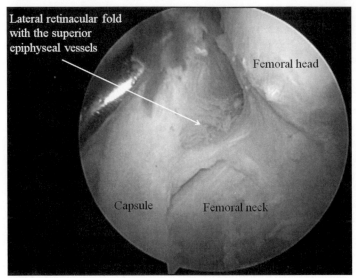

**Figure 6-9.** View of the lateral head/neck junction. The lateral retinacular fold contains the superior epiphyseal vessels.

compartment. A T-shaped capsulotomy is made with one limb along the acetabular rim and the other along the anterior femoral neck. Acetabular rim trimming and femoral head-neck osteochondroplasty are performed as necessary. A pneumatic leg holder will allow for moving the limb to gain access to different aspects of the femoral neck without the need for further portals. Arthroscopy is less invasive than surgical dislocation but is also technically demanding, and visualization may be limited compared to surgical dislocation. Arthroscopic treatment of FAI needs to respect the superior epiphyseal vessels and should be able to achieve the same surgical goals as would be achieved with an open procedure (Figures 6-9 and 6-10).

### Minimally Invasive Open Anterior Approach

A less invasive open approach has been advocated by some authors[30] because of the postoperative need for nonweight-bearing and possible morbidity of a trochanteric nonunion associated with the surgical dislocation. With the majority of FAI lesions occurring in the anterior and anterosuperior region of the hip, a modified Hueter approach can be used

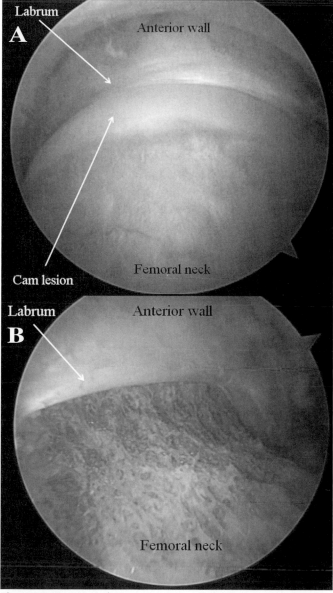

**Figure 6-10.** (A) Arthroscopic view of the head neck junction showing a mild cam deformity. (B) Arthroscopic view after osteo-chondroplasty showing the intact labrum adjacent to the femoral head/neck junction.

to address these lesions. Both a cam- or pincer-type lesion can be treated under direct visualization or with arthroscopic assistance.[30] Subluxation of the joint is also possible to treat cartilage lesions, but complete exposure of the hip joint is not possible, and this approach does not have the advantages of an arthroscopic procedure.

## CONCLUSION

FAI leads to the development of degenerative changes of the hip and has been implicated as the cause of OA in what was once considered to be idiopathic in origin. It has also been recognized to be the underlying cause of sports-related labral injuries. The diagnosis of FAI requires a complete history, a careful physical examination together, and correlating the findings with adequate radiographic imaging. Successful treatment of FAI can be achieved both with open or arthroscopic procedures with proper knowledge of the pathology and of the vascular anatomy of the proximal femur.

## REFERENCES

1. Beck M, Kalhor M, Leunig M, Ganz R. Hip morphology influences the pattern of damage to the acetabular cartilage: femoroacetabular impingement as a cause of early osteoarthritis of the hip. *J Bone Joint Surg Br.* 2005;87(7):1012-1018.
2. Beck M, Leunig M, Parvizi J, Boutier V, Wyss D, Ganz R. Anterior femoroacetabular impingement: part II. Midterm results of surgical treatment. *Clin Orthop Relat Res.* 2004;418:67-73.
3. Ganz R, Parvizi J, Beck M, Leunig M, Nötzli H, Siebenrock KA. Femoroacetabular impingement: a cause for osteoarthritis of the hip. *Clin Orthop Relat Res.* 2003;417:112-120.
4. Ito K, Minka MA II, Leunig M, Werlen S, Ganz R. Femoroacetabular impingement and the cam-effect: a MRI-based quantitative anatomical study of the femoral head-neck offset. *J Bone Joint Surg Br.* 2001;83-B:171-176.
5. Philippon MJ, Maxwell RB, Johnston TL, Schenker M, Briggs KK. Clinical presentation of femoroacetabular impingement. *Knee Surg Sports Traumatol Arthrosc.* 2007;15:1041-1047.
6. Philippon MJ, Schenker M, Briggs K, Kuppersmith D. Femoroacetabular impingement in 45 professional athletes: associated pathologies and return to sport following arthroscopic decompression. *Knee Surg Sports Traumatol Arthrosc.* 2007;15:908-914.

7. Philippon MJ, Stubbs AJ, Schenker ML, Maxwell RB, Ganz R, Leunig M. Arthroscopic management of femoroacetabular impingement: osteoplasty technique and literature review. *Am J Sports Med.* 2007;35:1571-1580.

8. Klaue K, Durnin CW, Ganz R. The acetabular rim syndrome: a clinical presentation of dysplasia of the hip. *J Bone Joint Surg Br.* 1991;73-B:423-429.

9. Byrd JWT, Jones KS. Diagnostic accuracy of clinical assessment, magnetic resonance imaging, magnetic resonance arthrography, and intra-articular injection in hip arthroscopy patients. *Am J Sports Med.* 2004;32:1668-1674.

10. Ganz R, Gill TJ, Gautier E, Krugel N, Berlemann U. Surgical dislocation of the adult hip: a technique with full access to the femoral head and acetabulum without the risk of avascular necrosis. *J Bone Joint Surg Br.* 2001;83(8):1119-1124.

11. Leunig M, Beck M, Kalhor M, Kim YJ, Werlen S, Ganz R. Fibrocystic changes at anterosuperior femoral neck: prevalence in hips with femoroacetabular impingement. *Radiology.* 2005;236:237-246.

12. Ganz R, Leunig M, Leunig-Ganz K, Harris WH. The etiology of osteoarthritis of the hip: an integrated mechanical concept. *Clin Orthop Relat Res.* 2008;466:264-272.

13. Kim YT, Azuma H. The nerve endings of the acetabular labrum. *Clin Orthop Relat Res.* 1995;320:176-181.

14. Siebenrock KA, Kalbermatten DF, Ganz R. Effect of pelvic tilt on acetabular retroversion: a study of pelves from cadavers. *Clin Orthop Relat Res.* 2003;407:241-248.

15. Jamali AA, Mladenov K, Meyer DC, et al. Anteroposterior pelvic radiographs to assess acetabular retroversion: high validity of the "Crossover-sign." *J Orthop Res.* 2007;25:758-765.

16. Meyer DC, Beck M, Ellis T, Ganz R, Leunig M. Comparison of six radiographic projects to assess femoral head/neck asphericity. *Clin Orthop Relat Res.* 2006;445:181-185.

17. Nötzli HP, Wyss TF, Stoecklin CH, Schmid MR, Treiber K, Hodler J. The contour of the femoral head-neck junction as a predictor for the risk of anterior impingement. *J Bone Joint Surg Br.* 2002;84(4):556-560.

18. Leunig M, Podeszwa D, Beck M, Werlen S, Ganz R. Magnetic resonance arthrography of labral disorders in hips with dysplasia and impingement. *Clin Orthop Relat Res.* 2004;418:74-80

19. Schmid MR, Nötzli HP, Zanetti M, Wyss TF, Hodler J. Cartilage lesions in the hip: diagnostic effectiveness of MR arthrography. *Radiology.* 2003;226:382-386.

20. Espinosa N, Rothenfluh DA, Beck M, Ganz R, Leunig M. Treatment of femoro-acetabular impingement: preliminary results of labral refixation. *J Bone Joint Surg Am.* 2006;88(5):925-935.

21. Beaulé PE, Le Duff MJ, Zaragoza E. Quality of life following femoral head-neck osteochondroplasty for femoroacetabular impingement. *J Bone Joint Surg Am.* 2007;89(4):773-779.

22. Peters CL, Erickson JA. Treatment of femoro-acetabular impingement with surgical dislocation and debridement in young adults. *J Bone Joint Surg Am.* 2006;88(8):1735-1741.

23. Gautier E, Ganz K, Krugel N, Gill TJ, Ganz R. Anatomy of the medial femoral circumflex artery and its surgical implications. *J Bone Joint Surg Br.* 2000;82(5):679-683.

24. Grose AW, Gardner MJ, Sussmann PS, Helfet DL, Lorich DG. The surgical anatomy of the blood supply to the femoral head: description of the anastomosis between the medial femoral circumflex and inferior gluteal arteries at the hip. *J Bone Joint Surg Br.* 2008;90(10):1298-1303.

25. Lavigne M, Parvizi J, Beck M, Siebenrock KA, Ganz R, Leunig M. Anterior femoroacetabular impingement: part I. Techniques of joint preserving surgery. *Clin Orthop Relat Res.* 2004;418:61-66.

26. Bare AA, Guanche CA. Hip impingement: the role of arthroscopy. *Orthopedics.* 2005;28:266-273.

27. Sampson TG. Arthroscopic treatment of femoroacetabular impingement. *Tech Orthop.* 2005;20:56-62.

28. Weiland DE, Philippon MJ. Arthroscopic technique of femoroacetabular impingement. *Oper Tech Orthop.* 2005;15:256-260.

29. Ilizaliturri VM, Orozco-Rodriguez L, Acosta-Rodriguez E, Camacho-Galindo J. Arthroscopic treatment of cam-type femoroacetabular impingement. *J Arthroplasty.* 2008;23:226-233.

30. Clohisy JC, McClure JT. Treatment of anterior femoroacetabular impingement with combined hip arthroscopy and limited anterior decompression. *Iowa Orthop J.* 2005;25:164-171.

7

# ABDUCTOR TEARS

*Asheesh Bedi, MD; RobRoy L. Martin, PhD, PT, CSCS;*
*and Bryan T. Kelly, MD*

## INTRODUCTION

Disorders of the peritrochanteric compartment of the hip, including trochanteric bursitis, external coxa saltans, and abductor tears, are common and have collectively been categorized as "greater trochanteric pain syndrome" (GTPS). While GTPS is mainly treated conservatively, open surgery has been recommended for individuals with intractable symptoms.[1-3] As surgeons are becoming increasing adept with minimally invasive techniques, arthroscopic treatment of peritrochanteric compartment disorders is becoming popular. This includes endoscopic repair of hip abductor tears.

Ranawat A, Kelly BT. *Musculoskeletal Examination of the Hip and Knee: Making the Complex Simple* (pp. 183-208).
© 2011 SLACK Incorporated

Bunker et al[4] and Kagan[3] first described tears of the gluteus medius and minimus tendons in the late 1990s. Bunker et al[4] reported a 22% incidence of concomitant medius tears in 50 patients treated for femoral neck fractures. The tears commonly occurred distally at the medius-minimus junction.[4] Kagan[3] performed an open medius tendon repair in 7 patients with recalcitrant GTPS and magnetic resonance imaging (MRI) evidence of a tear. In all cases, the tear was located anteriorly in the lateral facet portion of the insertion.[3] Additionally, Howell et al[2] reported that 22% of women and 16% of men who underwent total hip arthroplasty for osteoarthritis (n=176) had abductor tears. Generally, the incidence of abductors tears was found to increase with age and to be related to gender with approximately 25% of middle-aged women and 10% of middle-aged men developing a tear of the gluteus medius tendon.[2-5] In a recent report of 482 consecutive patients undergoing hip arthroscopy, 10 individuals (2%) were noted to have gluteus medius tears. Of these, 8 were women and 2 were men with an average age of 50 years (range: 33 to 66 years).[6] While this information provides some insight into the incidence of abductor tears, the true incidence in the athletic population has not been well-defined.

Tendinopathy and tendon tears of the gluteus medius and minimus can cause recalcitrant pain along the lateral side of the hip. Abductor involvement should be suspected in patients with intractable GTPS, particularly after conservative management fails. When the abductors are involved, pain is characteristically exacerbated by resisted hip abduction and single-limb weight-bearing on the involved extremity. Although the etiology is likely multifactorial, gluteus medius and minimus tears likely reflect a progressive degenerative process.[2,5,7] A precipitating traumatic event, such as a fall, may be noted, although many times patients describe an insidious onset.[6] The common complaint in individuals with abductor involvement consistently is debilitating lateral-sided hip pain that does not respond to corticosteroid injections, physical therapy, rest, and anti-inflammatory medication.[6] When lateral hip pain does not respond to conservative treatment, an MRI is indicated to rule out abductor tendon involvement.[7,8] Bird et al[1] used MRI to evaluate the integrity of the gluteus medius in 24 women with recalcitrant GTPS. It was noted that 46% of patients had a tear of the medius tendon insertion, while an additional 38% had gluteus medius tendonitis without an appreciable tear.[1] We find it difficult to differentiate high-grade partial tears from full-thickness abductor tears and rely on our knowledge of the anatomy of the abductor footprint on the greater trochanter.

The abductors have been likened to the "rotator cuff of the hip," with the medius and minimus being analogous to the supraspinatus and subscapularis muscles, respectively.[3,4,9] The medius tendon inserts on the lateral and posterosuperior facets, resulting in a moment arm similar in direction and force to the supraspinatus.[10] The minimus inserts on the anterior facet and can exert several different moments, including flexion, abduction, internal rotation, or external rotation, depending on the position of the femur. Based upon these observations, it follows that one of the primary functions of the minimus is to act as a femoral head stabilizer.[11] However, when the hip is flexed, the minimus provides a primary internal rotation force comparable to that of the subscapularis.[12] Similar to the rotator cuff, where supraspinatus tears are more common than tears of the subscapularis, the medius tears are more common than tears of the minimus.[13,14]

Gluteus medius tears can be characterized as interstitial, partial-thickness, or full-thickness.[4] Interstitial tears occur in parallel with the tendon fibers. Tears likely reflect a continuous spectrum of pathology with progression occurring over time. Initial medius tendon pathology probably begins as undersurface tendon degeneration, which progresses to a partial-thickness tear and finally to a full-thickness tear as it propagates posteriorly.[3,5,7,11] Most tears occur in the anterior portion of the tendon as it attaches into the lateral facet of the greater trochanter.[1]

In regard to operative treatment of medius tears, both open and arthroscopic techniques of repair can provide excellent symptomatic relief and restore abductor function. Kagan[3] performed an open medius tendon repair in 7 patients with recalcitrant GTPS and MRI evidence of a tear. At a median follow-up of 45 months, all patients were pain-free, and all but one returned to previous levels of activity.[3] Arthroscopic techniques provide a less invasive alternative and can be readily performed. However, an open repair may offer the best approach when complete avulsion of the abductor tendons from the greater trochanter with retraction present on MRI.[6]

Regardless of the technique, determining the anatomic gluteus medius footprint is critical and can often be difficult. Unlike the supraspinatus tendon, no articular margin is present to be used as a reference landmark.[5,10]

# History and Examination

Patients will typically present with a history of persistent lateral hip pain and abductor weakness despite extensive conservative measures, including physical therapy and anti-inflammatory drugs. These symptoms may be present in isolation or combination with groin pain arising from other intra-articular pathology. Patients often localize the discomfort to the lateral region of the hip overlying the greater trochanter and have variable pain to direct palpation of this region. Patients with significant abductor tears, however, will commonly have discomfort at the greater trochanter with resisted abduction. It is important to test patients in the lateral decubitus position with the knee both fully extended and flexed at 90 degrees. In the extended position, the tensor fascia lata and iliotibial band can contribute to abduction strength. Knee flexion, however, helps to isolate the abductors with resisted strength testing. It is important to note that lateral-sided discomfort from abductor injuries will not resolve with an intra-articular diagnostic injection. In contrast, however, ultrasound-guided corticosteroid injection of the trochanteric bursa can confer significant relief and confirm the diagnosis. Examine gait and one-leg standing position for both extremities to identify a Tredelenberg's sign. If the pelvis drops on the side opposite of the stance leg, it is positive and implies significant abductor insufficiency on the side of the stance leg (Table 7-1).

# Pathonatomy

The peritrochanteric space is a well-defined compartment between the greater trochanter and iliotibial band. Its borders are defined by proximal sartorius and tensor fascia lata muscles anteriorly, vastus lateralis inferomedially, anterior tendon of the gluteus maximus insertion into the iliotibial

**Table 7-1**

## METHODS FOR EXAMINING ABDUCTOR TEARS

*Examination*

*Illustration*

Complete a thorough examination of the hip in the supine position to identify concomitant intra-articular pathology of the hip, including femoroacetabular impingement, abral tears, or osteoarthritis.

Examine the abductors and peritrochanteric space in the lateral decubitus position.

Pain with direct palpation over the muscles and greater trocharter may help to confirm diagnosis if reproductive of patient's lateral-sided symptoms.

(continued)

**Table 7-1 (continued)**

## *METHODS FOR EXAMINING ABDUCTOR TEARS*

*Examination*

*Illustration*

Resisted strength testing of abduction strength
with the knee in flexion is important to isolate the
abductor muscles of the hip. Testing in full extension is confounded by contribution of the tensor
fascia lata and iliotibial band.

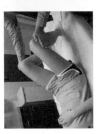 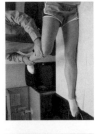

Examine gait and one leg standing position for both
extremities to identify a Tredelenberg's sign. If the
pelvis drops on the side opposite of the stance leg,
it is positive and implies significant abductor insufficiency on the side of the stance leg.

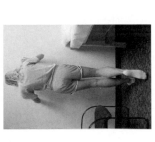

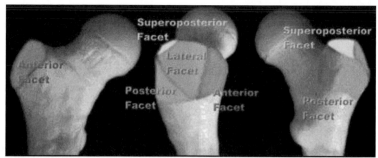

**Figure 7-1.** The 4 facets of the greater trochanter. (Reprinted from *Magn Reson Imaging Clin N Am*, 13(4), Dwek J, Pfirrmann C, Stanley A, Pathria M, Chung CB, MR imaging of the hip abductors: normal anatomy and commonly encountered pathology at the greater trochanter, pp. 691-704, copyright 2005, with permission from Elsevier.)

band distally, and the gluteus medius and minimus tendons superomedially. The trochanteric bursa is contained within the peritrochanteric space.

To assist in standardizing the MRI approach to assess for abductor tears, the greater trochanter has been divided into 4 facets: posterosuperior, lateral, anterior, and posterior (Figure 7-1).[7,8] The posterior facet (Figure 7-2) is covered by the trochanteric bursa and is the only facet without a distinct tendon insertion. The gluteus medius tendon has 2 separate entheses on the greater trochanter. The posterior fibers attach to the posterosuperior facet (PSF), whereas the central and anterior fibers insert on the lateral facet (LF) of the trochanter (Figure 7-3).[10] The tendinous portion inserting into the PSF is robust, having a circular insertion site with an approximate radius and area of 8.5 mm and 200 mm$^2$, respectively.[10] The lateral facet insertion is more rectangular in shape, with an approximate 440 mm$^2$ surface area.[10] MRI can be used to distinguish normal insertional anatomy of the medius (Figure 7-4) from tendon tears on the LFs (Figure 7-5) and PSFs (Figure 7-6).

The anatomical insertions and fiber orientation for posterior, central, and anterior gluteus medius are thought to correlate with their function.[10] The posterior gluteus medius stabilizes the femoral head in the acetabulum during heel strike while the central portion, with fibers that run more vertically, functions to initiate hip abduction.

**Figure 7-2.** Axial MRI demonstrating the posterior facet (curved, white arrow).

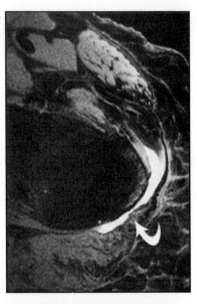

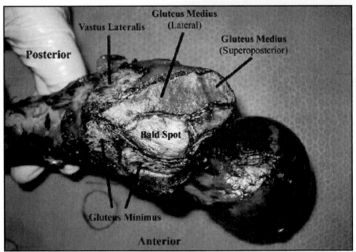

**Figure 7-3.** Cadaveric dissection of the greater trochanter demonstrating gluteus medius insertion footprints at the superoposterior (SP) and lateral facets and their relationship to the vastus tubercle and gluteus minimus insertion. Also demonstrated is the bald spot located between the insertion of the gluteus medius on the lateral facet and the insertion of the gluteus minimus on the anterior facet. (Reprinted from *Arthroscopy*, 24(2), Robertson WJ, Gardner MJ, Barker JU, Boraiah S, Lorich DG, Kelly BT, Anatomy and dimensions of the gluteus medius tendon insertion, pp. 130-136, copyright 2008, with permission from Elsevier.)

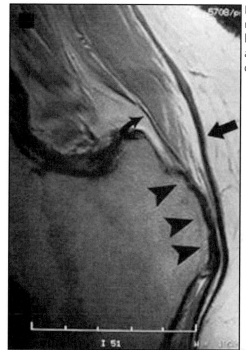

**Figure 7-4.** Normal coronal MRI demonstrating the lateral facet (arrowheads) and inserting medius tendon (arrow).

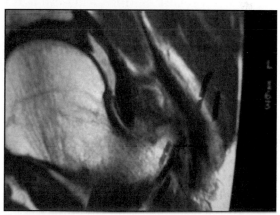

**Figure 7-5.** Coronal MRI demonstrating a partial tear of the gluteus medius tendon near its insertion on the lateral facet.

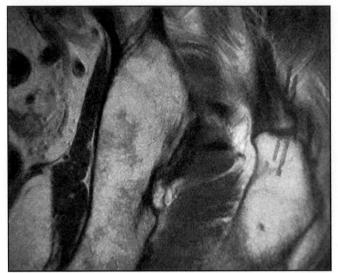

**Figure 7-6.** Coronal MRI demonstrating a partial tear of the most lateral gluteus medius tendon fibers near their insertion on the posterosuperior facet.

The anterior portion aids in abduction but also functions as a pelvic external rotator during swing-through phase of gait.[10,11]

The minimus attaches to the anterior facet (see Figure 7-3). The trochanteric insertion of the gluteus minimus is separated from the proximal portion of the LF footprint by the trochanteric bald spot. Near the midpoint of the LF footprint, the bald spot ends and the long head of the minimus begins. At this location, the medius footprint abuts and covers a portion of the gluteus minimus.[10] The trochanteric bald spot is circular in shape with a radius of approximately 11 mm. It combines with the gluteus medius to comprise the entire lateral facet of the greater trochanter.[10] It is critical not to overestimate the size of tendon detachment with an abductor tear by mistakenly incorporating the normal bald spot into the anatomic footprint of the medius tendon.[5] Similar to the gluteus medius, MR imaging can be used to distinguish normal attachment of the gluteus minimus (Figure 7-7) from a minimus tear (Figure 7-8).

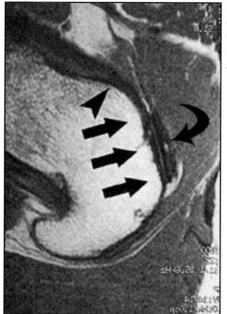

**Figure 7-7.** Axial MRI demonstrating the anterior facet (straight arrows) and inserting minimus tendon (curved arrow).

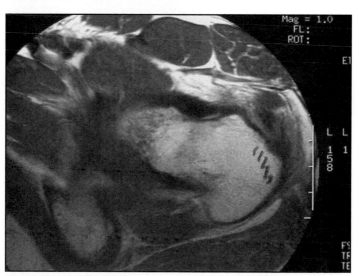

**Figure 7-8.** Axial MRI demonstrating abnormal signal characteristics in the inserting gluteus minimus tendon consistent with a high-grade partial tear.

# IMAGING

Ultrasonography or MRI can be utilized to confirm the diagnosis of abductors tears of the hip. With MRI, the studies are carefully reviewed to identify tendon discontinuity, elongation of the tendon, atrophy of gluteus medius and gluteus minimus muscles, or the presence of an area of high signal intensity superior or lateral to the greater trochanter on T2-weighted images.[15] As defined by Cvitanic et al,[15] tendon discontinuity is the distal tendon of the gluteus medius or gluteus minimus either replaced by intermediate or high signal (granulation tissue, fluid, or synovitis) or absent altogether. High signal intensity indicates the presence of fluid or bursitis near the abductor enthesis. Cvitanic showed 91% accuracy for the diagnosis of tears of the gluteus medius and gluteus minimus tendons on MRI and found that an area of T2 hyperintensity superior to the greater trochanter had the highest sensitivity and specificity for tears at 73% and 95%, respectively.[15] Ultrasonography may offer the advantage of imaging during dynamic, provocative maneuvers that elicit pain in patients. In addition, a diagnostic and/or therapeutic bursal injection may be administered at the time of ultrasonography.

# TREATMENT

Entry in the peritrochanteric space or lateral compartment typically follows routine evaluation and treatment of pathology in the central and peripheral compartment. Central compartment arthroscopy is performed in all patients who undergo peritrochanteric space endoscopy to document and treat any associated intra-articular pathology that may co-exist.

As with any arthroscopic procedure, portal placement is critical and dependent on accurate identification of the trochanter and anterior superior iliac spine (ASIS) for this procedure. We typically use 4 portals: anterior, mid-anterior, proximal anterolateral, and distal anterolateral accessory (Figure 7-9). The anterior and mid-anterior portals can afford access into the peritrochanteric space. The anterior portal is placed 1 cm lateral to the ASIS in the interval between the TFL and

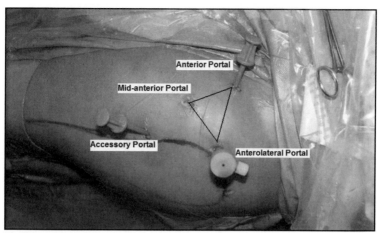

**Figure 7-9.** Portals used for peritrochanteric arthroscopy and medius tear arthroscopic repair. Note the equilateral triangular relationship between the direct anterior, mid-anterior, and anterolateral portals. The distal (accessory) portal (distal anterolateral accessory) is in line with the anterolateral portal and is placed midway between the tip of the greater trochanter and the vastus tubercle approximately 3 to 4 cm distal.

Sartorius with the proximal anterolateral portal being placed just proximal to the anterolateral tip of the greater trochanter. The mid-anterior portal is placed directly anterior to the lateral prominence of the greater trochanter at the distal point of an equilateral triangle formed using standard anterior and proximal anterolateral portals. This mid-anterior portal avoids potential injury to the proximal gluteus medius and distal vastus lateralis musculature while minimizing the risk of injuring the lateral femoral cutaneous nerve.[5] The use of fluoroscopic imaging can help confirm proper placement of the mid-anterior portal. Not only does the mid-anterior portal minimize the risk of injury to surrounding tissue, but it also offers an improved angle of approach to the peritrochanteric space when compared with the standard anterior portal.

From the mid-anterior portal, the peritrochanteric space is entered with the cannula directed in an anterior-to-posterior direction. The hip is held in 0 degrees of adduction, 10 degrees of flexion, and 15 degrees of internal rotation.[5] Traction is released prior to entry into the lateral space to relax tension on the iliotibial band. The hip can be abducted slightly if

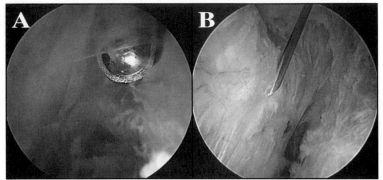

**Figure 7-10.** (A) Identifying the space between the iliotibial band and greater trochanter. (B) Once the space is developed and cleared of bursal tissue, the greater trochanter (being touched by the spinal needle) and iliotibial bands (right) can be clearly identified.

necessary to increase the space between the iliotibial band and the greater trochanter. Gentle axial load may be applied to help distinguish the muscular fibers of the gluteus medius from the overlying bursal tissue. For better access to the peritrochanteric space, the cannula is swept back and forth between the iliotibial band and trochanteric bursa, with a technique similar to that used for access into the subacromial space of the shoulder. When the appropriate plane is identified, a clear space between the iliotibial band and the greater trochanter can be easily identified (Figure 7-10A). The remaining bursal tissue present in the space can be easily removed with a motorized shaver to more clearly define the lateral (iliotibial band) and medial (greater trochanter and vastus lateralis) borders of peritrochanteric space (Figure 7-10B).

With the visualization of the camera directed distally, a distal anterolateral accessory (DALA) portal is established (see Figure 7-9). This DALA portal is approximately 4 to 5 cm directly distal to the anterolateral portal and can be located with the assistance of spinal need guidance. This portal can be used for diagnostic purposes and operative intervention as well as to provide outflow.[5] The standard proximal anterolateral portal can also be useful as a third working or viewing portal. This portal can improve distal visualization and can facilitate suture management with abductor repair.[5]

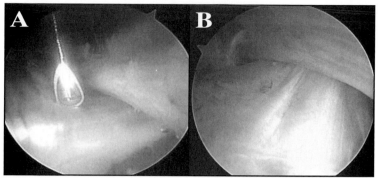

**Figure 7-11.** (A) Viewing from the anterolateral portal looking distal, the maximus tendon insertion can be cleared of tissue and serves as a distal landmark. (B) Viewing from the distal anterolateral accessory portal, the tendon insertion can be closely inspected.

Once the 4 portals are established, diagnostic arthroscopy is initiated with the 70 degree scope in the mid-anterior portal. The initial view identifies the so-called "sickle-band," or insertion of the gluteus maximus running posterior to the vastus lateralis toward the iliotibial band and posterior femur. The maximus tendon insertion can be cleared of tissue and serves as a distal landmark (Figure 7-11). This reproducible landmark should serve as a posterior stopping point as the sciatic nerve lays approximately 3 to 4 cm posterior to the maximus insertion. Instruments should not be placed posterior to the maximus insertion without direct visualization to make sure that the nerve is protected. Inspection then proceeds in a counterclockwise direction distally and posterior at the gluteus maximus insertion toward the vastus lateralis and gluteus minimus located more proximal and anterior.[5]

As the arthroscope is moved proximally, the longitudinal fibers of the vastus lateralis are identified and traced up to the vastus tubercle, immediately anterior to the lateral facet (Figure 7-12),[5] The gluteus medius tendon and muscle are best visualized at the lateral facet with the arthroscope in the proximal anterolateral portal with the light source rotated anterior and superior (Figure 7-13). Visualization of the gluteus minimus can be difficult as it is most often covered by muscle tissue of the gluteus medius. By gently sweeping away medius muscle, the tendinous insertion of the minimus onto the

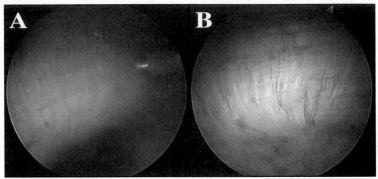

**Figure 7-12.** (A) The longitudinal fibers of the vastus lateralis identified by the arthroscope are moved proximally and traced up to the vastus tubercle (B), looking immediately anterior to the lateral facet.

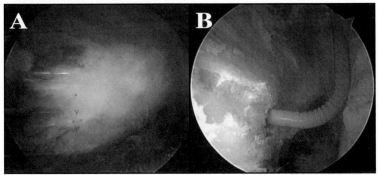

**Figure 7-13.** (A) The gluteus medius insertion onto the lateral facet with muscular fibers proximal to the tendon. (B) Probing the medius tendon insertion at the lateral and anterior facets.

anterior facet can be better identified. If fibrinous bands are noted in this area, they should be excised. Hemostasis can be obtained with either radiofrequency ablation or standard co-ablation. The fibers of the medius lie posterior to the minimus and should be carefully inspected for a tear. When evaluating the tendon insertion, the entire lateral and anterior facets should be carefully probed. A partial tear typically occurs as an undersurface injury and may be difficult to visualize directly. Correlation with the MRI is important during this inspection process.

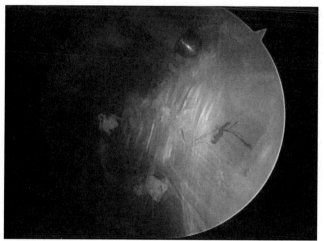

**Figure 7-14.** Arthroscopic view of the iliotibial band.

Finally, the arthroscope should be directed toward the iliotibial band (Figure 7-14). The posterior one-third of the iliotibial band may demonstrate abrasive changes if a symptomatic coxa saltans externus is present. An arthroscopic iliotibial band release can be performed at this time if necessary as previously described.[16]

The technique for assessing and repairing a full-thickness tear of the abductor tendons is similar to that described for the rotator cuff. A thorough débridement of the trochanteric bursae is performed first to decompress the compartment and improve visualization (Figures 7-15A and B). The edges of the tear should be débrided, and clear margins around the tear should be demarcated. As with the rotator cuff, an acute tear may be more amenable to repair than a chronic tear. Therefore, an assessment of reparability should be performed by assessing the mobility of the torn edge and the quality of the tissue (Figures 7-15C and D).

If the tear is repairable, the edges should be clearly identified and débrided to healthy, viable tissue. Débridement of residual tissue can be done using a motorized shaver and electrocautery (Figure 7-16A). Similarly, the anatomic footprint on the lateral facet should be clear of soft tissue debris and decorticated to bleeding, cancellous bone with a burr (Figure 7-16B).

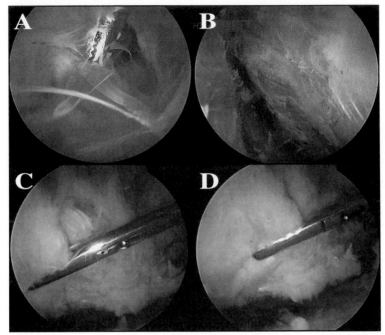

**Figure 7-15.** (A) Thickened bursa impairing visualization and inspection of the medius tendon. (B) Visualization after the bursa is excised with the assistance of a motorized shaver. (C) A full-thickness tear with retraction of the medius tendon is appreciated. (D) The tear edges need to be clearly demarcated, and the mobility of the tendon edge is tested.

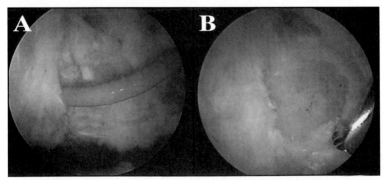

**Figure 7-16.** (A) The tear footprint prepared for arthroscopic repair by electrocautery. (B) The bed débrided to bleeding, cancellous bone in preparation for anchor insertion.

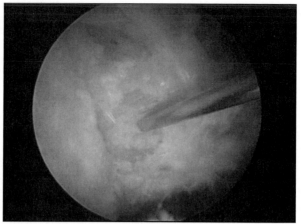

**Figure 7-17.** The ideal trajectory for anchor insertion is determined using percutaneous insertion of a spinal needle.

Suture anchors are then placed into the footprint using standard arthroscopic technique, typically through a small stab incision. A spinal needle or curved snap can be used to determine the ideal location and trajectory for anchor insertion. The location for anchor insertion can be confirmed with fluoroscopy. Placement of the anchor should be done under direct arthroscopic visualization. The ideal trajectory of anchor insertion is determined using percutaneous insertion of a spinal needle (Figure 7-17). Once the anchor is in place, its location and angle of insertion should be checked using fluoroscopy (Figure 7-18). Typically, 2 anchors will be sufficient to repair the anatomic footprint of the medius tendon from the lateral facet. Adequate spacing of the anchors should allow for good bone stock between anchors (Figure 7-19). Metallic anchors are frequently used to repair gluteus medius tears because of the good bone quality of the trochanter.

After anchors are placed, the sutures are passed sequentially through the free tendon edge using a suture-passing device (Figure 7-20). Typically, the free edges of the tendon can be captured with a needle-penetrating device entering from the distal anterolateral accessory portal with the suture being entered from the mid-anterior portal. The second limb of the suture can

**Figure 7-18.** Anchor position along the facet can be confirmed with intraoperative fluoroscopy.

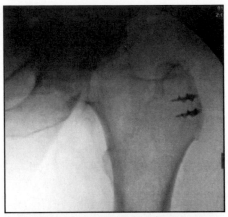

**Figure 7-19.** Two anchors have been placed in the lateral facet, each loaded with 2 sutures.

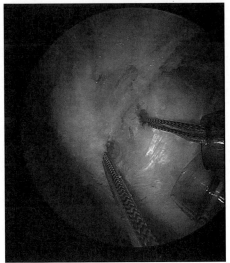

be passed through the more distal fibers bordering on the edge of the vastus ridge using a standard suture-penetrating device. Careful suture management needs to be exercised to avoid their entanglement and the entrapment of overlying soft tissue. Once the sutures have been passed and separated, sequential tying is performed using a standard arthroscopic knot-tying technique. Careful and complete evaluation of the tendon repair should be performed to confirm anatomic restoration of the tendon footprint and security of the repair.

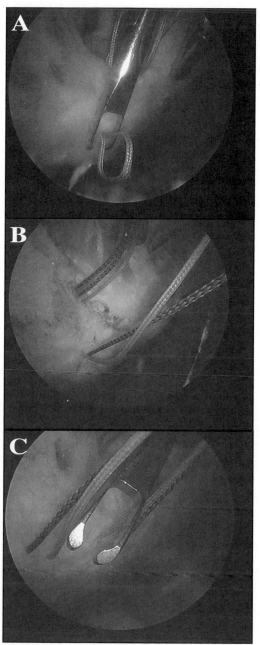

**Figure 7-20.** After the free edge of the tear is mobilized, a suture-passing device is used to grasp the retracted tendon edge.

Undersurface, partial-thickness tears in the anterior medius tendon should be carefully assessed. If they are high-grade lesions, they may be converted into full-thickness tears with a full-radius shaver and repaired using the technique as described above. A trans-tendon repair is also an option to avoid completion of the tear. However, anchor placement and suture passage may be more difficult in these cases as visualization is impaired by the intact tendon.

## POSTOPERATIVE REHABILITATION

Postoperative rehabilitation can be divided into 3 phases: 1) Maximum protection (immediately postoperatively to 4 to 6 weeks postoperatively); 2) moderate protection (from 6 to 12 weeks postoperatively); and 3) minimal protection (from 12 to 24 weeks postoperatively). The goal during the maximal protection phase is to allow the repair to heal without introducing any harmful stresses. Therefore, active hip abduction and internal rotation as well as passive hip adduction and external rotation are not permitted. Additionally, hip flexion is limited to 90 degrees. A lateral hinged hip abduction brace is used for 6 weeks postoperatively to allow hip flexion and extension for normal gait while preventing abduction and adduction movements. Additionally, to help protect the repair, weight-bearing is limited to 20 pounds. During this maximum protection phase, range of motion within the previously described limits is encouraged. Therefore, use of a continuous passive motion (CPM) device 4 hours per day and low resistance stationary biking 20 minutes per day are included as part of rehabilitation. Passive hip abduction, extension, external rotation, and hip flexion less than 90 degrees is also included as part of treatment in this phase. Once the portals are healed, scar massage can be initiated. At 2 weeks postoperatively, isometric hip extension, adduction, external rotation, quadriceps, and hamstrings exercise are initiated. For individuals with significantly weak knee extension, neuromuscular electrical stimulation for the quadriceps can be included.

The moderate protection phase continues from 6 to 12 weeks postoperatively with goals of normalizing range of motion and increasing strength. Exercises for the trunk and entire lower extremity, including hip, are added and progressed as tolerated. This includes initiating sub-maximal isometric hip flexion, abduction, and internal rotation. During the next 4 weeks, strengthening exercises are progressed from isometric to isotonic as symptoms allow. Caution should be used when progressive hip abduction strengthening exercises use pain complaints as a limiting factor. At 6 to 8 weeks post-operatively, weight-bearing status is progressed from partial weight-bearing to weight-bearing as tolerated. The patient can be weaned from crutches and can discontinue their use once the patient has more than 3/5 strength and is able to ambulate without gait deviation. By 10 weeks postoperatively, the patient should be independent in a comprehensive trunk and lower extremity strengthening program. Criteria to progress from this phase include normal hip range of motion and 4/5 hip abduction strength.

The minimal protection phase continues from 12 weeks postoperatively to 24 weeks postoperatively with goals of normalizing strength and returning to previous level of activity. A progression of functional activities can begin and progress as tolerated. In addition to the activity being pain-free, progression is also dependent on the patient being able to complete the activities with adequate pelvic stability (ie, no Trendelenburg). At this point, the patient should be pain-free and should have quadriceps and hamstring peak torque strength within 15% of the contralateral extremity on isokinetic testing. Running can usually be initiated at around 16 weeks postoperatively, once hip abduction strength is symmetrical. Furthermore, by 24 weeks, the patient should demonstrate a normal step-down test and score at least 85% or greater on the single-leg cross-over triple hop for distance.

## OUTCOMES

Voos and colleagues recently reviewed the short-term clinical outcomes of endoscopic gluteus medius tendon tear repairs performed by Dr. Bryan T. Kelly.[6] Of 482 consecutive hip arthroscopies, 10 patients had gluteus medius tendon tears that were repaired endoscopically. There were 8 female and 2 male patients, with a mean age of 50 years. All 10 patients experienced persistent lateral hip discomfort and abductor weakness and failed nonoperative intervention. At the time of endoscopic tendon repair, 5 patients (50%) had full-thickness and 5 had high-grade partial-thickness tears that were converted to complete tears. At 2 years follow-up (average: 25 months), all patients were doing well and reported complete resolution of pain. Objectively, hip abduction strength with manual muscle testing was 5/5 with Modified Harris Hip Scores and Hip Outcomes Scores that averaged 94 and 93, respectively.[6]

## CONCLUSION

Tendinopathy and tendon tears of the gluteus medius and minimus can cause of recalcitrant pain along the lateral side of the hip. This chapter outlined the anatomy and function of the gluteus medius and minimus as well the diagnostic process used to identify those with abductor tears. Surgical techniques to endoscopically evaluate and treat those with abductor tears, along with the corresponding rehabilitation program, were also described. Table 7-2 outlines "Helpful Hints" discussed in this chapter for diagnosing and surgically treating individuals with abductor tears.

## REFERENCES

1. Bird PA, Oakley SP, Shnier R, Kirkham BW. Prospective evaluation of magnetic resonance imaging and physical examination findings in patients with greater trochanteric pain syndrome. *Arthritis Rheum.* 2001;44(9):2138-2145.
2. Howell GE, Biggs RE, Bourne RB. Prevalence of abductor mechanism tears of the hips in patients with osteoarthritis. *J Arthroplasty.* 2001;16(1):121-123.
3. Kagan A 2nd. Rotator cuff tears of the hip. *Clin Orthop Relat Res.* 1999;368:135-140.
4. Bunker TD, Esler CN, Leach WJ. Rotator-cuff tear of the hip. *J Bone Joint Surg Br.* 1997;79(4):618-620.
5. Voos JE, Rudzki JR, Shindle MK, Martin H, Kelly BT. Arthroscopic anatomy and surgical techniques for peritrochanteric space disorders in the hip. *Arthroscopy.* 2007;23(11):1246e1-5.
6. Voos JE, Shindle MK, Pruett A, Asnis PD, Kelly BT. Endoscopic repair of gluteus medius tendon tears of the hip. *Am J Sports Med.* 2009;37(4):743-747.

**Table 7-2**

# HELPFUL HINTS

## Diagnosis

- Lateral-sided hip pain and weakness with abduction is the hallmark of the diagnosis of abductor tears of the hip.
- Testing of abduction strength with the knee in flexion is important to isolate the abductor muscles of the hip.
- MRI is >90% sensitive to confirm the diagnosis, with increased T2-signal superior to the greater trochanter demonstrating a high sensitivity and specificity of abductor injury.
- Sonographic-guided injection of the trochanteric bursa can help to confirm the diagnosis and confer transient relief of symptoms.

## Surgical Treatment

- Initial entry into the peritrochanteric space should be performed using the mid-anterior portal. Fluoroscopy should be used to confirm that placement of the portal overlies the lateral prominence of the greater trochanter to avoid injury to the gluteus medius proximally and the vastus lateralis distally.
- Use of both the anterior and mid-anterior portals can risk injury to the lateral femoral cutaneous nerve. After the skin incision is made, blunt dissection down the portal tract will help minimize injury to this neurovascular structure.
- Fluid extravasation into the thigh must be monitored throughout the case as there is the potential for fluid accumulation distally. Fluid pressure should be minimized throughout the case as much as is feasible to allow for adequate visualization.
- Extra-long cannulas should be used to make sure that the surrounding soft-tissue structures are protected throughout the procedure. Typically, cannulas need to be between 90 and 110 mm in length.
- Postoperative adhesions can be minimized through the use of the CPM machine for the first 4 to 6 weeks.
- Early failure of the abductor repair can be minimized by cautious progression through the postoperative rehab protocol.

7. Dwek J, Pfirrmann C, Stanley A, Pathria M, Chung CB. MR imaging of the hip abductors: normal anatomy and commonly encountered pathology at the greater trochanter. *Magn Reson Imaging Clin N Am.* 2005;13(4):691-704, vii.

8. Pfirrmann CW, Chung CB, Theumann NH, Trudell DJ, Resnick D. Greater trochanter of the hip: attachment of the abductor mechanism and a complex of three bursae—MR imaging and MR bursography in cadavers and MR imaging in asymptomatic volunteers. *Radiology.* 2001;221(2):469-477.

9. LaBan MM, Weir SK, Taylor RS. "Bald trochanter" spontaneous rupture of the conjoined tendons of the gluteus medius and minimus presenting as a trochanteric bursitis. *Am J Phys Med Rehabil.* 2004;83(10):806-809.

10. Robertson WJ, Gardner MJ, Barker JU, Boraiah S, Lorich DG, Kelly BT. Anatomy and dimensions of the gluteus medius tendon insertion. *Arthroscopy.* 2008;24(2):130-136.

11. Gottschalk F, Kourosh S, Leveau B. The functional anatomy of tensor fasciae latae and gluteus medius and minimus. *J Anat.* 1989;166:179-189.

12. Beck M, Sledge JB, Gautier E, Dora CF, Ganz R. The anatomy and function of the gluteus minimus muscle. *J Bone Joint Surg Br.* 2000;82(3):358-363.

13. Connell DA, Bass C, Sykes CA, Young D, Edwards E. Sonographic evaluation of gluteus medius and minimus tendinopathy. *Eur Radiol.* 2003;13(6):1339-1347.

14. Kingzett-Taylor A, Tirman PF, Feller J, et al. Tendinosis and tears of gluteus medius and minimus muscles as a cause of hip pain: MR imaging findings. *AJR Am J Roentgenol.* 1999;173(4):1123-1126.

15. Cvitanic O, Henzie G, Skezas N, Lyons J, Minter J. MRI diagnosis of tears of the hip abductor tendons (gluteus medius and gluteus minimus). *Am J Roentgenol.* 2004;182(1):137-143.

16. Craig RA, Jones DP, Oakley AP, Dunbar JD. Iliotibial band Z-lengthening for refractory trochanteric bursitis (greater trochanteric pain syndrome). *ANZ J Surg.* 2007;77(11):996-998.

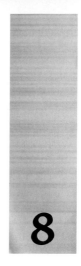

**8**

# CARTILAGE INJURIES

*Ryan G. Miyamoto, MD and Marc J. Philippon, MD*

## INTRODUCTION

The treatment of articular cartilage injuries in the hip continues to draw increasing interest as the ability to treat these injuries has improved during the past few decades. They are frequently associated with such pathologies as labral tears, loose bodies, femoroacetabular impingement, and hip dysplasia. Conditions such as hip instability and dislocation, femoral head osteonecrosis, slipped capital femoral epiphysis, and degenerative joint disease can also predispose a patient to have significant chondral damage about the hip. Osteochondral defects of the hip may be acute, chronic, or degenerative and may be partial thickness or full thickness.

Ranawat A, Kelly BT. *Musculoskeletal Examination of the Hip and Knee: Making the Complex Simple* (pp. 209-224). © 2011 SLACK Incorporated

In general, chondral injuries will not spontaneously heal either in acute, chronic, or degenerative conditions.[1] These cartilage injuries, which were previously treated with nonoperative measures or arthroplasty options, can now frequently be addressed with arthroscopic techniques in the appropriate setting.

# HISTORY

The patient's history provides much of the information necessary to diagnose intra-articular hip pathology. The onset of pain and exacerbating and alleviating symptoms should be identified. Patients with femoroacetabular impingement will often state they have groin pain with prolonged sitting or with activities that require hip flexion and internal rotation, such as skiing. A history of mechanical symptoms, such as clicking, locking, or catching, are common with labral pathology or with a loose body that often occurs in conjunction with osteochondral defects. The location of pain, character, frequency, and radiation should be determined. True hip pain is located within the groin region and is often referred to the knee. Occasionally, pain will be present only within the knee, and therefore every patient with unexplained knee pain should have a thorough evaluation of the hip. Pain in the low back, posterior aspect of the hip, thigh, or buttock pain that radiates distally may be related to a lumbar spine disorder.

A thorough medical and surgical history should also be obtained. Any history of previous brace use as a child, suggesting developmental dysplasia of the hip, should raise the examiner's suspicion for a degenerative hip process. A history of lower extremity trauma and the treatment rendered should be recorded. Current and previous sports participation can clue the examiner in to possible sources of pathology. Elite athletes are more likely to develop labral tears and chondral injuries. Those who participate in martial arts, soccer, rugby, or long distance running have a higher incidence of degenerative changes in the hip. Medically, patients should be screened for malignancy, coagulopathies, collagen disorders, inflammatory diseases, vascular disorders, alcohol abuse, and steroid treatment. The patient should also be asked about any medications or previous intra-articular injections used to treat his or her hip pain. Last, a detailed history of previous hip surgery should be obtained.

## EXAMINATION

Examination of the hip should start with inspection of both gait and the position of the hip at rest. An antalgic or Trendelenburg gait can suggest an intra-articular process or weakness of the muscles surrounding the hip joint. Synovitis or a hip effusion can often manifest itself as a hip positioned in a flexed, abducted, and externally rotated position, where the hip joint achieves the maximal capsular volume. The lumbar spine should be carefully evaluated with a full motor, reflex, and sensory exam of the lower extremities along with a straight leg-raise test to rule out spinal pathology. The presence of scoliosis and any leg length discrepancies should be documented as well.

The focused hip examination should be performed on both the symptomatic and asymptomatic hip. The examination begins with palpation of all bony prominences and documentation of range of motion (ROM). The pubic symphysis, greater trochanter, and ischial tuberosity should be examined for tenderness. Muscles prone to overuse and spasm such as the hip adductors, abductors, and iliopsoas should be palpated and stretched to examine for contractures and pain. ROM should be tested, including flexion, extension, abduction, adduction, internal rotation, and external rotation. Ranges in both the supine and prone positions should be recorded. Discrepancies between the symptomatic and asymptomatic hip may highlight potential areas of pathology. A patient with increased hip pain and decreased ROM with passive flexion and internal rotation may have avascular necrosis of the femoral head. Additionally, the FABER (flexion, abduction, external rotation) test can be used to assess guarding and limitation secondary to pain and inflammation of the hip capsule and surrounding musculature. Both anterior and posterior impingement tests should be performed to rule out associated pathology. During ROM testing, any clicking, catching, or popping is noted. While chondral injuries are frequently associated with mechanical symptoms, there is no specific exam maneuver for chondral injuries.

If an inflammatory process is suspected, laboratory studies should include HLA-B27 titers, C-reactive protein, erythrocyte sedimentation rate, rheumatoid factor, and an antinuclear antibody titer.

## PATHOANATOMY

Classically, chondral defects in the hip are related to trauma or to chronic progressive joint degeneration as seen in osteoarthritis and rheumatoid arthritis. The "lateral impact injury" mechanism occurs subsequent to a direct blow to the greater trochanter, which, because of its subcutaneous location, has a poor ability to absorb large forces. The energy imparted on this area is thus transferred to the joint surface, causing cartilage injury to the femoral head and acetabulum. This injury mechanism is prevalent in young active males who sustain impact loading during sports or activity. Arthroscopic findings by Byrd support this mechanism.[2]

There are a variety of other conditions that can also cause chondral lesions in the hip. The relationship between femoroacetabular impingment and chondral damage has been described in Chapter 6. McCarthy and Lee have described the most common location of acetabular cartilage lesions as the anterior quadrant (59%) in a series of 457 hip arthroscopies, and these frequently occurred with concomitant labral tears.[3] The superior quadrant was involved in 24% and the posterior acetabulum in 25% of chondral injuries. Advanced lesions (Grade III and Grade IV) were involved in the anterior acetabulum 70% of the time, 36% in the posterior acetabulum, and 27% in the superior acetabulum. They also noted that the extent of chondral damage had the most direct relationship to surgical outcomes. Acetabular cysts are frequently associated with chondral injuries as are labral separations from the articular surface at the chondro-labral junction.[4]

Avascular necrosis (AVN) of the hip is a problematic entity that results from compromised blood flow to the femoral head for a multitude of reasons. Necrosis of osteocytes can occur with decreased vascular flow, and this is followed by localized bony resorption and subsequent collapse of unsupported articular cartilage.[5]

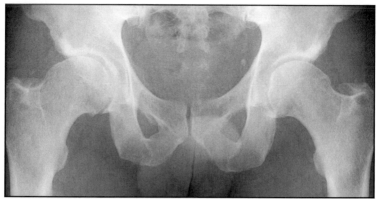

**Figure 8-1.** AP pelvis radiograph.

# IMAGING

Imaging studies should begin with plain radiographs of the pelvis and cross-table frog-leg lateral of the affected hip to evaluate for degenerative changes, dysplasia, bony lesions, calcified loose bodies, and impingement (Figure 8-1). Ultrasound can be used to check for an effusion or dynamic instability, and bone scan should be used if malignancy is suspected. Computed tomography can be performed to further evaluate bony structure; however, the cartilage surface and surrounding soft tissues are better evaluated with magnetic resonance imaging (MRI; Figure 8-2 and Table 8-1). Osteonecrosis, early degenerative changes, and soft tissue pathology are best detected with MRI.[4,6,7] The evaluation of osteochondral defects by MRI is somewhat limited, particularly with a low-resolution magnet. When compared with hip arthroscopy, Sekiya and colleagues showed that MRI is inadequate at evaluating the articular cartilage.[8] They recommended direct visualization or arthroscopy for accurate staging of cartilage lesions, especially in the late stages of osteonecrosis. One new technique currently being explored to evaluate cartilage lesions is MRI with traction applied. This technique, particularly in combination with a high-resolution magnet, appears to have promising early results.

**Figure 8-2.** MRI of chondral surface and soft tissues, demonstrating a labral tear.

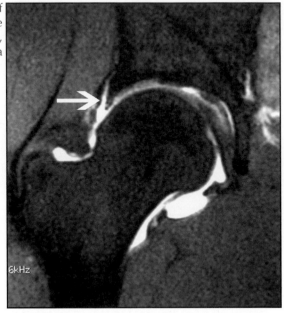

## Table 8-1

## METHODS FOR EXAMINING CHONDRAL DEFECTS IN THE HIP

| Exam | Results |
|------|---------|
| Radiographs | Show degenerative joint disease |
| | Identify bony lesions |
| | Show dysplastic changes |
| | Provide alpha angle measurement that correlates to size of chondral damage |
| | Show presence of loose bodies |
| | Shows rim fracture |
| | Identify bony defects |
| | |
| MRI | Identify chondral defects |
| | New protocols can identify the health of cartilage |
| | Radiologist dependent |

MRI arthrogram uses gadolinium injected intra-articularly to distend the capsule and allow for better visualization of articular cartilage and labral tears. Keeney and co-workers compared MRI arthrograms with articular cartilage findings on hip arthroscopy and noted correlation only 62.7% of the time.[9] This study reported that MRI arthrogram had a sensitivity of 47%, specificity of 89%, positive predictive value of 84%, and negative predictive value of 59%. While this may be an improvement in visualization of cartilage lesions over non-arthrogram MRIs, the high false negative rate limits its use in ruling out chondral defects.[7,9]

# TREATMENT

## Conservative (Nonarthroscopic)

The initial treatment of chondral lesions of the hip frequently includes the use of anti-inflammatory medications, intra-articular injections, as well as physical therapy. Physical therapy should focus on maintaining hip ROM as well as stretching and strengthening the musculature around the hip and core.

Arthroscopic contraindications to treat chondral injuries also include advanced osteoarthritic changes or ankylosis, which would preclude manipulation of arthroscopic instruments. Additionally, the presence of infection, superficial or deep, is a contraindication to arthroscopic intervention. Patients with advanced degenerative changes with deformation of the proximal femur and acetabulum may be better served with arthroplasty options.

## Surgical Treatment—Chondral Lesions (Arthroscopic)

The indications for surgical treatment of an osteochondral defect of the hip are similar to that of the knee. Shaving chondroplasty is used for the treatment of partial-thickness lesions and for débridement of partial-thickness chondral flaps that may cause mechanical symptoms (Figure 8-3). The lesion is first trimmed with a motorized shaver to smooth the surface, and then a gliding radiofrequency probe is used to further contour the cartilage surface.

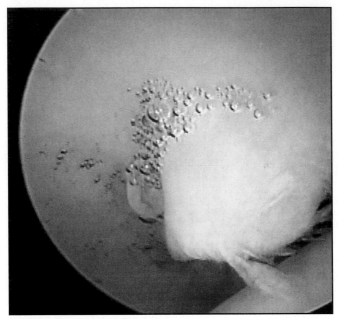

**Figure 8-3.** Chondral flap.

Microfracture can be used for focal and contained lesions less than 4 cm in size (Figure 8-4 and Table 8-2). Steadman and colleagues have noted improved responses to microfracture of full-thickness lesions less than 400 mm$^2$ versus larger lesions.[10] The defect should be full thickness in character and have a surrounding rim of stable full-thickness cartilage. Indications for microfracture also include full-thickness cartilage loss in weight-bearing areas and unstable chondral flaps overlying intact subchondral bone. Patients with degenerative joint disease may be candidates if there are focal chondral defects and the patient's age and activity level do not warrant arthroplasty options.

After identifying a lesion amenable to microfracture, the size and depth of the lesion is noted. The bed of the lesion is then prepared using a motorized shaver to remove any soft tissue debris and unstable cartilage neighboring the full-thickness lesion. A curette or motorized burr is used to remove the calcified cartilage layer and expose but not penetrate the subchondral plate.[11,12] A ring curette is then used

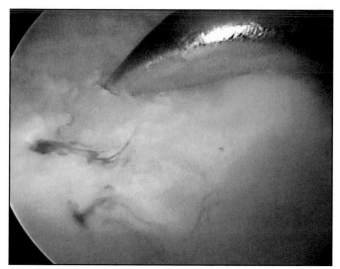

**Figure 8-4.** Micro-fracture technique using awl to induce punctate bleeding on the surface of the cartilage.

## Table 8-2

## *HELPFUL HINTS*

### *Indications*

- Good borders to contain clot
- Typically size less than 4cm
- Stable surrounding cartilage
- Intact subchondral bone

### *Contra-indications*

- Degenerative lesions with thin surrounding cartilage
- Lesions larger than 4 cm in most cases
- Unstable surrounding cartilage
- Bony defects associated with chondral lesions
- Patient's inability or unwillingness to comply with postoperative protocol

to create a perpendicular rim of normal cartilage around the periphery of the lesion. Arthroscopic awls are then used to create multiple holes in the lesion bed, initially at the periphery and then in the center of the lesion. The holes should be 3 to 4 mm apart and 2 to 4 mm deep. Place as many holes as possible without them collapsing into one another. The femoral side cartilage is typically thinner than on the acetabular side; therefore, the creation of a perpendicular rim is crucial to stabilize the clot formed. After the microfracture process is completed, the pump pressure is decreased in order to verify the efflux of blood and marrow elements into the defect.

Only a few small series have been published regarding the outcomes of arthroscopically treated chondral defects in the hip. Philippon and colleagues reviewed 9 cases of acetabular chondral defects treated with microfracture and evaluated with revision arthroscopy.[13] The average percentage fill of those defects was 91% with 8 of 9 patients having 95% to 100% coverage. Each of those 8 patients had a Grade 1 or 2 appearance of cartilage at an average of 20 months of follow-up. The patient with only 25% coverage and a Grade 4 appearance of the lesion had diffuse osteoarthritis.

Byrd and Jones published a prospective evaluation of 38 hip arthroscopies with a modified Harris hip score at 2 years post-operatively.[14] Of the 38 patients, 15 had a diagnosis of chondral injuries. Those patients had a median improvement of 18 points while the complete cohort had a median improvement of 28 points. The type of treatment rendered for the chondral defects was not detailed. Byrd also evaluated 9 patients with an inverted acetabular labrum, of which 3 underwent microfracture. At 2-year follow up, those 3 patients were the only ones in the cohort to return to high-level athletic activities, including martial arts, horseback riding, and fitness activities.[15]

Microfracture is contraindicated in partial-thickness defects and chondral defects associated with bony lesions. Additionally, patients who are likely to be noncompliant with postoperative rehabilitation protocols or those unable to use crutches or bear weight on the contralateral extremity are not good candidates for microfracture. It is also contraindicated in patients with immune-mediated diseases or systemic disease-induced arthritis or cartilage injury.[4,10,16]

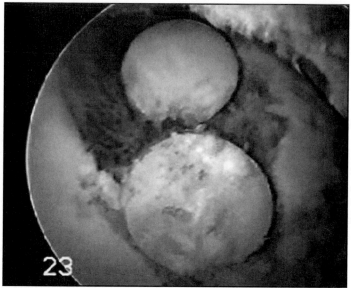

**Figure 8-5.** Mosaicplasty demonstrating chondral plugs transplanted from donor site to areas of large chondral defects.

Larger lesions within the weight-bearing surface of either the acetabulum or femoral head may be treated successfully with mosaicplasty (Figure 8-5). We consider mosaicplasty in cases of large (>400 mm²) defects with a healthy donor bed within the nonweight-bearing chondral surface of the femoral head. In the case of a contained osseous defect associated with a cartilage lesion, mosaicplasty may be the best option.

For mosaicplasty, the lesion is defined with a full radius shaver, and a healthy cartilaginous rim is defined. The lesion is measured to determine the size and number of osteochondral plugs needed. The osteochondral plugs can be harvested from the peripheral nonweight-bearing zone of the femoral head anteriorly. This area of cartilage is often removed with removal of a cam lesion in FAI. The appropriate size plugs are harvested from the donor site, and the recipient bed is prepared with the appropriate size drill inserted to the appropriate depth (approximately 12 mm in the femoral head). The plugs are then inserted into the recipient bed using a press-fit technique. Bone harvested from the recipient bed is then placed into the donor bed to fill the defect created. In the event that full coverage of the osteochondral defect is not obtained by the plugs, the exposed subchondral bone is microfractured using the technique described above. The use of mosaic-plasty in the hip has only been described in the form of a case report.[17] In this report, an open technique was used to treat a large osteochondral defect in the femoral head with a good result at 6 months of follow-up.

Autologous chondrocyte implantation may be considered for larger lesions without bony deficiency; however, we have no experience with this technique in the hip. The technique requires separate harvesting and implantation procedures and is performed in the open fashion in the knee. In the future, this technique may be a useful alternative to the treatment of chondral defects in the hip.

Frequently, full-thickness cartilage defects are found in the peripheral portion of the acetabulum, particularly in a patient with pincer, cam, or mixed-type femoroacetabular impingement. A delamination of this peripheral cartilage can manifest itself as a wave sign upon arthroscopic inspection.[18] In these instances, a resection of the delaminated cartilage and trimming the eburnated rim of bone back to a healthy region can be performed. First, the labrum is elevated from the damaged articular surface, and a shaver is used to débride soft tissue from the acetabular rim. An arthroscopic burr is then used to trim the rim back to a healthy osteochondral junction. After the rim trimming is complete, the labrum is reattached to the healthy osteocartilaginous rim. This technique can be employed in patients with a center edge angle greater than 25 degrees without creating a dysplastic or unstable hip.

The initial postoperative management of the above procedures is the similar. Patients can be discharged home the same day or stay overnight for maximum pain control. Cold therapy is initiated in the recovery room. A continuous passive motion (CPM) machine is used for all patients. For those undergoing abrasion chondroplasty or peripheral rim trimming, CPM is used for 2 weeks. For patients undergoing microfracture or mosaicplasty, CPM is used for 6 to 8 weeks. Crutch-assisted touchdown weight-bearing is used for 2 weeks for patients after abrasion chondroplasty or peripheral rim trimming and is used for 6 to 8 weeks for patients after microfracture or mosaicplasty. Patients are allowed full weight-bearing after 8 weeks. Physical therapy begins immediately and focuses on early motion with strength emphasized later in the rehabilitative protocol. Passive ROM commences in the early stages advancing to active assisted ROM and active ROM to regain hip internal rotation and extension. A stationary bike can be used immediately without resistance. After 4 to 6 months of rehabilitation and after full ROM, strength, and functional agility have been restored, patients are permitted to gradually return to high-impact activities.[4,10]

## Surgical Treatment—AVN (Arthroscopic)

The use of hip arthroscopy for the treatment of AVN has helped to accurately classify patients with late-stage disease as well as function as an adjunct to open techniques, such as core decompression and vascularized or nonvascularized bone grafting[19] (Figure 8-6). Crucial to the treatment of AVN is to accurately stage the disease process. Sekiya and colleagues have described an arthroscopic staging system for AVN in addition to the previous staging systems described by Ficat as well as Steinberg and associates.[8,20,21]

After thorough inspection of the femoral head from all portals, an arthroscopically directed core decompression can be performed in isolation or augmented with graft material or autologous bone marrow cells in a retrograde fashion.[22,23] Additionally, Sekiya and Wojtys have described a mini open technique through a modified Smith-Peterson approach that allows for both arthroscopic examination as well as a rapid transition to open procedures.[24] Distraction of the hip is facilitated with the limited dissection, allowing an improved operative window for manipulation about the joint.

## CONCLUSION

Correct diagnosis and treatment of chondral injuries of the hip relies on a thorough history and physical as well as appropriate imaging. The surgeon has multiple options for the arthroscopic treatment of osteochondral lesions in the hip including abrasion chondroplasty, peripheral rim trimming,

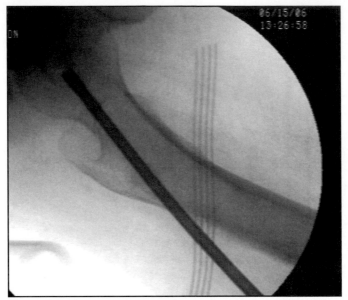

**Figure 8-6.** Fluoroscopic view of core decompression for AVN.

microfracture, and mosaicplasty. For partial-thickness defects in the acetabulum or on the femoral head, abrasion chondroplasty is appropriate. Peripheral rim trimming is appropriate for peripheral full-thickness defects in the region of the acetabular rim. Full-thickness defects located in other weight-bearing portions of the articular cartilage can be treated with microfracture or mosaicplasty depending on the size of the lesion and bone quality. The use of ACI in the hip has not been used by our group, but there is potential for its benefit. Microfracture and mosaicplasty have been shown to be effective methods to treat osteochondral defects in the knee; however, their long-term benefit in the hip has yet to be demonstrated.

## REFERENCES

1. Buckwalter JA. Articular cartilage: injuries and potential for healing. *J Orthop Sports Phys Ther.* 1998;28:192-202.
2. Byrd JW. Lateral impact injury: a source of occult hip pathology. *Clin Sports Med.* 2001;20(4):801-815.

3. McCarthy JC, Lee JA. Arthroscopic intervention in early hip disease. *Clin Orthop Relat Res.* 2004;429:157-162.

4. McCarthy JC. The diagnosis and treatment of labral and chondral injuries. *AAOS Instructional Course Lectures.* 2004;53:573-577.

5. Mont MA, Hungerford DS. Non-traumatic avascular necrosis of the femoral head. *J Bone Joint Surg Am.* 1995;77:459-474.

6. DeAngelis NA, Busconi BD. Assessment and differential diagnosis of the painful hip. *Clin Orthop Relat Res.* 2003;406:11-18.

7. Newberg AH, Newman JS. Imaging the painful hip. *Clin Orthop Relat Res.* 2003;406:19-28.

8. Sekiya JK, Ruch DS, Hunter DM, et al. Hip arthroscopy in staging avascular necrosis of the femoral head. *J South Orthop Assoc.* 2000;9(4):254-261.

9. Keeney JA, Peelle MW, Jackson J, Rubin D, Maloney WJ, Clohisy JC. Magnetic resonance arthrography versus arthroscopy in the evaluation of articular hip pathology. *Clin Orthop Relat Res.* 2004;429:163-169.

10. Steadman JR, Briggs KK, Rodrigo JJ, Kocher MS, Gill TJ, Rodkey WG. Outcomes of microfracture for traumatic chondral defects of the knee: average 11-year follow-up. *Arthroscopy.* 2003;19(5):477-484.

11. Steadman JR, Rodkey WG, Rodrigo JJ. Microfracture: surgical technique and rehabilitation to treat chondral defects. *Clin Orthop Relat Res.* 2001;391 Suppl:S362-S369.

12. Steadman JR, Rodkey WG, Briggs KK. Microfracture to treat full-thickness chondral defects: surgical technique, rehabilitation, and outcomes. *J Knee Surg.* 2002;15(3):170-176.

13. Philippon MJ, Schenker ML, Briggs KK, Maxwell RB. Can microfracture produce repair tissue in acetabular chondral defects? *Arthroscopy.* 2008;24(1):46-50.

14. Byrd JWT, Jones KS. Prospective analysis of hip arthroscopy with 2-year follow-up. *Arthroscopy.* 2000;16(6):578-587.

15. Byrd JWT, Jones KS. Osteoarthritis caused by an inverted acetabular labrum: radiographic diagnosis and arthroscopic treatment. *Arthroscopy.* 2002;18:741-747.

16. Steadman JR, Miller BS, Karas SG, Schlegel TF, Briggs KK, Hawkins RJ. The microfracture technique in the treatment of full-thickness chondral lesions of the knee in national football league players. *J Knee Surg.* 2003;16(2):83-86.

17. Hart R, Janecek M, Visna P, Bucek P, Kocis J. Mosaicplasty for the treatment of femoral head defect after incorrect resorbable screw insertion. *Arthroscopy.* 2003;19(10):E1-E5.

18. Philippon MJ, Schenker ML. Arthroscopy for the treatment of femoroacetabular impingement in the athlete. *Clin Sports Med.* 2006;25(2):299-308, ix.

19. Rockwood JH, Whiddon DR, Sekiya JK. Arthroscopic management of avascular necrosis. *Oper Tech Orthop.* 2005;15:273-279.

20. Ficat RP. Idiopathic bone necrosis of the femoral head: early diagnosis and treatment. *J Bone Joint Surg Br.* 1985;67:3-9.

21. Steinberg ME, Hayken GD, Steinberg DR. A quantitative system for staging avascular necrosis. *J Bone Joint Surg Br.* 1995;77:34-41.

22. Ruch D, Satterfield W. The use of arthroscopy to document accurate position of core decompression of the hip. *Arthroscopy*. 1998;14:617-619.
23. Gangi V, Hauzeur JP, Matos C. Treatment of osteonecrosis of the femoral head with implantation of autologous bone-marrow cells—a pilot study. *J Bone Joint Surg Am*. 2004;86:1153-1160.
24. Sekiya JK, Wojtys EM, Loder RT, Hensinger RN. Hip arthroscopy using a limited anterior exposure: an alternative approach for arthroscopic access. *Arthroscopy*. 2000;16(1):16-20.

# 9

# SNAPPING HIP SYNDROMES

*Victor M. Ilizaliturri Jr, MD*

## INTRODUCTION

The snapping hip syndromes are conditions of diverse origin that are grouped in a single "family" because they present a snapping phenomenon around the hip joint. Allen and Cope[1] classified them as 3 different types: 1) external snapping hip syndrome; 2) internal snapping hip syndrome; and 3) intra-articular snapping hip syndrome. The third type, intra-articular snapping hip syndrome, is no longer referred to as a snapping hip syndrome because diagnosis of intra-articular hip pathology is now more specific and precise.[2]

The internal and external snapping hip syndromes are more frequent in women and usually present between the ages

Ranawat A, Kelly BT. *Musculoskeletal Examination of the Hip and Knee: Making the Complex Simple* (pp. 225-251).
© 2011 SLACK Incorporated

of 15 and 40 years. An increased incidence in ballet dancers has been reported.[3]

Even though these conditions share a common "family" name, they have very different etiologies that should be clearly identified to establish an adequate treatment, both conservative and surgical.

A detailed and specific clinical history and specific clinical tests are necessary for accurate diagnosis of both conditions.

Because the snapping hip syndromes may be associated with other hip pathology, a complete examination of the hip joint is always necessary, including a precise assessment of gait, range of motion, impingement tests, etc.

Low back symptoms should always be assessed as well as the inguinal area. Inguinal hernias may mislead the examiner to think symptoms are originated by the hip joint. It is also important to remember that hip pathology may co-exist with some of these conditions, including sports hernias.

Our protocol of specific examination techniques for the external and internal snapping hip syndromes is presented next (Table 9-1).

# HISTORY

## External Snapping Hip Syndrome

The external snapping hip syndrome is produced by the posterior iliotibial band snapping over the posterior aspect of the greater trochanter.[1] Clinical presentation of this phenomenon is typical in 2 different forms. The first clinical form is the "hip dislocator." The patient usually refers to the ability to dislocate the hip joint, which is usually not related to pain. This is always reproducible, and patients often volunteer to demonstrate it by standing with bilateral weight-bearing while doing a tilting and rotating motion of the pelvis with lateral displacement of the affected side. The snapping phenomenon can be visible or palpable around the area of the greater trochanter. As mentioned, this phenomenon occurs without pain and usually does not interfere with the performance of sporting activities or activities of daily living. Stretching exercises of the iliotibial band may be indicated to treat this condition.

# Table 9-1

## HELPFUL HINTS

| Type of Snapping Hip | Origin of Snapping | Typical Patient Complaint |
|---|---|---|
| Internal snapping hip | Iliopsoas tendon snapping over the iliopectineal eminence and in some cases the femoral head. May be associated with femoroacetabular impingement | Snapping phenomenon present at the front of the groin while extending the hip from a flexed position of more than 90 degrees<br><br>The phenomenon is voluntary, the patient may volunteer to reproduce it, it is not visible through the skin, it may be audible, and it may be palpated at the groin area |
| External snapping hip | The posterior aspect of the iliotibial band over the posterior margin of the greater trochanter | Two clinical forms:<br><br>1) The "hip dislocator"; the phenomenon is usually reproduced while the patient is standing. A combination of pelvic tilting and rotation will reproduce the snapping. This form is usually not painful. The snapping is not reproduced by passive motion<br><br>2) Snapping present with flexion and extension. The posterior iliotibial band "dislocates" over the posterior margin of the greater trochanter with flexion and "relocates" during extension. This is usually associated with pain and tenderness behind the tip of the greater trochanter. The patients often volunteer to reproduce this phenomenon actively and it may also be reproduced with passive motion |
| Intra-articular snapping hip | Intra-articular pathology, loose bodies, labral tears, condral flaps | This is more related to unvoluntary mechanical hip symptoms like catching and locking. The term intra articular snapping hip is no longer in use because we are now more precise in the diagnosis of intra-articular hip pathology |

The second clinical form is a "true" external snapping hip, characterized by a snapping phenomenon at the area of the greater trochanter that occurs while flexing and extending the hip. Patients often complain of the snapping occurring during stair climbing, exercising, or while sitting or standing from a chair. The phenomenon is frequently associated with pain and tenderness around the greater trochanter.[4]

## Internal Snapping Hip Syndrome

The internal snapping hip syndrome is produced by the iliopsoas tendon snapping over the iliopectineal eminence or the femoral head.[1] In the case of the internal snapping hip syndrome, patients feel the snapping phenomenon at the groin. The snapping may be a normal occurrence (without pain) in 5% to 10% of the general population.[2] In symptomatic patients, there is always pain related to the snapping phenomenon. In general, the snapping phenomenon is voluntary and reproducible by extending the hip from a position of flexion of more than 90 degrees. The patients complain of snapping during activities of daily living that involve flexion and extension, like climbing stairs or moving into or out of a sitting position. The snapping may also be present during sporting activity.

## EXAMINATION

## External Snapping Hip Syndrome

Our clinical assessment of the patient starts by evaluating the gait pattern. A Trendelenburg gait may be related to gluteus medius or gluteus minimus tendonosis or tears associated with or not associated with the external snapping hip syndrome (especially in chronic cases). After gait assessment, a formal Trendelenburg test is performed.[5] Next, we proceed to the decubitus evaluation of the patient. At this time, leg length is clinically evaluated along with any differences in the relaxed posture of both lower limbs. Increased external rotation is commonly found and may be associated with hip instability, increased anteversion, or other skeletal deformities of the proximal femur. Our routine evaluation of range of motion, the iliopsoas tendon, and impingement tests is performed.

Specific assessment of the iliotibial band is better per-formed in the lateral decubitus position. We start by evaluat-ing the strength of the hip abductors by performing a straight lateral rise of the lower extremity. The patient should be able to sustain the elevation of the lower limb against force applied by the examiner. If the limb drops to the table or if there is pain while performing the test, tendonosis or a hip abduc-tor tear should be suspected. Incapacity to perform a straight leg raise should warn the examiner about the possibility of a massive hip abductor tear. Pain may also indicate the pres-ence of trochanteric bursitis. Ober's test[6] is very sensitive to detect tightness of the iliotibial band. It is performed in the lateral decubitus position with the examined leg on the upper side. The contralateral leg is supported by the examining table in slight flexion of the hip and knee joints to increase the patient's stability and decrease lumbar lordosis. The tested leg is abducted, and the knee is flexed 90 degrees. The lower limb is allowed to fall into adduction on the examining table. If the examined leg does not fall down, the test is positive for ilio-tibial band contracture. After the Ober's test, we always evalu-ate the snapping phenomenon. Even though many patients are able to demonstrate the snapping in the standing position by actively flexing and extending the hip, the best way to evaluate it is in the lateral decubitus position. With the affected hip on the upper side, the patient is asked to actively reproduce the snapping phenomenon by flexing and extending the hip. Next, the snapping is reproduced by passive motion, as described previously. Many times, it is a visible phenomenon on the greater trochanteric area, but in some cases, it may be detected by palpation of the greater trochanteric area with the fully extended hand. Tenderness frequently corresponds to the area of the snapping phenomenon, just posterior to the posterior aspect of the greater trochanter. A FABER test[7] may produce an uncomfortable feeling of tension behind the greater tro-chanter. This can also be reproduced by performing a FABER test in a sitting position.

## Internal Snapping Hip Syndrome

As it is the case with the external snapping hip syndrome, the internal snapping hip syndrome may be associated with diverse intra-articular pathology. A complete examination of the hip joint should be performed.

Specific iliopsoas evaluation starts by examining flexion contractures with the patient supine. The Thomas test[6] is the most sensitive test to detect a flexion contracture. A straight leg raise with and without resistance by the examiner should always be performed. Incapacity for leg raising or associated pain may be related to iliopsoas tendonosis. The snapping phenomenon is better evaluated with the patient supine. It is reproduced by bringing the hip to extension from a flexion position of more than 90 degrees. The snapping occurs at the groin, and it is usually not visible. It is frequently audible or referred by the patient when it is reproduced by the examiner. The patient may also volunteer to reproduce the snapping phenomenon by performing flexion to extension actively. The snapping phenomenon may be accentuated by starting with the hip in a flexed position of more than 90 degrees adding external rotation and abduction. As the hip is brought to extension, it is also abducted and internally rotated. The snapping phenomenon may be palpated by placing the examiner's hand over the groin of the affected side while performing the examining maneuver.

Adductor tendonitis may confuse the examiner and is a differential diagnosis for iliopsoas tendonitis. It is important to detect whether pain is originated at the adductor tendons. An adduction against resistance test is a useful tool to evaluate this. It is also important to look for tenderness at the adductor tendons and around the pubic region (Table 9-2).

## PATHOANATOMY

In the case of the external snapping hip syndrome, the problem is originated by tightness of the iliotibial band. This generates the snapping phenomenon as the hip is flexed or extended when the iliotibial band translates anteriorly and posteriorly over the greater trochanter. A chronic case may be associated with greater trochanteric bursitis and/or tears of the gluteus medius or minimus tendons.[1,4]

**Table 9-2**

## METHODS FOR EXAMINING THE SNAPPING HIP

| Examination | Technique | Illustration | Grading | Significance |
|---|---|---|---|---|
| Hip abductor strength<br>Trendelenburg<br><br>Fatigue Trendelenburg | Active; patient single limb stand | 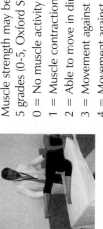 | Positive when pelvis falls to the unsupported limb side<br><br>Fatigue Trendelenburg, single limb standing over measured time periods (10, 15, and 20 seconds). Comparative, positive is pelvis falls over time | Hip abductor muscle insufficiency may be secondary to intrinsic abductor muscle pathology or superior gluteal nerve injury |
| Hip abductor strength<br>Straight leg rise (Lateral) | Active; against resistance from examiner; straight leg raise in lateral decubitus | | Muscle strength may be evaluated in 5 grades (0-5, Oxford Scale)<br>0 = No muscle activity<br>1 = Muscle contraction; no movement<br>2 = Able to move in direction of gravity<br>3 = Movement against gravity<br>4 = Movement against resistance<br>5 = Movement against full resistance | Evaluation of strength of hip abductor muscles |

*(continued)*

**Table 9-2 (continued)**

## METHODS FOR EXAMINING THE SNAPPING HIP

| Examination | Technique | Illustration | Grading | Significance |
|---|---|---|---|---|
| Tightness of iliotibial band | Passive; the patient does a lateral raise of the lower limb while in lateral decubitus, the knee is flexed while the hip is abducted and the patient is told to stop abducting, the flexed knee should fall over the opposite knee when negative. If the hip remains abducted, it suggests tightness of the iliotibial band | 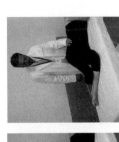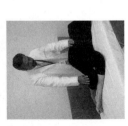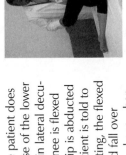 | | Evaluates tension of the iliotibial band |
| Ober's test | | | | |

(continued)

**Table 9-2 (continued)**

## METHODS FOR EXAMINING THE SNAPPING HIP

| Examination | Technique | Illustration | Grading | Significance |
|---|---|---|---|---|
| Tightness of iliotibial band<br><br>Reproduction of snapping phenomenon | Passive in lateral decubitus; the snapping may be observed under the skin at the area of the greater trochanter or in some cases palpated by positioning the extended palm over the trochanteric region | 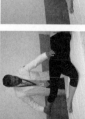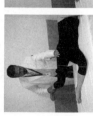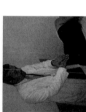 | | Evaluates tension of the iliotibial band and the presence of snapping |
| Pain in the trochanteric region | Passive; palpation of the trochanteric region looking for tenderness | | | May be related with abductor muscle pathology and greater trochanteric bursistis |

*(continued)*

**Table 9-2 (continued)**

## METHODS FOR EXAMINING THE SNAPPING HIP

| Examination | Technique | Illustration | Grading | Significance |
|---|---|---|---|---|
| FABER (flexion, abduction, and external rotation) test | Passive; hip is brought to flexion, abduction, and external rotation, the distance from the examining table to the knee is measured and compared to the test in contralateral side | 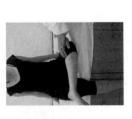 | Differences in the distance between the knee and examining table may be measured | May indicate intra-articular hip pathology<br><br>Iliotibial band tightness<br><br>Pathology of the Sacroiliac joint (when pain is referred to sacroiliac joint) |
| FABER modified | Passive; same as the FABER test but performed with the patient in a sitting position. The examiner applies a down force on the knee of the examined side | | | May reproduce pain or the feeling of tightness behind the greater trochanter<br><br>Iliotibial band tightness |

*(continued)*

**Table 9-2 (continued)**

## METHODS FOR EXAMINING THE SNAPPING HIP

| Examination | Technique | Illustration | Grading | Significance |
|---|---|---|---|---|
| Thomas test Flexion contracture | Passive; the Thomas test is performed to detect flexion contracture of the hip. The patient lies supine and flexes the opposite hip to full flexion (more than 90 degrees). The examiner looks for "lifting" of the examined hip from the table. The test can also be performed with the knee flexed, hanging the leg over the edge of the table | 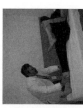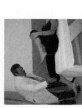 | | Flexion contracture of the hip |
| Supine leg raise | Active; the test is performed first against gravity and then against resistance from the examiner | 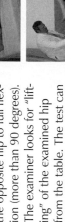 | 0-5, Oxford Scale<br>0 = No muscle activity<br>1 = Muscle contraction; no movement<br>2 = Able to move in direction of gravity<br>3 = Movement against gravity<br>4 = Movement against resistance<br>5 = Movement against full resistance | Examination of hip flexion strength |

(continued)

**Table 9-2 (continued)**

## METHODS FOR EXAMINING THE SNAPPING HIP

| Examination | Technique | Illustration | Grading | Significance |
|---|---|---|---|---|
| Reproduction of internal snapping hip phenomenon | Passive; the test is performed with the patient supine. The hip is flexed more than 90 degrees with abduction and external rotation. To reproduce the snapping phenomenon, it is then brought to extension, neutral abduction, and rotation. The snapping occurs while going from flexion to extension. The snapping may be referred by the patient or may be audible. The examiner may palpate the snapping by placing a hand on the groin while performing the test | 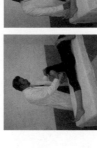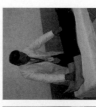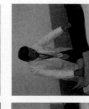 | | The presence of the snapping phenomenon means there is hypertension in the iliopsoas tendon |

*(continued)*

**Table 9-2 (continued)**

## METHODS FOR EXAMINING THE SNAPPING HIP

| Examination | Technique | Illustration | Grading | Significance |
|---|---|---|---|---|
| Adduction against resistance | Active; with the patient supine the hips and knees are flexed as the feet are put together, the patient is asked to abduct and then to adduct against resistance from the examiner | | 0-5, Oxford Scale<br>0 = No muscle activity<br>1 = Muscle contraction; no movement<br>2 = Able to move in direction of gravity<br>3 = Movement against gravity<br>4 = Movement against resistance<br>5 = Movement against full resistance | Examination of hip abduction strength |

In the case of the external snapping hip syndrome, it has been traditionally described that the snapping phenomenon is produced by the iliopsoas tendon snapping over the iliopectineal eminence of the pelvis.[1] More recently, it has been hypothesized that an acetabular overcoverage and a prominence of the femoral head-neck junction secondary to impingement may also contribute to the problem by increasing the bone volume under the iliopsoas tendon as it passes anterior to the hip joint.[2]

# IMAGING

## External Snapping Hip Syndrome

Diagnosing external snapping hip syndrome is mainly clinical, but imaging studies are important to look for associated hip joint pathology, to evaluate the hip abductors, and to confirm the diagnosis (Table 9-3).

### Simple Radiographs

Radiologic evaluation of the external snapping hip syndrome should always include an anteroposterior view of the pelvis and a lateral view of the affected hip. We use the frog-leg lateral view. Both of these radiographic projections serve as screening tools for intra-articular pathology or abnormalities of the bony anatomy of the hip joint that may co-exist with the external snapping hip syndrome. The greater trochanter should always be carefully inspected, looking for osteophytes or calcifications around it.

### Dynamic Ultrasound

It is possible to detect the snapping phenomenon using dynamic ultrasound.[8,9] The best way to reproduce the snapping phenomenon in the case of the external snapping hip is with the patient in the lateral decubitus position, as described in the physical examination section of this chapter. The ultrasound transducer is positioned over the area of snapping to detect this phenomenon. A transverse orientation of the transducer is usually the best way to detect it (Figure 9-1). It is possible to detect tendon pathology using ultrasound, but the method is very dependent on the observer's experience.

# Table 9-3

## IMAGING

| Image | Pertinent Image Views | Findings |
|---|---|---|
| Simple x-rays | AP pelvis, lateral views (frog leg, cross table, Dunn view, etc) | Effective screening for osteoarthritis (the presence of osteoarthritis may contraindicate any form of hip preserving surgery) |
| | | Diagnosis of femoroacetabular impingement deformities |
| | | Other skeletal pathology such as stress fractures, tumors, etc |
| Ultrasound scan | Dynamic ultrasound | May detect the presence of the snapping phenomenon, both internal and external. May detect abductor pathology such as tears. It is operator dependant |
| Magnetic resonance imaging (MRI) | Axial, coronal | Very sensitive to detect abductor muscle problems and hip pathology such as avascular necrosis, stress fractures, tumors, etc. Ideal if abductor muscle pathology is suspected in association with external snapping hips |
| Arthro-magnetic resonance imaging (MRA) | Axial, coronal, radial | Better sensitivity than MRI in diagnosing intra-articular pathology such as labral tears, chondral flaps, and ligamentum teres pathology. Very useful in the case of internal snapping hip because more than half of the cases are associated with intra-articular pathology |

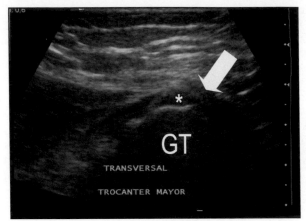

**Figure 9-1.** Photograph obtained from a dynamic ultrasound study of a right hip. In this image, the patient had hip flexion of more than 90 degrees and produced the snapping phenomenon. The transducer is in a transversal position. The greater trochanter (GT) is indicated. The white arrow points to the iliotibial band. The greater trochanteric bursa (*) is observed under the iliotibial band presenting increased fluid content.

## *Magnetic Resonance Imaging*

Magnetic resonance imaging (MRI) is the best method to detect hip abductor muscle tears, tendonitis, and greater trochanteric bursitis (Figure 9-2).[10,11] When our physical examination suggests there is hip abductor muscle pathology, we always perform an MRI study.

# Internal Snapping Hip Syndrome

Clinical diagnosis of internal snapping hip syndrome is less evident than it is for external snapping hip syndrome.

A detailed clinical history and physical exam are very reliable and can greatly contribute to the adequate diagnosis of internal snapping hip syndrome. Simple radiographs are always important, and it is essential to have a good-quality anteroposterior pelvis and a hip lateral radiograph. Our preference is the frog-leg lateral because it is reproducible by almost every x-ray technician. Abnormalities of the bony anatomy of the hip joint or the presence of hip osteoarthritis are easy to detect with simple radiographs.

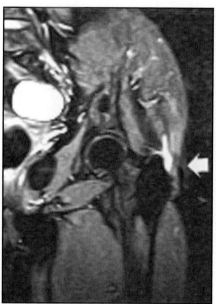

**Figure 9-2.** MRI of a left hip in a coronal plane, short tau inversion recovery (STIR) sequence. The white arrow points to a complete rupture of the gluteus medius from its insertion at the greater trochanter with retraction of muscle fibers. Fluid is observed at the insertion site of the gluteus medius. (Reprinted with permission from Dr. Isabel Ramirez-Mora.)

Iliopsoas bursography has been used to assist in the diagnosis of internal snapping hip syndrome. If the iliopsoas tendon is observed using radiographic contrast, the snapping phenomenon may be detected in fluoroscopy. This method requires a precise technique for infiltrating the iliopsoas bursa, and the radiologist performing the examination should be able to use the maneuver to reproduce the snapping within the constraint of the C-arm from the image intensifier. One should also consider that this is an invasive technique.

The snapping phenomenon may also be detected with dynamic ultrasound. The ultrasonographer should also know the maneuver that reproduces the snapping and be able to detect the snapping tendon using the ultrasound transducer.

Because internal snapping hip syndrome is very frequently associated with intra-articular hip pathology, our preference is to use magnetic resonance arthrography (MRA) to assist in precise diagnosis of intra-articular problems. It is impossible to detect the snapping phenomenon using MRA, but some findings related to iliopsoas tendonitis or bursitis may be occasionally reported (Figure 9-3).

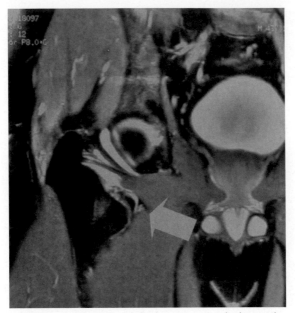

**Figure 9-3.** MRA of a right hip in coronal plane. The gray arrow points to the insertion of the iliopsoas tendon on the lesser trochanter. There is hyperintensity on the lesser trochanter compatible with bone edema, associated with heterogeneous signal of the insertion of the iliopsoas tendon, probably because of partial avulsion. Contrast is observed in the iliopsoas bursa from a communication with the hip capsule. (Reprinted with permission from Dr. Isabel Ramirez-Mora.)

# TREATMENT

There is more peer-review literature regarding treatment for the internal snapping hip syndrome, both open and endoscopic variants. Treatment is initially conservative with physical therapy, nonsteroidal anti-inflammatory therapy and corticosteroid injections. If there is no positive response to conservative treatment, surgical treatment is indicated.[4]

Traditionally, open surgical release or lengthening of the iliopsoas tendon has been the standard procedure for the symptomatic internal snapping hip syndrome.[12-15] Recently, successful endoscopic iliopsoas tendon release has been reported in the literature.[2,16-18] Results of endoscopic release of the iliopsoas tendon for internal snapping hip syndrome compare well with results reported for open release or open lengthening techniques (Table 9-4).

Endoscopic iliopsoas release is always performed in conjunction with hip arthroscopy. It has been demonstrated that almost half of the patients with internal snapping hip syndrome present associated intra-articular pathology.[2,16,17] Endoscopic release can be performed accessing the iliopsoas bursa through an anterior hip capsulotomy. The capsulotomy may be performed at different levels:

- From the central compartment[19] with the hip under traction at the level of the separation between the femoral head and the acetabulum (separation produced by traction). A cut is performed at the anterior hip capsule, immediately anterior to the anterior labrum between geographic zones 1 and 2 or 3 o'clock in a right hip,[20] the iliopsoas tendon is found in close relationship with the hip capsule at the most anterior aspect of the capsulotomy. The tendon is identified and released with a radiofrequency hook in a retrograde fashion. The iliacus muscle is left intact behind the tendon (Figure 9-4).

- Through the anterior hip capsule from the hip periphery, the hip without traction at the level of the inferior femoral head. A communication between the hip capsule and the iliopsoas bursa is established by doing an anterior hip capsulotomy between the anterior labrum and zona orbicularis. This provides access from the hip capsule into the iliopsoas bursa. The iliopsoas tendon is identified at this level and released (a radiofrequency hook is frequently used) leaving the iliacus muscle intact behind it (Figure 9-5).[18,21]

An alternative technique is to release the tendon from its insertion at the level of the lesser trochanter. Only the tendinous portion is released, leaving some muscle fibers intact. Access is gained through accessory portals that are directed to the psoas bursa by aiming to the area above the lesser trochanter navigating with an image intensifier. The procedure is done without traction and with hip external rotation to further expose the lesser trochanter at the image intensifier. A radiofrequency hook is frequently used to perform the release (Figure 9-6).[2,16,17]

**Table 9-4**

## RESULTS OF SURGICAL TREATMENT OF INTERNAL SNAPPING HIP SYNDROME (OPEN AND ENDOSCOPIC)

| Author | Number of Hips | Technique | Follow-up | Pain | Re-snapping |
|---|---|---|---|---|---|
| Taylor[13] | 17 | Open release | 17 months | 0 | 5 cases |
| Jacobson[12] | 20 | Open Z-plasty | 20 months | 2 cases (re-operated) | 6 cases |
| Dobbs[14] | 11 | Open Z-plasty | 4 years | 0 | 1 case |
| Gruen[15] | 11 | Open Z-plasty | 3 years | 0 | 0 |
| Byrd[2] | 9 | Endoscopic release at lesser trochanter | 20 months | 0 | 0 |
| Ilizaliturri[16] | 7 | Endoscopic release at lesser trochanter | 21 months | 0 | 0 |
| Wettstein[18] | 9 | Endoscopic release (preserving iliacus muscle) trans-capsular | 3 months (Technique report) | 0 | 0 |
| Flanum[17] | 6 | Endoscopic release at lesser trochanter | 1 year | 0 | 0 |
| Contreras[19] | 7 | Endoscopic release, capsulotomy from central compartment (hip with traction) | 2 years | 0 | 0 |

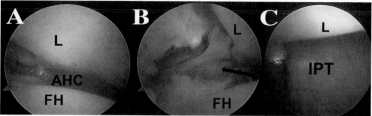

**Figure 9-4.** Arthroscopic series of photographs demonstrating transcapsular release of the iliopsoas tendon from the central compartment in a left hip (the hip is with traction). (A) A radiofrequency hook is used to perform a cut on the anterior hip capsule (AHC), parallel to the free margin of the anterior labrum (L). The femoral head is at the bottom. (B) A shaver is used to remove capsular tissue from around the iliopsoas tendon (black arrow). The anterior labrum (L) is at the top, the femoral head (FH) is at the bottom. (C) Once the capsule has been removed, the iliopsoas tendon (IPT) is clearly visible and ready for release with a radiofrequency hook. The labrum (L) is at the top.

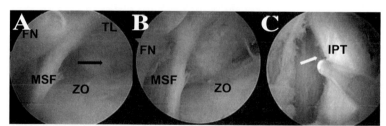

**Figure 9-5.** Sequence of arthroscopic photographs demonstrating a transcapsular iliopsoas tendon release from the peripheral compartment in a right hip (the hip is without traction). (A) The black arrow demonstrates the site of the capsulotomy on the anterior inferior hip capsule. Behind this area, the iliopsoas tendon will be located. The femoral neck (FN) is at the top left, the medial synovial fold (MSF) is at the center and the zona orbicularis (ZO) is at the bottom of the photograph. (B) An arthroscopic knife is used to perform the capsulotomy. The relation of the cut with the femoral neck (FN), medial synovial fold (MSF), and zona orbicularis (ZO) is demonstrated. (C) Once the capsulotomy has been performed, a radiofrequency hook is used to cut the iliopsoas tendon (IPT) in a retrograde fashion. The white arrow points to the iliacus muscle behind the iliopsoas tendon (IPT). This muscle is preserved intact.

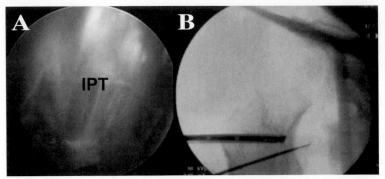

**Figure 9-6.** The photographs demonstrate a release of the iliopsoas tendon at its insertion on the lesser trochanter (bursoscopic release). (A) Endoscopic view of the iliopsoas tendon (IPT) at its insertion on the lesser trochanter. (B) Fluoroscopy photograph demonstrating the arthroscope and the radiofrequency hook probe in position for release of the iliopsoas tendon on the lesser trochanter.

Treatment for the external snapping hip syndrome is also conservative initially. If there is no positive response, surgical release is indicated. Open surgical release and lengthening techniques have been described in the literature.[22-25] More recently, endoscopic techniques have been introduced. To date, the only results that have been published of endoscopic treatment of the external snapping hip is our own series.[4] Our original report included 11 hips treated for external snapping hip syndrome using an endoscopic technique consisting in creating a diamond shaped window on the iliotibial band, allowing the greater trochanter to freely rotate within the window. At an average follow-up of 25 months, all of the patients were free of pain and one presented mild re-snapping that was treated successfully with further physical therapy. These results compare well with those of open surgical techniques utilized for this pathology (Table 9-5).

The diamond shape release of the iliotibial band was initially used to treat the external snapping hip syndrome. More recently, we have used the technique to provide access to the peritrochanteric space. The release itself is used to relieve pressure from the iliotibial band over the area of the greater trochanter. The resulting defect on the iliotibial band provides access to the greater traochanteric bursa. After resection of the

**Table 9-5**

## RESULTS OF SURGICAL TREATMENT OF EXTERNAL SNAPPING HIP SYNDROME (OPEN AND ENDOSCOPIC)

| Author | Number of Hips | Technique | Follow-up | Pain | Re-snapping |
|--------|----------------|-----------|-----------|------|-------------|
| Fery[22] | 35 | Open, cruss-cut and inverted flap suture | 7 years | 21 cases | 10 cases |
| Faraj[23] | 11 | Open Z-plasty | 1 year | 3 cases | 0 |
| Provencher[24] | 9 | Open Z-plasty | 22 months | 1 case | 0 |
| White[25] | 17 | Open vertical incision and multiple transverse cuts | 32.5 months | 0 | 2 cases (re-operated) |
| Ilizaliturri[4] | 11 | Diamond shape defect | 25 months | 0 | 1 case, improved with physical therapy |

bursa, the gluteus medius tendon is accessible for inspection. Internal rotation will provide access to the area of the short external rotators. Next we describe the surgical technique.

We position the patient lateral similar to the setup for total hip replacement. Surgical drapes most allow for free range of motion of the lower extremity to reproduce the snapping phenomenon during surgery. No traction is necessary to access the greater trochanteric bursa and the iliotibial band. The greater trochanter is marked on the skin using a skin marker as it is the main landmark for portal establishment. We utilize 2 portals—a proximal trochanteric and distal trochanteric. The area of snapping should be between both portals and is also marked on the skin. We start by infiltrating the space under the iliotibial band with 40 to 50 cc of saline.

Next the inferior trochanteric portal is established using a standard arthroscopic cannula that is introduced under the skin and directed proximally to the site of the superior trochanteric portal using the blunt obturator to develop a working space above the iliotibial band. The site of the proximal trocanteric portal is identified arthroscopically using a needle inserted at the portal landmark. The skin incision is made and a shaver is introduced to dissect subcutaneous tissue from the iliotibial band situated between the portals. Hemostasia is performed in this step to allow clear visualization of the iliotibial band. Then, a radiofrequency hook probe is introduced from the proximal trocanteric portal and a 4 to 5 cm vertical retrograde cut is performed on the iliotibial band starting at the level of the inferior trochanteric portal, which is the viewing portal. The pump pressure should be kept low while working on the subcutaneous space to avoid complications with the skin. Once the vertical cut on the iliotibial band is complete, the pump pressure can be increased and a transverse anterior cut of 2 cm in length is performed starting at the middle of the vertical cut. The resulting superior and inferior anterior flaps are resected using a shaver, developing a triangular defect on the anterior iliotibial band that will provide access to the posterior iliotibial band. Next, a transverse posterior cut is started at the same level of the transverse anterior cut. This is the most important release and should be carried out until the snapping phenomenon is solved. Finally, the superior and inferior posterior flaps are resected, which results in a diamond shape defect on the iliotibial band. The greater trochanter will rotate freely within the defect without snapping. The greater trochanteric bursa should be removed through the defect on the iliotibial band and the abductor tendons inspected for tears (Figure 9-7).

When hip arthroscopy is also necessary, we start with the patient positioned lateral and perform arthroscopy of the central and peripheral compartment of the hip. After hip arthroscopy is complete, the foot is released from the traction device and the endoscopic iliotibial band release is performed as described.

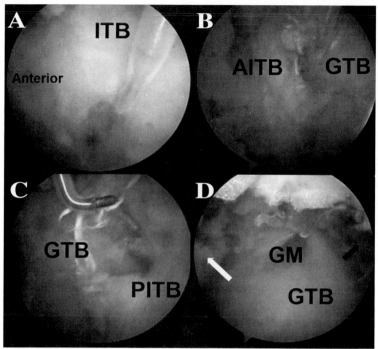

**Figure 9-7.** The sequence demonstrates endoscopic iliotibial band release in a right hip. (A) A vertical cut is performed on the iliotibial band (ITB). The arthroscope is in the inferior trochanteric portal. A radiofrequency hook probe is introduced through the superior trochanteric portal and is used to perform the above mentioned cut in a retrograde fashion. (B) The anterior transverse cut is performed at the mid-portion of the anterior edge of the iliotibial band cut (AITB). The greater trochanteric bursa (GTB) is observed through the cut. (C) The posterior transverse release is performed at the mid-portion of the posterior edge of the original vertical release on the iliotibial band (PITB). The greater trochanteric bursa is observed through the cut. (D) The greater trochanteric bursa (GTB) is removed through the defect on the iliotibial band. The gluteus medius muscle is observed under the bursa. The white arrow indicates the limit of the anterior release on the iliotibial band. The black arrow indicates the posterior limit of the resection on the iliotibial band. Fibers of the gluteus maximus are observed in this area.

# CONCLUSION

Most of the patients presenting to an orthopedic evaluation because of a snapping hip syndrome will generally be able to perform activities of daily living and only have symptoms with high range of motion or during exercise. The examiner should be very aware of the etiology and clinical presentation of the snapping hips and be careful to look for specific details in clinical history and very specific findings at the clinical examination. Once the diagnosis is established, the clinician should always think of and look for associated pathology.

# REFERENCES

1. Allen WC, Cope R. Coxa saltans: the snapping hip revisited. *J Am Acad Orthop Surg.* 1995;3:303-308.
2. Byrd JWT. Evaluation and management of the snapping iliopsoas tendon. *Tech in Ortho.* 2005;20:45-51.
3. Winston P, Awan R, Cassidy JD, Bleakney RK. Clinical examination and ultrasound of self-reported snapping hip syndrome in elite ballet dancers. *Am J Sports Med.* 2007;35:118-126.
4. Ilizaliturri VM Jr, Martinez-Escalante FA, Chaidez PA, Camacho-Galindo J. Endoscopic iliotibial band release for external snapping hip syndrome. *Arthroscopy.* 2006;22:505-510.
5. Youdas JW, Mraz ST, Norstad BJ, Schinke JJ, Hollman JH. Determining meaningful changes in pelvic-on-femoral position during the Trendelenburg test. *J Sport Rehabil.* 2007;16:326-335.
6. Teitz CC, Garrett WE Jr, Miniaci A, Lee MH, Mann RA. Tendon problems in athletic individuals. *Instr Course Lect.* 1997;46:569-582.
7. Martin RL, Sekiya JK. The interrater reliability of 4 clinical tests used to assess individuals with musculoskeletal hip pain. *J Orthop Sports Phys Ther.* 2008;38:71-77.
8. Pelsser V, Cardinal E, Hobden R, Aubin B, Lafortune M. Extraarticular snapping hip: sonographic findings. *AJR Am J Roentgenol.* 2001;176:67-73.
9. Choi YS, Lee SM, Song BY, Paik SH, Yoon YK. Dynamic sonography of external snapping hip syndrome. *J Ultrasound Med.* 2002;21:753-758.
10. Wunderbaldinger P, Bremer C, Schellenberger E, Cejna M, Turetschek K, Kainberger F. Imaging features of iliopsoas bursitis. *Eur Radiol.* 2002;12:409-415.
11. Cvitanic O, Henzie G, Skezas N, Lyons J, Minter J. MRI diagnosis of tears of the hip abductor tendons (gluteus medius and gluteus minimus). *AJR Am J Roentgenol.* 2004;182:137-143.

12. Jacobson T, Allen WC. Surgical correction of the snapping iliopsoas tendon. *Am J Sports Med.* 1990;18:470-474.
13. Taylor GR, Clarke NM. Surgical release of the "snapping iliopsoas tendon." *J Bone Joint Surg Br.* 1995;77:881-883.
14. Dobbs MB, Gordon JE, Luhmann SJ, Szymanzki DA, Schoenecker PL. Surgical correction of the snapping iliopsoas tendon in adolescents. *J Bone Joint Surg Am.* 2002;84:420-424.
15. Gruen GS, Scioscia TN, Lowenstein JE. The surgical treatment of internal snapping hip. *Am J Sports Med.* 2002;30:607-613.
16. Ilizaliturri VM Jr, Villalobos FE, Chaidez PA, Valero FS, Aguilera JM. Internal snapping hip syndrome: treatment by endoscopic release of the iliopsoas tendon. *Arthroscopy.* 2005;21:1375-1380.
17. Flanum ME, Keene JS, Blankenbaker DG, Desmet AA. Arthroscopic treatment of the painful "internal" snapping hip: results of a new endoscopic technique and imaging protocol. *Am J Sports Med.* 2007;35:770-779.
18. Wettstein M, Jung J, Dienst M. Arthroscopic psoas tenotomy. *Arthroscopy.* 2006;22(8):907.e1-907.e4.
19. Contreras MEK, Dani WS, Endges WK, De Araujo LCT, Berral FJ. Arthroscopic treatment of the snapping iliopsoas tendon trough the central compartment of the hip. A pilot study. *J Bone Joint Surg.* 2010;92: 777-780.
20. Ilizaliturri VM Jr, Byrd JWT, Sampson TG, et al. A geographic zone method to describe intra-articular pathology in hip arthroscopy: cadaveric study and preliminary report. *Arthroscopy.* 2008;24:534-539.
21. Ilizaliturri VM Jr., Chaidez C, Villegas P, Briseño A, Camacho-Galindo J. Prospective randomized study of 2 different techniques for endoscopic iliopsoas tendon release in the treatment of internal snapping hip syndrome. *Arthroscopy.* 2009;25:159-163.
22. Fery A, Sommelet J. The snapping hip. Late results of 24 surgical cases. *Int Orthop.* 1988;12:277-282.
23. Faraj AA, Moulton A, Sirivastava VM. Snapping iliotibial band. Report of ten cases and review of the literature. *Acta Orthop Belg.* 2001;67:19-23.
24. Provencher MT, Hofmeister EP, Muldoon MP. The surgical treatment of external coxa saltans (the snapping hip) by Z-plasty of the iliotibial band. *Am J Sports Med.* 2004;32:470-476.
25. White RA, Hughes MS, Burd T. A new operative approach in the correction of external coxa saltans. *Am J Sports Med.* 2004;32:1504-1508.

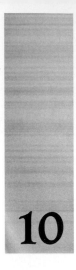

**10**

# FEMORAL DEFORMITIES AND HIP OSTEOTOMIES

*Robert L. Buly, MD*

## INTRODUCTION

There are a number of anatomic anomalies of the femur. Some may be genetically predetermined, such as coxa valga, some types of femoroacetabular impingement, or abnormalities of femoral version (Table 10-1). Others may develop after birth and may be the result of injury, damage to the capital physis, or infection. These skeletal aberrations can lead to a host of problems, including gait abnormalities, leg length inequality, restricted range of motion, limp, patellofemoral maltracking, damage to the labrum and articular cartilage, and ultimately osteoarthritis.[1-5] These may occur in isolation or may be associated with pelvic abnormalities, such as acetabular dysplasia, coxa profunda, protrusion, or acetabular retroversion.[6,7]

Ranawat A, Kelly BT. *Musculoskeletal Examination of the Hip and Knee: Making the Complex Simple* (pp. 252-273).
© 2011 SLACK Incorporated

**Table 10-1**

## *HELPFUL HINTS*

*Imaging*

| DIAGNOSIS | CLINICAL FINDINGS | RADIOGRAPHIC FINDINGS | FIGURES | SUGGESTED TREATMENT |
|---|---|---|---|---|
| Coxa valga | Increased internal rotation and (+) external rotation apprehension sign if associated with increased femoral anteversion<br><br>Increased external rotation if associated with femoral retroversion | Neck-shaft angle >140 degrees | 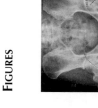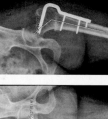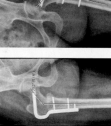 | Varus-producing intertrochanteric osteotomy, ± derotation |

(continued)

**Table 10-1 (continued)**

*HELPFUL HINTS*

| DIAGNOSIS | CLINICAL FINDINGS | RADIOGRAPHIC FINDINGS | FIGURES | SUGGESTED TREATMENT |
|---|---|---|---|---|
| Coxa vara | Leg shortening, (+) Trendelenburg limp | Neck-shaft angle <125 degrees | 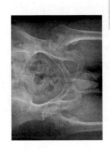 | Valgus-producing intertrochanteric osteotomy, ± derotation |

(continued)

**Table 10-1 (continued)**

## HELPFUL HINTS

| DIAGNOSIS | CLINICAL FINDINGS | RADIOGRAPHIC FINDINGS | FIGURES | SUGGESTED TREATMENT |
|---|---|---|---|---|
| Excessive femoral anteversion | In-toeing gait with "squinting" patellae. May be associated with compensatory external tibial torsion leading to an out-toeing gait | Normal = 15 to 20 degrees anteversion (Tönnis)<br><br>Normal = 10 degrees anteversion (Toogood) | 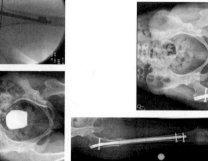 | Derotation femoral osteotomy, ± varus or valgus correction |

(continued)

**Table 10-1 (continued)**

*HELPFUL HINTS*

| DIAGNOSIS | CLINICAL FINDINGS | RADIOGRAPHIC FINDINGS | FIGURES | SUGGESTED TREATMENT |
|---|---|---|---|---|
| Trochanteric overgrowth and short femoral neck | Short leg, decreased range of motion, especially internal rotation and abduction. (+) Trendelenburg limp | Short femoral neck with high greater trochanter. Significant leg length inequality | 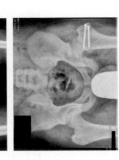 | 1) Advancement of the greater trochanter<br>2) "Relative lengthening" of the femoral neck with trochanteric advancement and surgical dislocation |

*(continued)*

**Table 10-1 (continued)**

*HELPFUL HINTS*

| DIAGNOSIS | CLINICAL FINDINGS | RADIOGRAPHIC FINDINGS | FIGURES | SUGGESTED TREATMENT |
|---|---|---|---|---|
| Femoral retroversion | Out-toeing gait. Lack of internal rotation at 90 degrees hip flexion. (+) impingement sign | Normal = 15 to 20 degrees anteversion (Tönnis)<br><br>Normal = 10 degrees anteversion (Toogood)<br><br>Completely normal-appearing femoral neck or cam lesion. With or without Pincer lesion (acetabular retroversion)<br><br>May have normal or altered neck-shaft angle |  | For pure femoral retroversion: derotation intertrochanteric or subtrochanteric osteotomy. Blade-plate with varus or valgus correction as well if necessary |

*(continued)*

## Table 10-1 (continued)

### HELPFUL HINTS

| DIAGNOSIS | CLINICAL FINDINGS | RADIOGRAPHIC FINDINGS | FIGURES | SUGGESTED TREATMENT |
|---|---|---|---|---|
| SCFE deformity | Out-toeing gait. Lack of internal rotation at 90 degrees hip flexion. (+) impingement sign. With large SCFE deformity; also leg shortening and limited flexion | SCFE "Pistol-grip" deformity, femoral cam lesion or completely normal-appearing femoral neck. With or without pincer lesion (acetabular retroversion) | 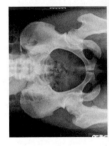 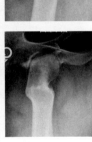 | For large SCFE deformity in younger patients, intertrochanteric or femoral neck osteotomy. For cam lesion and lesser SCFE angulation, femoral neck osteochondroplasty |

The optimal treatment includes establishing the correct diagnosis and executing the proper surgical technique to reduce pain, improve function, and hopefully provide the opportunity for a hip to last the patient's lifetime.

# HISTORY

Patients may present with a host of problems that have been present since infancy: breech birth, prematurity, congenital dislocation, and gait abnormalities. Alternatively, other patients may not be aware of a problem until the insidious onset of pain as an adolescent or young adult, or there may have been some dramatic event such as Perthes disease, a slipped capital femoral epiphysis, or infection.

A limp may be present at all times or may only occur with long walks due to fatigue. Often, there are associated gait abnormalities such as in-toeing or out-toeing. Others may report that they never had good range of motion or had difficulty sitting "Indian style" with the hips flexed and externally rotated or "W style" with the hips flexed and internally rotated. Some claim that they have never felt right with activities such as biking because of awkward joint positioning. There may also be a history of knee pain or leg length inequality. Ultimately, as joint deterioration progresses, there may be increasing mechanical pain from labral tears or increased walking pain associated with osteoarthritis.

# EXAMINATION

A careful history and physical examination are critical. It is helpful to start with an observation of the gait. Is there a limp? If so, is it antalgic in nature or due to abductor weakness with an associated positive Trendelenburg sign? Patients with excessive anteversion tend to walk with an in-toeing type gait with "squinting" of the patellae, while those with femoral retroversion tend to walk with an external foot progression angle instead.[8] It is important to measure leg lengths. Conditions such as slipped epiphysis, Perthes disease, coxa vara, and proximal femoral growth arrest may lead to shortening of the affected leg. Muscle strength of all groups should be assessed, along with range of motion measurements. A positive impingement test may give a false indication of a lack of internal rotation; this may not be a bony block, but pain-induced inhibition. It is useful to assess the range of motion immediately after an intra-articular injection containing local anesthetic, not only to confirm an intra-articular source for the pain but also to get a better assessment of the true range of motion.

Patients with excessive femoral anteversion often have more internal rotation than external rotation. External rotation may be nearly absent in severe cases. Conversely, with femoral retroversion, there may be a complete lack of internal rotation.[9] This lack of internal rotation is found with almost all forms of femoroacetabular impingement. It may be helpful to assess rotation in the prone position as well to remove the elements of a positive impingement test.

The findings associated with coxa valga may mimic those of acetabular dysplasia, in which there is increased pain with extension combined with external rotation, as this leads to subluxation of the head against the rim of the socket. This is often referred to as the apprehension sign.

Hip abduction may be blocked if there is overgrowth of the greater trochanter, which leads to impingement against the lateral ilium.

Range of motion assessment is important for osteotomy preoperative planning. It is important to remember that a varus intertrochanteric osteotomy is also referred to as "adduction osteotomy" and vice versa for a valgus osteotomy. Therefore, it is important to ensure that enough residual abduction will be present after a varus osteotomy. It is possible to simulate a femoral osteotomy with abduction/adduction and/or rotation of the leg. The patient should be more comfortable when the head is placed in the corrected position. Functional radiographs should also be performed to ascertain whether the head actually rotates within the acetabulum with abduction as opposed to hinging. It should also be noted whether coverage of the femoral head and the joint space looks better in the simulated position.

Certainly, not all hip pain is intrinsic to the joint itself. It is important to rule out referred lumbosacral pain as well as conditions such as inguinal hernia or the so-called "sports hernia" or "athletic pubalgia," which is a chronic disruption of the pectineus or adductor muscle origins on the pelvis.[10] If in doubt, selective local anesthetic injections, either intra- or extra-articular, will often allow the determination of the painful source.

## PATHOANATOMY

Coxa valga is a problem because the steep neck-shaft angle causes a relative uncovering of the femoral head. The contact area between the acetabulum and femoral head is diminished, subjecting the articular cartilage to higher loads. Contributing to cartilage overload is the fact that there may be concomitant acetabular dysplasia, usually with anterior and lateral socket deficiency. The labrum, overloaded and subjected to shear stress, undergoes degeneration and tearing. Coxa valga may be associated with normal version or excessive femoral anteversion or retroversion.[9] Compounding the problem is that a valgus neck-shaft angle decreases the abductor lever arm, raising joint reaction forces. Adding insult to injury, there may be coexisting femoroacetabular impingement due to either a femoral cam lesion or acetabular pincer lesion.

Abnormalities of femoral version can affect not only the hip joint but the patellofemoral joint and gait.[11] Excessive anteversion overloads the front of the acetabulum and can result in labral degeneration. Femoral retroversion can create havoc, similar to the problems that occur if the femoral component of a hip replacement is retroverted. Femoral retroversion causes femoroacetabular impingement with resultant damage to the labrum and articular cartilage.[9,12,13] The femur and acetabulum can have completely different version measurements, either compounding the problem or offsetting each other. Diminished anteversion of the acetabulum or femur appears to be both more common and more damaging than excessive anteversion.[9] These abnormalities may appear as isolated entities or as part of a constellation of anatomic deformities.[6,7]

In cases of slipped capital femoral epiphysis, the deformity also creates hip impingement and ultimately osteoarthritis with more damage occurring with larger deformities.[3,14]

A growth arrest of the capital femoral physis in infancy leads to a short femoral neck, a deformed femoral head, and overgrowth of the greater trochanter.[15-18] This condition is associated with abductor weakness and fatigue with ambulation, along with impingement of the greater trochanter against the ilium with abduction, but there may be considerable intra-articular deformities as well.[19]

With Perthes disease, there is often a resultant "coxa magna" deformity, which is analogous to a square peg and a round hole.[20,21] This deformity may also be associated with acetabular dysplasia along with premature cartilage degeneration, labral tears, and osteoarthritis.

# IMAGING

## Plain Radiographs

Most hip abnormalities are readily apparent on plain radiographs. The radiographic protocol that the author employs is as follows: 1) an AP pelvis radiograph including the iliac crests, without rotation or excessive caudad or cephalad tilt,[22] 2) an "elongated neck" or Dunn lateral of both femoral necks,[23] and 3) a false profile view of both hips.[24] The reason both hips are imaged is that there is a high incidence of bilateral abnormalities, and the contralateral side may be asymptomatic. It is important to know the condition of the other hip for prognosis and future planning. An additional AP radiograph of the pelvis is obtained with the legs abducted if a periacetabular or varus derotation osteotomy is contemplated to assess femoral head rotation and joint appearance.[25]

Long-leg films may be obtained if there is concern about the overall mechanical axis of the leg or leg length inequality. Knee films should be obtained if there is symptomatology. Radiographs should be assessed for the presence of osteoarthritis (Tönnis classification) and joint space narrowing.[26] The radiographic parameters to be measured may include but are not limited to center edge angle of Wiberg,[27] anterior center edge angle,[24] neck-shaft angle,[26] roof slope angle,[28] and the alpha angle.[29] The presence of osteophytes and a "cross-over sign" indicative of pincer impingement should be noted as well.[30] Os acetabuli may be present in cases of either hip impingement or dysplasia.[31]

## Magnetic Resonance Imaging Scanning

Magnetic resonance imaging (MRI) scans provide useful adjunct information about the status of the articular cartilage, labrum, synovium, and joint fluid. This is especially important as patients approach middle age, as there may be far more cartilage degeneration than is apparent on plain radiographs; these patients may be better off waiting for a total hip arthroplasty. In addition, extra-articular structures, such as muscles, tendons, ligaments, neurovascular structures, tumors, cysts, and fluid, are all readily visible. Excellent diagnostic results have been obtained with or without the use of intra-articular gadolinium.[32,33] Scout views of the entire pelvis should be obtained along with high-resolution images of the hip in all 3 planes with the use of a surface coil.

## Computed Tomography Scan

Computed tomography (CT) scanning allows visualization not only of the axial slices, but also coronal and sagittal reformations as well. Improved software packages can also provide beautiful 3-D reformations that may be viewed from various angles. 3-D imaging is helpful in viewing and understanding the more subtle forms of hip impingement.[34] It is possible from the scans to measure the alpha and beta angles of the femoral neck as well as femoral version, acetabular version, and neck-shaft angle.[7]

# TREATMENT

## Surgical Techniques

The surgical correction of femoral abnormalities must take into account many factors: age, activity, coexisting problems, leg length, and the degree of joint damage. Changing one problem may create another. The goal of any surgical correction is to relieve pain, improve biomechanics, provide a more functional range of motion, and reduce the joint reaction forces on the articular cartilage.

With coxa valga, the goal is to improve femoral head coverage. This is best performed with a varus-producing intertrochanteric osteotomy. It is important not to overdo correction with excessive varus, which can lead to increased shortening of the leg and abductor weakness. A Trendelenburg limp may persist for many months after a varus osteotomy until hip abductor strength returns. Coxa valga and dysplasia are typically associated with excessive anteversion.[35-37] However, femoral version may have a wide range, from excessive anteversion to femoral retroversion. Tönnis reported that 47% of patients with coxa valga had diminished femoral version (less than 15 degrees).[9] It is important to make that determination as part of the preoperative plan with either a CT or MRI scan that includes slices through the knees as well as hips. Historically, the 90 degree AO blade plate has been used, which not only provides correction of the neck-shaft angle but produces medial displacement of the distal fragment, thought to be important in the maintenance of a leg mechanical axis that passes through the center of the knee joint. The blade plate comes with 10, 15, or 20 mm of offset, depending upon the degree of medial displacement desired.[25] At times, the other blade plates with angles of 95, 100, 110, 120, or 130 degrees may be more appropriate. The blade plates with angles at the upper end of the spectrum were often used with valgus, producing intertrochanteric osteotomies.[38] They may also be used in the correction of coxa vara with or without the correction of femoral version (Figure 10-1).

At times when coxa valga coexists with acetabular dysplasia, it may be difficult to ascertain whether the correction should be performed on the pelvis, femur, or both.[39,40] A periacetabular pelvic osteotomy is certainly more invasive but provides very powerful correction of the dysplastic socket. Another benefit is less shortening of the leg and less distortion of the femoral canal should it be necessary to perform a hip replacement in the future. The decision making should lean toward the femoral side if the acetabulum has no or minimal dysplasia. A varus derotation intertrochanteric osteotomy should be performed if that is the site of major deformity. Another benefit of a periacetabular osteotomy is the ability to perform an anterior hip arthrotomy to assess and treat coexisting conditions such as cam impingement, labral tears, and cartilage defects. If a femoral osteotomy is to be performed, it may be desirable to perform an arthroscopic débridement before or at the same setting.

For abnormalities of femoral version, it is possible to perform the correction with a blade plate. Prior to plate application, rotation marks or preferably Steinmann pins placed

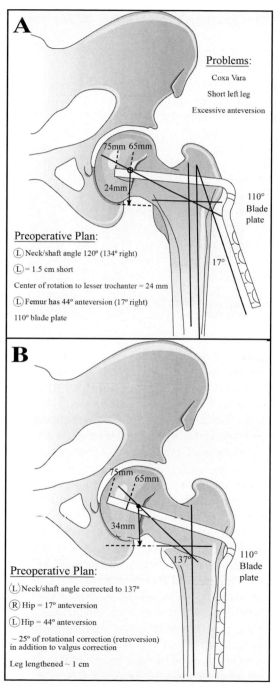

**A**

Problems:

Coxa Vara

Short left leg

Excessive anteversion

75mm 65mm

24mm

110°
Blade
plate

17°

Preoperative Plan:

Ⓛ Neck/shaft angle 120° (134° right)

Ⓛ = 1.5 cm short

Center of rotation to lesser trochanter = 24 mm

Ⓛ Femur has 44° anteversion (17° right)

110° blade plate

**B**

75mm 65mm

34mm

137°

110°
Blade
plate

Preoperative Plan:

Ⓛ Neck/shaft angle corrected to 137°

Ⓡ Hip = 17° anteversion

Ⓛ Hip = 44° anteversion

~ 25° of rotational correction (retroversion)
in addition to valgus correction

Leg lengthened ~ 1 cm

**Figure 10-1.** (A, B) Preoperative planning for a valgus derotation intertrochanteric osteotomy of the left hip to simultaneously correct varus and excessive anteversion *(continued)*.

**Figure 10-1 (continued).** (C) Postoperative radiograph of the left hip demonstrating correction of the neck-shaft angle to 135 degrees along with removal of 25 degrees of anteversion.

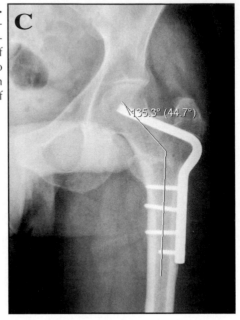

proximal and distal to the osteotomy are used to monitor rotation correction. If the neck-shaft angle is normal and varus or valgus correction is not required, it may be sufficient to perform a pure derotation. Rotation should be corrected to normal, in the range of 12 to 20 degrees.[9] To correct excessive anteversion, the distal fragment is externally rotated, with the converse for femoral retroversion. Rather than a more invasive blade plate approach, it is possible to use a locked intramedullary nail with a small incision for the subtrochanteric osteotomy or even a purely intramedullary osteotomy performed with a Winquist saw.[41]

In the rare cases with a simple greater trochanteric overgrowth, a simple advancement of the greater trochanter may provide better abductor power and relieve impingement.[18] The operation may provide little benefit if performed alone for the sequelae of Perthes disease.[16,17,42] In addition, most of these cases also have a shortened femoral neck and femoroacetabular impingement. To correct this, Ganz and coworkers have devised a "relative lengthening" of the femoral neck along with cam débridement and greater trochanteric advancement that is performed with a surgical dislocation.[19]

With Perthes disease, the problem is not only a dysplastic socket but also a head that is too large and not congruent with the acetabulum. Because of this, a salvage-type procedure has often been used, such as the Chiari osteotomy.[43-46] Ganz and coworkers have devised a novel approach, which is a "head reduction" osteotomy in which a portion of the femoral head is removed to reduce the overall volume and permit containment by the acetabulum. This is performed as well with a surgical dislocation.[19]

The problem with slipped capital femoral epiphysis is convex deformity that is left at the anterosuperior head-neck junction of the femur. At times, this deformity can be quite severe. Historically, corrective intertrochanteric osteotomies, such as the Imhauser, have been performed at a distance from the femoral neck to avoid avascular necrosis of the femoral head that has been associated with an intra-articular femoral neck osteotomy.[47,48] Fish has described the use of a cuneiform femoral neck osteotomy for slips greater than 30 degrees with mostly good results.[49] With better delineation of the anatomy of the femoral head blood supply, Ganz et al proposed a more powerful correction of the deformity right at its location on the femoral neck.[50] If done carefully via a surgical dislocation with careful attention paid to the retinacular vessels, the chance of avascular necrosis should be minimized. For more mild deformities that seem to be a cause of cam-type femoroacetabular impingement, it may be sufficient to débride the femoral neck by means of an open or arthroscopic osteochondroplasty. Care must be taken to avoid excessive débridement to compensate for a large deformity, as this may lead to a femoral neck fracture. If the débridement is inadequate, an open correction should be performed.

## Rehabilitation

Following corrective osteotomy of the femur, braces and/or cast immobilization should not be necessary provided there is adequate internal fixation. Range of motion is encouraged with care taken if an arthrotomy was performed, which is almost always anterior. Protective toe-touch weight-bearing is necessary for 6 to 8 weeks to prevent loss of correction and/or hardware fracture or displacement. If a pure derotation femoral osteotomy was performed with a locked intramedullary nail, weight-bearing is encouraged with dynamic locking to hasten bone union.

## Complications

Nonunion can occur but is rare if proper technique and internal fixation are used. An articulated tensioning device applied to the plate before screw placement increases compression at the osteotomy site and promotes healing. Avoid over-correction or under-correction by using intraoperative fluoroscopy and radiographs. With derotation osteotomies, it is possible to assess the range of motion both before and after correction. Smoking is to be discouraged as it makes it more difficult for bone healing to occur. Patients should be warned that a varus osteotomy will produce shortening and an abductor limp that may persist for months until the abductors regain their power. Hardware may need to be removed after healing of the osteotomy if it causes pain. This is especially true with blade plates.

## Results

Several long-term studies have demonstrated the utility of these joint-sparing procedures. Voos reported on 45 hips in 40 patients who underwent a varus-producing intertrochanteric osteotomy for coxa valga at an average follow-up of 22.6 years (range: 15 to 34 years). At 10 years, approximately one-third of patients had undergone total hip replacement. This figure increased to two-thirds by 20 years. However, better results and survivorship occurred in patients with a better initial HSS hip score, younger age, or minimal osteoarthritis and subluxation.[51]

A recurring theme in hip preservation surgery is that earlier intervention, before the onset of significant articular cartilage damage, leads to better long-term success. Haverkamp and Marti reported the long-term results of bilateral varus intertrochanteric osteotomy for coxa valga in 26 patients.[52] In this study, the painful hip was done first (the "therapeutic" group), and patients were encouraged to have the contralateral side done early, even if minimally symptomatic ("early" osteotomy group). There were no significant differences in center-edge angle or neck-shaft angle in the 2 groups.

Follow-up was 20 years, with a range of 15 to 26 years. In the therapeutic group, 15-year survivorship was 56%, with 14 of 26 undergoing hip replacement at an average of 9.9 years. In the early group, survivorship was 76%, with 6 hip replacements. The results were significant. Results were also better in those of younger age, with a lower Tönnis arthritis score, and with a better Merle d'Aubigne score.[52]

Ito et al studied 55 varus femoral osteotomies in 46 coxa valga patients at an average follow-up of 17 years (range: 6 to 28 years).[53] Using hip replacement or a Harris Hip Score of 70 or less as a marker for failure, the survivorship was 81% at 10 years, 60% at 20 years, and 50% at 25 years. Better results were obtained in patients with Tönnis grades 0, 1, or 2; spherical heads; and mild dysplasia at the time of osteotomy.[53]

Iwase et al published the study results of 52 varus femoral osteotomies at an average follow-up of 21 years and 58 valgus osteotomies at an average of 20 years.[54] The 10- and 15-year survivorships were 89% and 87%, respectively, for varus osteotomies. The 10- and 15-year survivorships for valgus osteotomies were 66% and 38%, respectively.[54]

Ansari and colleagues reported on 26 varus rotational osteotomies in 24 patients at an average follow-up of 5 years (range: 1.6 to 23 years).[55] The average Harris Hip Score increased from 72 to 97. There were no reoperations and one nonunion.[55]

The results of the Imhäuser intertrochanteric osteotomy in 51 slipped capital femoral epiphysis patients followed for an average of 24 years (range: 20 to 29 years) was investigated by Schai and Exner.[47] At latest follow-up, 55% were clinically asymptomatic with minimal adverse radiographic changes, while 28% had moderate changes and 17% had advanced changes.[47]

Leunig et al reported on subcapital corrective osteotomies performed for severe slipped epiphysis deformities in 30 hips at an average of 55 months of follow-up (range: 24 to 96 months).[56] The posterior slip angle ranged from 30 to 70 degrees. The average age for girls was 12 years, and the average age for boys was 14 years. There were no cases of avascular necrosis. There were 3 revisions for hardware failure and one case of heterotopic ossification that restricted motion.[56] This series was updated to a minimum 3-year follow-up in 2009 with maintenance of the good results reported in the earlier publication.[19]

The technique of "relative lengthening" of the femoral neck for greater trochanter overgrowth and neck shortening from growth arrest of the proximal femoral physis was devised by Ganz. From 1998 to 2004, there were 132 lengthenings performed using a surgical dislocation and an extended retinacular soft tissue flap. There was one hip replacement following fracture and 3 re-fixations of the greater trochanter. There were no cases of avascular necrosis.[19]

Ganz also reported on 11 femoral head reductions performed for Perthes disease, avascular necrosis, or high dislocation with follow-up ranging from 6 months to 7 years. All improved with no cases of avascular necrosis.[19]

## CONCLUSION

In the management of hip disorders in young patients, it is imperative to make the correct diagnosis. It is important to know the natural history of various anatomic abnormalities and the likelihood of osteoarthritis of the hip if left untreated. Surgical management should not only provide pain relief and functional improvement but should also have a long-term goal of hip preservation. It should be kept in mind that conditions such as dysplasia, coxa valga, coxa vara, excessive femoral anteversion, femoral retroversion, and hip impingement may exist as isolated entities or may coexist in varying degrees. A recurring theme seen throughout published series is that the results are better with earlier intervention and when less joint destruction is present at the time of surgical treatment.

## REFERENCES

1. Boyer DW, Mickelson MR, Ponseti IV. Slipped capital femoral epiphysis. Long-term follow-up study of one hundred and twenty-one patients. *J Bone Joint Surg Am.* 1981;63(1):85-95.
2. Ganz R, Parvizi J, Beck M, Leunig M, Notzli H, Siebenrock KA. Femoroacetabular impingement: a cause for osteoarthritis of the hip. *Clin Orthop.* 2003;417:112-120.
3. Goodman DA, Feighan JE, Smith AD, Latimer B, Buly RL, Cooperman DR. Subclinical slipped capital epiphysis. Relationship to osteoarthrosis of the hip. *J Bone Joint Surg Am.* 1997;79:1489-1497.

4. Harris WH. Etiology of osteoarthritis of the hip. *Clin Orthop.* 1986;213:20-33.

5. Harris WH. The correlation between minor or unrecognized developmental deformities and the development of osteoarthritis of the hip. *Instr Course Lect.* 2009;58:257-259.

6. Allen D, Beaule PE, Ramadan O, Doucette S. Prevalence of associated deformities and hip pain in patients with cam-type femoroacetabular impingement. *J Bone Joint Surg Br.* 2009;91(5):589-594.

7. Moya LE, Molisani D, Henn F, Ma Y, Kelly BT, Buly RL. Femoral retroversion in patients with femoroacetabular impingement: a cofactor in the development of hip osteoarthritis. Paper presented at: Orthopaedic Research Society 55th Annual Meeting;  February 22-24, 2009; Las Vegas, NV.

8. Crane L. Femoral torsion and its relation to toeing-in and toeing-out. *J Bone Joint Surg Am.* 1959;41A(3):421-428.

9. Tönnis D, Heinecke A. Acetabular and femoral anteversion: relationship with osteoarthritis of the hip. *J Bone Joint Surg Am.* 1999;81(12):1747-1770.

10. Meyers WC, McKechnie A, Philippon MJ, Horner MA, Zoga AC, Devon ON. Experience with "sports hernia" spanning two decades. *Ann Surg.* 2008;248(4):656-665.

11. Eckhoff DG, Montgomery WK, Kilcoyne RF, Stamm ER. Femoral morphometry and anterior knee pain. *Clin Orthop Relat Res.* 1994;302:64-68.

12. Tönnis D, Heinecke A. Decreased acetabular anteversion and femur neck antetorsion cause pain and arthrosis. 2: Etiology, diagnosis and therapy. *Z Orthop Ihre Grenzgeb.* 1999;137(2):160-167.

13. Tönnis D, Heinecke A. Diminished femoral antetorsion syndrome: a cause of pain and osteoarthritis. *J Pediatr Orthop.* 1991;11(4):419-431.

14. Cooperman DR, Charles LM, Pathria M, Latimer B, Thompson GH. Post-mortem description of slipped capital femoral epiphysis. *J Bone Joint Surg Br.* 1992;74(4):595-599.

15. Iwersen LJ, Kalen V, Eberle C. Relative trochanteric overgrowth after ischemic necrosis in congenital dislocation of the hip. *J Pediatr Orthop.* 1989;9(4):381-385.

16. Lloyd-Roberts GC, Wetherill MH, Fraser M. Trochanteric advancement for premature arrest of the femoral capital growth plate. *J Bone Joint Surg Br.* 1985;67(1):21-24.

17. Macnicol MF, Makris D. Distal transfer of the greater trochanter. *J Bone Joint Surg Br.* 1991;73(5):838-841.

18. Wagner H. Treatment of osteoarthritis of the hip by corrective osteotomy of the greater trochanter. In: Schatzker J, ed. *The Intertrochanteric Osteotomy.* Berlin, Germany: Springer-Verlag; 1984:179-201.

19. Ganz R, Huff TW, Leunig M. Extended retinacular soft-tissue flap for intra-articular hip surgery: surgical technique, indications, and results of application. *Instr Course Lect.* 2009;58:241-255.

20. McAndrew MP, Weinstein SL. A long-term follow-up of Legg-Calve-Perthes disease. *J Bone Joint Surg Am.* 1984;66(6):860-869.

21. Stulberg SD, Cooperman DR, Wallensten R. The natural history of Legg-Calve-Perthes disease. *J Bone Joint Surg Am.* 1981;63(7):1095-1108.

22. Tannast M, Zheng G, Anderegg C, et al. Tilt and rotation correction of acetabular version on pelvic radiographs. *Clin Orthop Relat Res.* 2005;438:182-190.

23. Meyer DC, Beck M, Ellis T, Ganz R, Leunig M. Comparison of six radiographic projections to assess femoral head/neck asphericity. *Clin Orthop Relat Res.* 2006;445:181-185.

24. Lequesne M, de Seze S. La faux profil du bassin: nouvelle incidence radiographique pour l'etude de la hanche. Son utilite dans les dysplasies et les differentes coxopathies. *Rev Rhum.* 1961;28:643-652.

25. Muller ME. Intertrochanteric osteotomy: indication, preoperative planning, technique. In: Schatzker J, ed. *The Intertrochanteric Osteotomy.* Berlin, Germany: Springer-Verlag; 1984:25-66.

26. Tönnis D. General radiology of the hip joint. In: Tönnis D, ed. *Congenital Dysplasia and Dislocation of the Hip in Children and Adults.* Berlin, Germany: Springer-Verlag; 1987:100-142.

27. Wiberg G. Studies on the dysplastic acetabulum and congenital subluxation of the hip joint. *Acta Chir Scand.* 1939;83(Suppl. 58):1-135.

28. Tönnis D. Normal values of the hip joint for the evaluation of X-rays in children and adults. *Clin Orthop Relat Res.* 1976;119:39-47.

29. Notzli HP, Wyss TF, Stoecklin CH, Schmid MR, Treiber K, Hodler J. The contour of the femoral head-neck junction as a predictor for the risk of anterior impingement. *J Bone Joint Surg Br.* 2002;84(4):556-560.

30. Reynolds D, Lucas J, Klaue K. Retroversion of the acetabulum. A cause of hip pain. *J Bone Joint Surg Br.* 1999;81(2):281-288.

31. Martinez AE, Li SM, Ganz R, Beck M. Os acetabuli in femoro-acetabular impingement: stress fracture or unfused secondary ossification centre of the acetabular rim? *Hip Int.* 2006;16(4):281-286.

32. Mintz DN, Hooper T, Connell D, Buly R, Padgett DE, Potter HG. Magnetic resonance imaging of the hip: detection of labral and chondral abnormalities using noncontrast imaging. *Arthroscopy.* 2005;21(4):385-393.

33. Toomayan GA, Holman WR, Major NM, Kozlowicz SM, Vail TP. Sensitivity of MR arthrography in the evaluation of acetabular labral tears. *AJR Am J Roentgenol.* 2006;186(2):449-453.

34. Beaule PE, Zaragoza E, Motamedi K, Copelan N, Dorey FJ. Three-dimensional computed tomography of the hip in the assessment of femoroacetabular impingement. *J Orthop Res.* 2005;23(6):1286-1292.

35. Jacobsen S. Adult hip dysplasia and osteoarthritis. Studies in radiology and clinical epidemiology. *Acta Orthop Suppl.* 2006;77(324):1-37.

36. Anda S, Terjesen T, Kvistad KA, Svenningsen S. Acetabular angles and femoral anteversion in dysplastic hips in adults: CT investigation. *J Comput Assist Tomogr.* 1991;15(1):115-120.

37. Argenson JN, Ryembault E, Flecher X, Brassart N, Parratte S, Aubaniac JM. Three-dimensional anatomy of the hip in osteoarthritis after developmental dysplasia. *J Bone Joint Surg Br.* 2005;87(9):1192-1196.

38. Maistrelli GL, Gerundini M, Fusco U, Bombelli R, Bombelli M, Avai A. Valgus-extension osteotomy for osteoarthritis of the hip. Indications and long-term results. *J Bone Joint Surg Br.* 1990;72(4):653-657.

39. Steppacher SD, Tannast M, Ganz R, Siebenrock KA. Mean 20-year followup of Bernese periacetabular osteotomy. *Clin Orthop Relat Res.* 2008;466(7):1633-1644.
40. Trousdale RT, Ekkernkamp A, Ganz R, Wallrichs SL. Periacetabular and intertrochanteric osteotomy for the treatment of osteoarthrosis in dysplastic hips. *J Bone Joint Surg Am.* 1995;77(1):73-85.
41. Winquist RA. Closed intramedullary osteotomies of the femur. *Clin Orthop.* 1986;212:155-164.
42. Joo SY, Lee KS, Koh IH, Park HW, Kim HW. Trochanteric advancement in patients with Legg-Calve-Perthes disease does not improve pain or limp. *Clin Orthop Relat Res.* 2008;466(4):927-934.
43. Bennett JT, Mazurek RT, Cash JD. Chiari's osteotomy in the treatment of Perthes' disease. *J Bone Joint Surg Br.* 1991;73(2):225-228.
44. Cahuzac JP, Onimus M, Trottmann F, Clement JL, Laurain JM, Lebarbier P. Chiari pelvic osteotomy in Perthes disease. *J Pediatr Orthop.* 1990;10(2):163-166.
45. Koyama K, Higuchi F, Inoue A. Modified Chiari osteotomy for arthrosis after Perthes' disease. 14 hips followed for 2-12 years. *Acta Orthop Scand.* 1998;69(2):129-132.
46. Reddy RR, Morin C. Chiari osteotomy in Legg-Calve-Perthes disease. *J Pediatr Orthop B.* 2005;14(1):1-9.
47. Schai PA, Exner GU. Corrective Imhauser intertrochanteric osteotomy. *Oper Orthop Traumatol.* 2007;19(4):368-388.
48. Imhauser G. Late results of Imhauser's osteotomy for slipped capital femoral epiphysis (author's transl). *Z Orthop.* 1977;115(5):716-725.
49. Fish JB. Cuneiform osteotomy of the femoral neck in the treatment of slipped capital femoral epiphysis. A follow-up note. *J Bone Joint Surg Am.* 1994;76(1):46-59.
50. Ganz R, Gill TJ, Gautier E, Ganz K, Krugel N, Berlemann U. Surgical dislocation of the adult hip: a technique with full access to the femoral head and acetabulum without the risk of avascular necrosis. *J Bone Joint Surg Br.* 2001;83(8):1119-1124.
51. Voos JE, Ranawat AS, Pellicci PM, Buly RL, Salvati EA. Varus rotational osteotomies for adults with hip dysplasia: a 20-year followup. *Clin Orthop Relat Res.* 2007;457:138-143.
52. Haverkamp D, Marti RK. Bilateral varus osteotomies in hip deformities: are early interventions superior? A long-term follow-up. *Int Orthop.* 2007;31(2):185-191.
53. Ito H, Matsuno T, Minami A. Intertrochanteric varus osteotomy for osteoarthritis in patients with hip dysplasia: 6 to 28 years followup. *Clin Orthop Relat Res.* 2005;433:124-128.
54. Iwase T, Hasegawa Y, Kawamoto K, Iwasada S, Yamada K, Iwata H. Twenty years' followup of intertrochanteric osteotomy for treatment of the dysplastic hip. *Clin Orthop.* 1996;331:245-255.
55. Ansari A, Jones S, Hashemi-Nejad A, Catterall A. Varus proximal femoral osteotomy for hip dysplasia in adults. *Hip Int.* 2008;18(3):200-206.
56. Leunig M, Slongo T, Kleinschmidt M, Ganz R. Subcapital correction osteotomy in slipped capital femoral epiphysis by means of surgical hip dislocation. *Oper Orthop Traumatol.* 2007;19(4):389-410.

**11**

# Dysplasia in
# the Adult

*Martin Beck, MD*

## Introduction

Untreated acetabular dysplasia is the second most common cause of secondary osteoarthrosis of the hip after femoroacetabular impingement. Dysplasia of the hip involves morphologic alterations of the hip joint including both the acetabulum and the proximal femur. Typically, the acetabulum is too small and too steep, but often the femoral head also is affected. The insufficient cover and malorientation of the acetabulum causes overload with high shearing forces at the acetabular rim that lead to damage of the labrum and acetabular cartilage and eventually lead to osteoarthrosis (OA) of the hip.[1,2] Often, unfavorable leverages contribute to the overload and are

Ranawat A, Kelly BT. *Musculoskeletal Examination of the Hip and Knee: Making the Complex Simple* (pp. 274-290).
© 2011 SLACK Incorporated

responsible for fatiguing of the abductor musculature. There is general agreement that all dysplastic hips with subluxation evolve into OA in the second to third decade.[1] The natural history of the dysplastic hip without subluxation is not well known, but it is estimated that 40% to 50% of the patients develop OA before the age of 50 and approximately 50% have their first reconstructive surgery before the age of 60.[1,3] It was shown that hips with a lateral center-edge (LCE) angle of less than 16 degrees or an acetabular roof angle of more than 15 degrees will develop end-stage OA.[4] Surgical interventions aim to alter the natural course of degeneration.[5] Pelvic and periacetabular reorienting osteotomies have proven their efficacy in the long term.

# HISTORY

Generally, the patients are young adults with symptoms of labral pathology and pain related to overload and fatigue of the abductor musculature. Labral pathology presents as groin pain, often a sharp, knife-like pain that subsides as acutely as it presents. Mechanical symptoms like catching or blocking of the hip occur occasionally. Blocking most often is relieved by shaking or twisting the leg. Often, groin pain has an aching, more chronic character. Long sitting or walking can worsen the pain. The pain can be exacerbated by activities that involve flexion, adduction, and internal rotation of the hip, such as entering or exiting a motor vehicle or breaststroke swimming, rock climbing, and sporting activities with cutting and twisting movements. Symptoms of muscular overload range from early fatigue to apparent weakness of the abductors, with irritation at the tendinous insertion on the greater trochanter and limp.

# EXAMINATION

Physical examination of the hip includes assessment of gait, limb length, range of motion, muscle power, and some special tests (Table 11-1). Abductor strength is assessed with the Trendelenburg test and leg raise against resistance in the lateral position. Range of motion, particularly for internal rotation,

**Table 11-1**

## METHODS FOR EXAMINING THE DYSPLASTIC HIP

| Examination | Technique | Illustration | Grading | Significance |
|---|---|---|---|---|
| Impingement test | Supine patient. Passive flexion to 90 degrees, combined with adduction and internal rotation of the hip | 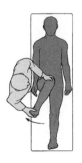 | Positive when maneuver reproduces the groin pain the patient is complaining about | Unspecific test for pathology of the acetabular rim. During the maneuver, the labrum is squeezed between the femoral neck and the bony rim. A damaged labrum will cause the typical pain |
| Apprehension test | Supine patient. The buttock is placed at the end of the examination table. The contralateral leg is maximally flexed and held to the chest by the patient. The extended leg then is externally rotated by the examiner | 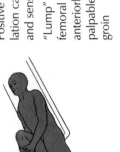 | Positive when manipulation causes discomfort and sense of instability "Lump" sign when femoral head subluxes anteriorly and becomes palpable/visible in the groin | Sign of anterior instability due to lack of anterior cover |

*(continued)*

**Table 11-1 (continued)**

## METHODS FOR EXAMINING THE DYSPLASTIC HIP

| Examination | Technique | Illustration | Grading | Significance |
|---|---|---|---|---|
| Bicycle test | Patient in lateral position. The upper leg is moved like driving a bicycle. The hand of the examiner palpates for areas of tenderness or snapping hip | | Positive when early fatigue and/or pain at the postero-superior part of the greater trochanter that can extend more proximal into the body of gluteus medius | Indicates overload of abductors as they are trying to keep the femoral head stable in the acetabulum |

often is increased in hip dysplasia. A snapping psoas tendon often is present. A lesion of the labrum is suspected if the impingement test is positive. With the patient supine, the hip is flexed to 90 degrees and, with additional internal rotation and adduction, the labrum is squeezed between the femoral neck and the acetabular rim. In the presence of a damaged labrum, this will cause the groin pain that is typical in these patients. The apprehension test may be possible in the presence of symptomatic anterior instability secondary to deficient anterior acetabular coverage. In this test, the patient lies supine, and the hip is extended, adducted, and externally rotated. Discomfort and a sense of instability are felt as the femoral head is subluxing anteriorly. In a very thin patient, the subluxing femoral head can produce a palpable and visible prominence in the inguinal region.

## PATHOANATOMY

Most often, the acetabulum not only is undersized but also maloriented with a steep acetabular roof. This results in a small inclined plane and leads to instability and migration of the femoral head, which leads to high load and shear stresses at the acetabular rim. The labrum initially hypertrophies in order to maintain the femoral head within the joint. The chronic stress may lead to fatigue failure of the labrum, which eventually is torn off the acetabular rim, sometimes with an osseous fragment.[6] Acetabular rim fractures usually occur only in the presence of bone cysts that have weakened the bony rim.[7] Histomorphologically, the labrum shows myxoid degeneration. Often, ganglion formation within the adjacent bone or soft tissues is observed. The avulsed labrum, often combined with an inside-out lesion where part of the adjacent joint cartilage is pulled off together with the labrum, leads to an increase of femoral head instability. Additionally, the joint-sealing function, which is required for cartilage lubrication and distribution of joint pressures, is also lost. This mechanically adverse situation causes an increase of joint contact pressures at the acetabular rim and is directly related to cartilage degeneration. As adaptation to the increased load, an increase of the subchondral bone density at the anterolateral acetabular rim can be observed.

# IMAGING AND DIAGNOSTIC STUDIES

## Conventional Radiography

An AP pelvic radiograph, a lateral cross-table view, and a false-profile view of the pelvis are required. The AP pelvis allows visualization of acetabular cover and version. Quite frequently, the dysplastic acetabuli additionally are retroverted. This is the case in up to one-third of the hip, and its recognition is important for planning the correction.[8] The LCE angle and the acetabular roof angle are measured. The former normally is 20 to 25 degrees, and the latter is 0 to 10 degrees. Superolateral migration of the femoral head can be seen by the increasing distance from the tear drop compared to the other side and a break of Shenton's line. This is suspicious for femoral head instability; however, Shenton's line can also be broken in the presence of a deformed femoral head (eg, with Perthes-like deformities). The false-profile view permits evaluation of the anterior acetabular coverage (anterior center edge angle, normally 20 to 25 degrees) and anterior migration or subluxation of the femoral head. The lateral cross-table view gives information about femoral torsion and head-neck offset (Table 11-2). Finally, anteroposterior abduction radiographs are necessary to assess the joint congruency that can be achieved with reorientation of the acetabulum and the potential need for a concomitant femoral osteotomy.[4]

## Magnetic Resonance Arthrography

Magnetic resonance arthrography (MRA) currently is the method of choice for imaging soft tissue structures of the hip joint. The application of intra-articular gadolinium-diethylenetriamine penta-acetic acid (DTPA) as a contrast agent allows improved visualization of the acetabular labrum and the cartilage surface of the hip. The technique includes high-field-strength magnetic resonance imaging and use of surface coils. In addition to standard T1- and T2-weighted sagittal oblique and coronal oblique images, MRA includes proton-weighted radial sequencing in the axis of the femoral neck. This has the advantage that the acetabular and femoral articular cartilage, as well as the labrum, is visualized orthogonally at any point around the circumference of the acetabular rim and femoral head.[9]

**Table 11-2**

## *HELPFUL HINTS*

*Imaging*

| VIEW | TECHNICAL ASPECTS | FINDINGS | RADIOGRAPH | MEASUREMENTS |
|------|-------------------|----------|------------|--------------|
| AP pelvis | Center beam pointed at mid-distance between line connecting anterior superior iliac spines and symphysis pubis | Estimation of acetabular cover<br><br>Anterior, posterior wall<br><br>Version of acetabulum | 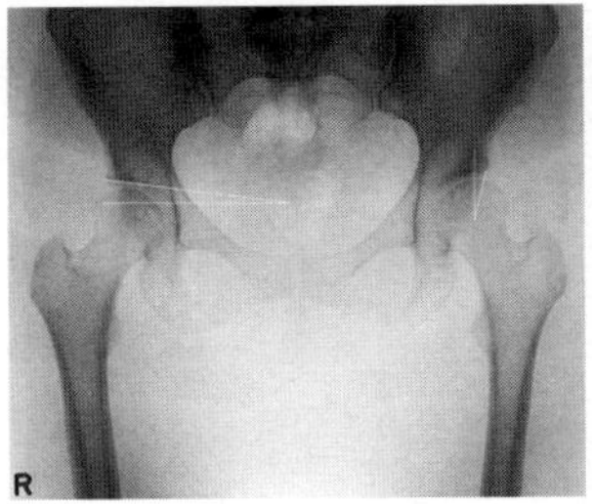 | Lateral center edge (LCE) angle (left hip) between vertical line and line between center of rotation and lateral end of the roof. Dysplastic LCE <20 degrees, borderline 20 to 25 degrees, normal 25 degrees<br><br>Acetabular roof angle (right hip) between a horizontal line and line passing through the most medial and most lateral end of the subchondral sclerosis of the roof (sourcil). Dysplastic >10 degrees, normal 0 to 10 degrees |

*(continued)*

**Table 11-2 (continued)**

## HELPFUL HINTS

| VIEW | TECHNICAL ASPECTS | FINDINGS | RADIOGRAPH | MEASUREMENTS |
|------|-------------------|----------|------------|--------------|
| False profile (faux profile or Lequesne view) | Patient standing obliquely as shown in the schematic below. The affected hip is adjacent to the x-ray plate, the foot parallel to it. The beam is directed to the femoral head 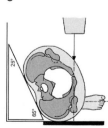 | Estimation of anterior acetabular cover<br><br>In a correct false profile, the distance between the 2 femoral heads approximately corresponds to the size of one head | 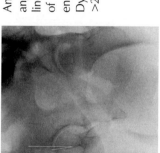 | Anterior centre edge (ACE) angle: Angle between vertical line and line from the center of rotation and the anterior end of the sclerosis of the roof. Dysplastic <25 degrees, normal >25 degrees |

(continued)

## Table 11-2 (continued)

### HELPFUL HINTS

| VIEW | TECHNICAL ASPECTS | FINDINGS | RADIOGRAPH | MEASUREMENTS |
|---|---|---|---|---|
| Lateral cross-table view | Patient supine. Affected hip extended, with patella pointing upward. Other leg is lifted and placed on a holder to permit the oblique course of the x-ray beam | Estimation of anterior offset problems Visualization of antetorsion | | A value for anterior offset is the so-called angle α. It is formed by a line in the axis of the femoral neck and a line from the center of rotation to the point where the femoral neck extrudes the circle around the femoral head. The normal value is between 43 and 50 degrees Antetorsion is the angle between the femoral shaft axis and the femoral neck axis |

Besides the analysis for cartilage defects of the femoral head and acetabulum, the presence of labral lesions, inside-out lesions, and subluxation of the femoral head that allows crescent-shaped pooling of the contrast agent between femoral head and posterior acetabulum are evaluated. Inside-out lesions are lesions of the acetabular rim, where a variable part of the acetabular cartilage is torn off the acetabular rim together with the labrum. Depending on the size of the cartilage damage, the prognosis can be impaired.

# TREATMENT

The goal of pelvic osteotomy is to change the acetabular orientation to optimize the joint mechanics by increasing the weight-bearing area and by transforming shearing forces into compressive forces.[5,10] Coverage of the femoral head can be increased either by augmentation of the acetabular roof or by changing spatial orientation of the acetabulum. Augmentation procedures such as the Chiari osteotomy and the shelf procedure reduce joint-loading forces by augmenting the weight-bearing area of the joint. With both methods, lateral osseous coverage can be improved; however, the posterior aspect of the femoral head often remains uncovered. The interposed capsule undergoes metaplastic transformation to fibrocartilage. The labrum remains within the main weight-bearing area, and a high failure rate was reported when the labrum was torn. Compared with hyaline cartilage, fibrocartilage has inferior mechanical properties for withstanding axial loading. While augmentation procedures can provide reliable pain relief for some years, they should be regarded as salvage procedures in cases where congruency of the joint cannot be achieved. Today, reorienting acetabular procedures are the treatment of choice for the dysplastic hip. Reorienting procedures change the orientation of the acetabular articular surface, thereby correcting the area of deficiency. This provides greater surface area for load transmission while re-establishing or maintaining stability of the joint. In reorientation procedures, coverage is achieved with hyaline cartilage supported by subchondral bone, which has optimal mechanical

**Figure 11-1.** After completing the approach, the first step is the osteotomy of the ischium from anterior. As part of the modified Smith-Petersen approach, the anterior superior iliac spine is osteotomized.

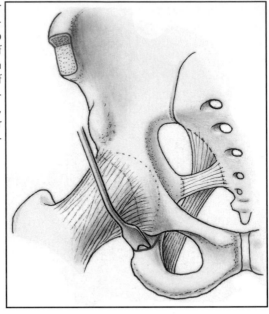

qualities for weight-bearing. Reorientation procedures include single, double, and triple osteotomies as well as spherical and periacetabular osteotomies.[5] Inherent drawbacks of those osteotomies are limited range of displacement, potential narrowing of the pelvic cavity, and the need for substantial internal fixation as some techniques create a discontinuity of the pelvic ring. Medialization of the joint is difficult to achieve, and some have an intra-articular course. To avoid these disadvantages, the Bernese periacetabular osteotomy was developed[10] (Figures 11-1 through 11-3). The polygonally shaped juxta-articular osteotomy respects the vascular blood supply to the acetabular fragment.[11,12] It facilitates extensive acetabular reorientation, including correction of version and mediolateral displacement. The posterior column remains intact, which protects the sciatic nerve and enables minimal internal fixation (Figures 11-4 and 11-5). The dimensions of the true pelvis remain unchanged, permitting unimpaired vaginal delivery. All steps of the acetabular osteotomy are performed with use of the modified Smith-Petersen approach.

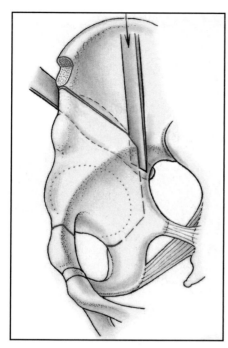

**Figure 11-2.** After completion of the partial ischial and the pubic osteotomy, the supra-acetabular and the retroacetabular osteotomy are performed.

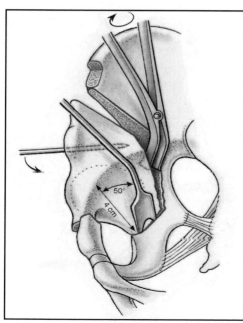

**Figure 11-3.** After completion of the infra-acetabular osteotomy that connects the first ischial osteotomy with the retroacetabular osteotomy, the acetabular fragment is completely mobile and can be maneuvered into the desired position. Note that the posterior column remains intact.

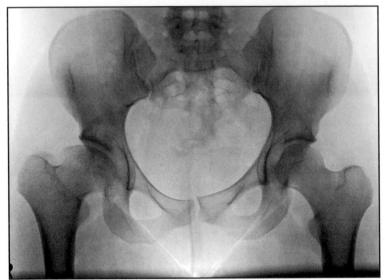

**Figure 11-4.** Preoperative radiograph of a 22-year-old woman with a dysplastic right hip and Perthes-like deformity of her right hip.

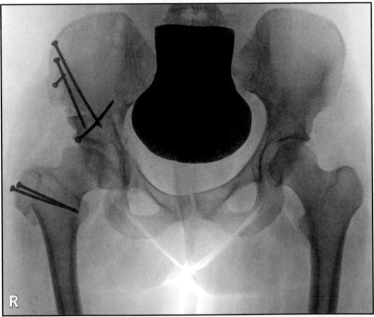

**Figure 11-5.** Same patient after right PAO and surgical dislocation of the hip with osteochondroplasty of the head-neck junction and advancement of the greater trochanter.

In addition, the Smith-Petersen approach allows an anterior capsulotomy for inspection and correction of labral pathology and for a potential femoroacetabular impingement.[13]

## POSTOPERATIVE REHABILITATION

The leg is positioned in a foam splint. Mobilization is started at the first or second postoperative day with 2 crutches. Touch-down weight-bearing of approximately 10 to 15 kg is maintained for 8 weeks. At this time, physiotherapy is limited to instruction and surveillance of proper gait and partial weight-bearing. Lifting of the leg while in a supine position is not allowed for 6 weeks (reattached hip flexors). After 8 weeks, when signs of bony union are present, progressive weight-bearing is started together with strengthening exercises of hip abductors. Physiotherapy now is directed to gain back normal strength and coordination. Three months postoperatively, walking without a limp and a cane should be possible.

## RESULTS

Long-term outcome depends on the preoperative stage of joint degeneration and the congruency present after the correction.[14-16] In hip joints with Grade 0 or 1 degeneration (Tönnis classification), good to excellent outcome was reported in 88%.[15] There is general agreement that unfavorable outcome is associated with older age of the patient, moderate to severe joint degeneration at surgery, labral lesions, and suboptimal correction that may cause femoroacetabular impingement. The presence of joint degeneration is correlated with a significantly worse outcome.[15-17]

There are several short-term outcome reports from various centers.[17-20] The results are remarkably consistent and can be summarized as follows: patients with minimal to moderate arthritic changes usually achieve pain relief and improved function. However, patients with advanced radiographic degenerative changes have less predictable success.

## COMPLICATIONS

Besides the usual surgical risks, such as bleeding, thrombosis, embolism, and infection, there are some additional risks related to the surgical approach, the osteotomy, and the after treatment.[21,22]

Risks associated with the approach include avulsion of reattached muscles (sartorius, rectus femoris), injury to vessels (obturator artery, medial femoral circumflex artery) and nerves (lateral femorocutaneous nerve, obturator nerve, femoral nerve, sciatic nerve), and heterotopic ossification. The most common complication is some damage to the lateral femorocutaneous nerve, because of its highly variable course in the area of the ASIS. The patient has to be advised that numbness of the proximal lateral thigh may occur. Other nerve lesions are rare. Heterotopic ossification is observed around the origin of the rectus femoris muscle. This ossification may cause an extra-articular impingement with painful limitation of flexion.

Complications associated with the osteotomy include intra-articular osteotomy, fracture of the posterior column, under- or overcorrection, loss of fixation, and delayed or nonunion.

Proud screw heads at the iliac crest may cause tenderness and may have to be removed.

In the postoperative course, premature weight-bearing can lead to loss of correction. Surgical revision is advised as soon as possible to realign the acetabular fragment. A slight decrease in the overall range of motion occurs not as a complication but as a consequence of the increased coverage of the femoral head.

## CONCLUSION

The suspicion of the diagnosis of hip dysplasia is based on good history and correct examination seeking for symptoms and signs for dysplasia. The diagnosis is confirmed by conventional radiography, and MRA is the method of choice to visualize intra-articular soft tissue pathologies. The Bernese periacetabular osteotomy is currently the most powerful technique for the correction of the dysplastic hip.

# REFERENCES

1. Cooperman DR, Wallensten R, Stulberg SD. Acetabular dysplasia in the adult. *Clin Orthop Rel Res.* 1983;175:79-85.
2. Weinstein SL. Natural history of congenital hip dislocation (CDH) and hip dysplasia. *Clin Orthop Rel Res.* 1987;225:62-76.
3. Harris WH. Etiology of osteoarthritis of the hip. *Clin Orthop Rel Res.* 1986;213:20-33.
4. Murphy SB, Ganz R, Müller ME. The prognosis in untreated dysplasia of the hip. A study of radiographic factors that predict the outcome. *J Bone Joint Surg Am.* 1995;77:985-989.
5. Leunig M, Siebenrock KA, Ganz R. Rationale of periacetabular osteotomy and background work. *J Bone Joint Surg Am.* 2001;83:438-448.
6. Klaue K, Durnin CW, Ganz R. The acetabular rim syndrome. A clinical presentation of dysplasia of the hip. *J Bone Joint Surg Br.* 1991;73:423-429.
7. Mast JW, Mayo KA, Chosa E, Berlemann U, Ganz R. The acetabular rim fracture: a variant of the acetabular rim syndrome. *Sem Arthroplasty.* 1997;8:97-101.
8. Mast JW, Brunner RL, Zebrack J. Recognizing acetabular version in the radiographic presentation of hip dysplasia. *Clin Orthop Rel Res.* 2004;418:48-53.
9. Werlen S, Leunig M, Ganz R. Magnetic resonance arthrography of the hip in femoroacetabular impingement: technique and findings. *Oper Tech Orthop.* 2005;15:191-203.
10. Ganz R, Klaue K, Vinh TS, Mast JW. A new periacetabular osteotomy for the treatment of hip dysplasias. Technique and preliminary results. *Clin Orthop Rel Res.* 1988;232:26-36.
11. Beck M, Leunig M, Ellis T, Sledge JB, Ganz R. The acetabular blood supply: implications for periacetabular osteotomies. *Surg Radiol Anat.* 2003;25:361-367.
12. Hempfing A, Leunig M, Nötzli HP, Beck M, Ganz R. Acetabular blood flow during Bernese periacetabular osteotomy: an intraoperative study using laser Doppler flowmetry. *J Orthop Res.* 2003;21:1145-1150.
13. Myers SR, Eijer H, Ganz R. Anterior femoroacetabular impingement after periacetabular osteotomy. *Clin Orthop Rel Res.* 1999;363:93-99.
14. Sharifi E, Sharifi H, Morshed S, Bozic K, Diab M. Cost-effectiveness analysis of periacetabular osteotomy. *J Bone Joint Surg Am.* 2008;90:1447-1456.
15. Siebenrock KA, Schöll E, Lottenbach M, Ganz R. Bernese periacetabular osteotomy. *Clin Orthop Rel Res.* 1999;363:9-20.
16. Steppacher SD, Tannast M, Ganz R, Siebenrock KA. Mean 20-year followup of Bernese periacetabular osteotomy. *Clin Orthop Rel Res.* 2008;466:1633-1644.
17. Murphy S, Deshmukh R. Periacetabular osteotomy: preoperative radiographic predictors of outcome. *Clin Orthop Rel Res.* 2002;405:168-174.

18. Clohisy JC, Barrett SE, Gordon JE, Delgado ED, Schoenecker PL. Periacetabular osteotomy for the treatment of severe acetabular dysplasia. *J Bone Joint Surg Am.* 2005;87:254-259.
19. Crockarell J Jr, Trousdale RT, Cabanela ME, Berry DJ. Early experience and results with the periacetabular osteotomy. The Mayo Clinic experience. *Clin Orthop Rel Res.* 1999;363:45-53.
20. Trousdale RT, Ekkernkamp A, Ganz R, Wallrichs SL. Periacetabular and intertrochanteric osteotomy for the treatment of osteoarthrosis in dysplastic hips. *J Bone Joint Surg Am.* 1995;77:73-85.
21. Davey JP, Santore RF. Complications of periacetabular osteotomy. *Clin Orthop Rel Res.* 1999;363:33-37.
22. Hussel JG, Rodriguez JA, Ganz R. Technical complications of the Bernese periacetabular osteotomy. *Clin Orthop Rel Res.* 1999;363:81-92.

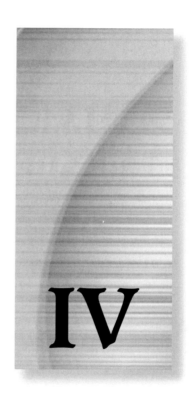

# IV

## Common Conditions of the Knee

# 12

# ANTERIOR CRUCIATE LIGAMENT INJURIES

*Andrew K. Wong, MD; Eric J. Kropf, MD;*
*and Freddie H. Fu, MD, DSc(Hon), DPs(Hon)*

Anterior cruciate ligament (ACL) injury is extremely common, with estimates of more than 200,000 injuries and 100,000 ACL reconstructions performed annually in the United States. With an ever-increasing number of young participants in athletic activities, a comprehensive understanding of the pathophysiology and treatment options of the injured ACL is crucial. Management of ACL injuries is an evolving discipline that continues to improve through basic science and clinical research focused on more accurately defining ACL anatomy, advancing surgical techniques, and detailed assessment of clinical outcomes.

Although the history and physical examination remain the key elements of the clinical evaluation, more sophisticated

Ranawat A, Kelly BT. *Musculoskeletal Examination of the Hip and Knee: Making the Complex Simple* (pp. 292-310).
© 2011 SLACK Incorporated

imaging techniques have aided physicians in more precise diagnosis and proper management of ACL injuries. Specifically, high-resolution magnetic resonance imaging (MRI) can be used to accurately diagnose partial injuries or single-bundle (anteromedial [AM] or posterolateral [PL]) tears.[1] Similarly, treatment approaches have evolved significantly during the past few decades. Traditionally, single-bundle ACL reconstruction has been performed using allograft or autograft via a single-incision, transtibial drilling technique. Recent literature has suggested that this method of ACL reconstruction commonly positions the graft in a "high" or nonanatomic position within the femoral notch.[2-4] Biodynamic studies of knees during functional activities have revealed that this technique does not restore normal knee kinematics.[5] Further, a long-term meta-analysis and prospective clinical control study suggest that traditional single-bundle techniques result in residual instability, pain, and development of degenerative arthritis.[6,7] The shortcomings of traditional single-bundle surgery have led to the development of double-bundle surgery to attempt to more accurately restore the anatomy of the native ACL. Studies have suggested that double-bundle ACL reconstruction more closely restores normal knee biomechanics when compared to single-bundle ACL reconstruction.[8,9] Recent emphasis in the field of ACL reconstruction has been placed on the concept of anatomic ACL reconstruction, which better restores the anatomy and kinematics of the normal knee.[10-12] Anatomic reconstruction techniques (either single- or double-bundle) emphasize close attention to the unique anatomy of each individual, allowing the surgeon to reconstruct the ACL in the exact anatomic position of the native uninjured ligament.

Drawing from the most recent literature, this chapter will describe the current evaluation and management principles of ACL injury.

# HISTORY

Like most other illnesses and injuries, a detailed history and meticulous physical exam are vital for the diagnosis and treatment planning of ACL injuries. The ACL is most commonly injured via low-energy noncontact motions of the knee such as cutting, rotation, and deceleration. ACL injuries may also result from direct trauma. The mechanism of injury is important to discern, as certain mechanisms will be strongly associated with injury to other structures, such as the medial and lateral collateral ligaments, menisci, and/or patella. The classic presentation of ACL rupture is an audible "pop" followed by pain and swelling of the knee joint. Instability is a common complaint for patients with a chronically ACL-deficient knee joint. Locking or "catching" of the knee does not suggest ACL rupture, but is more commonly associated with meniscal injury.

## EXAMINATION

Physical examination should begin with a general assessment of the patient's body habitus and continue toward a focus on the affected knee joint (Table 12-1). The lower extremity examination should begin with gait analysis and assessment of varus-valgus alignment. Following this, a general knee exam may be performed including visual inspection, palpation for abnormalities and tenderness, active and passive range of motion, and neurovascular testing. Effusion and pain may limit the range of motion in an acute setting. However, the clinician should be aware of possible mechanical obstructions such as a displaced bucket-handle meniscal tear, loose osteochondral fragments, or ACL remnant tissue.

Following the general examinations above, ACL-specific examinations may be performed. Using the uninjured contralateral knee as reference, several tests are performed to assess the integrity of the ACL. The Lachman test is considered the most reliable and sensitive test for evaluation of ACL injury. The Lachman test is performed with the knee at 20 to 30 degrees of flexion and neutral rotation. One hand should stabilize the femur, while the other hand applies an anterior translation force on the proximal tibia. A grade for this test is assigned based on the degree of anterior translation of the tibial plateau:

- Grade I: <5 mm anterior displacement
- Grade II: 5 to 10 mm anterior displacement
- Grade III: >10 mm anterior displacement

**Table 12-1**

## METHODS FOR EXAMINING THE ANTERIOR CRUCIATE LIGAMENT

| Examination | Technique | Illustration | Grading | Significance |
|---|---|---|---|---|
| Lachman | Anterior transla-tion of the tibia at 30 degrees of knee flexion | 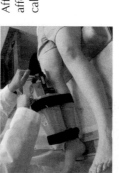 | I: <5 mm anterior dis-placement<br>II: 5 to 10 mm anterior displacement<br>III: >10 mm anterior dis-placement<br><br>A: Firm endpoint<br>B: Soft endpoint | Increased displacement compared to the normal contralateral knee is suggestive of ACL injury. Additionally, a soft end-point also contributes to a diagnosis of ACL injury |
| KT-2000 Arthrometer | Anterior transla-tion of the tibia at 30 degrees of knee flexion | | Affected side to non-affected side difference calculated in mm | <3 mm side-to-side difference is considered normal |

(continued)

**Table 12-1 (continued)**

## METHODS FOR EXAMINING THE ANTERIOR CRUCIATE LIGAMENT

| Examination | Technique | Illustration | Grading | Significance |
|---|---|---|---|---|
| Anterior drawer | Anterior translation of the tibia at 90 degrees of knee flexion with the foot secured | 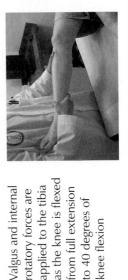 | I: <5 mm anterior displacement<br>II: 5 to 10 mm anterior displacement<br>III: >10 mm anterior displacement<br><br>A: Firm endpoint<br>B: Soft endpoint | Increased displacement compared to the normal contralateral knee is suggestive of ACL injury. Additionally, a soft endpoint also contributes to a diagnosis of ACL injury |
| Pivot shift | Valgus and internal rotatory forces are applied to the tibia as the knee is flexed from full extension to 40 degrees of knee flexion | | I: Glide<br>II: Shift<br>III: Transient lock with gross shift | Positive test is indicative of rotational instability, suggesting injury to the PL bundle of the ACL |

*(continued)*

**Table 12-1 (continued)**

## METHODS FOR EXAMINING THE ANTERIOR CRUCIATE LIGAMENT

| Examination | Technique | Illustration | Grading | Significance |
|---|---|---|---|---|
| Range of motion | Examine at full flexion and full extension | 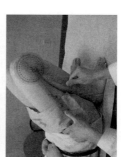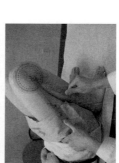 | Measured in degrees using a goniometer | Restoration of nearly normal ROM is recommended before surgery |

The quality of the endpoint should also be determined. A firm endpoint is assigned Grade A, while a soft endpoint is given Grade B. So, by convention, if a patient has 5 to 10 mm of translation and a soft endpoint, the Lachman test is graded IIB. A quantitative and standardized measure of anteroposterior knee laxity may also be performed using a KT-2000 arthrometer. With the knee at 20 to 30 degrees of flexion, a side-to-side difference of 2 mm or less is considered normal.[13]

The anterior drawer test is performed with the knee at 90 degrees of flexion. With the patient's foot stabilized, an anterior translation force is applied to the proximal tibia. The degree of translation and quality of the endpoint is again determined. The anterior drawer test is graded similar to the Lachman test (I, II, III; A or B).

The pivot-shift test begins with the hip held in slight abduction and the knee in full extension. A valgus and internal rotation force is applied to the knee as it is passively flexed. When the ACL-deficient knee is flexed to approximately 20 degrees, the tibia reduces from its anteriorly subluxed and internally rotated position, thus producing the "pivot shift." Note that this maneuver may be difficult to perform on the patient in the clinical setting due to guarding and hamstring spasm. During examination under anesthesia, the pivot shift test is an invaluable and sensitive tool.[14,15] Grading for the pivot-shift test is as follows:

- Grade I: Glide
- Grade II: Shift
- Grade III: Transient lock with gross shift

Range of motion is also important to assess both before and after knee ligament surgery. If surgery is performed during the acute phase when the patient's knee is still severely swollen and motion is restricted, the risk of postoperative complications and delayed rehabilitation is greatly increased. It is generally recommended that patients undergo preoperative physical therapy to reduce joint effusion, improve range of motion, and strengthen quadriceps and hamstring musculature prior to proceeding with ligament reconstruction.[16]

# PATHOANATOMY

Anatomy is the basis of orthopedic surgery. Whether evaluating ACL injury or considering ACL reconstruction, a thorough understanding of normal anatomy is critical. The femoral origin of the ligament is located on the posterior aspect of the medial wall of the lateral femoral condyle. The ligament inserts on the tibia between the medial and lateral tibial spines. Importantly, the ACL fibers fan out as they course from the mid-substance of the ligament toward the femoral and tibial insertions. Thus, the insertion site cross-sectional areas are significantly larger than that of the mid-substance ligament.[17]

Anatomic studies have shown that the ACL consists of 2 distinct bundles: the anteromedial (AM) and posterolateral (PL) bundles, named for their relative insertion locations on the tibia (Figure 12-1).[17] Additionally, each bundle exhibits varying tension at different knee flexion angles. The AM bundle is taught in flexion, while the PL bundle is taught in extension.[18] Though the 2 bundles work in conjunction to provide anteroposterior and rotational stability to the knee joint, the PL bundle has been found to largely contribute to the rotational stability of the knee (Table 12-2).[18]

To ensure anatomic tunnel positioning during ACL reconstruction surgery, it is necessary to identify the insertion sites of the ACL (Figure 12-2). On the femoral side, with the knee in 90 degrees of flexion, the insertion site is located in the lower one-third of the medial wall of the lateral condyle. Two bony prominences provide landmarks for identifying the insertion area. First, the lateral intercondylar ridge marks the superior border of the femoral insertion area. Second, the lateral bifurcate ridge separates the AM and PL bundles. On the tibial side, the ACL insertion area lies between the medial and lateral tibial spines, anterior to the retroeminence ridge, and medial to the anterior horn of the lateral meniscus.[19]

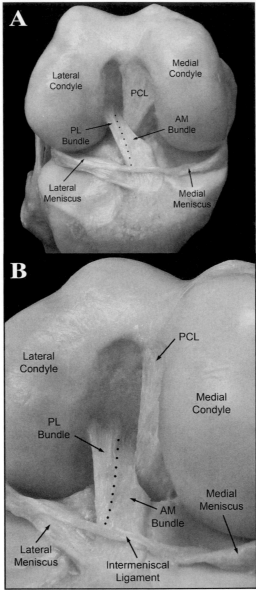

**Figure 12-1.** Cadaveric dissection of the right knee, depicting normal anatomy of the ACL and surrounding structures from (A) anterior and (B) anteromedial views. The AM and PL bundles are separated by a dotted line.

## Table 12-2

### HELPFUL HINTS: ANTERIOR CRUCIATE LIGAMENT AND SURROUNDING ANATOMY

| Anatomical Structure | Function |
| --- | --- |
| AM bundle | Predominantly restricts anterior translation of the tibia relative to the femur |
| PL bundle | Predominantly restricts internal rotation of the tibia relative to the femur |
| Lateral intercondylar ridge | Serves as the anterior border of the ACL on the medial wall of the lateral condyle |
| Lateral bifurcate ridge | Serves as the border between the AM and PL bundle insertions on the medial wall of the lateral condyle |

### Imaging

| IMAGE | FUNCTION | FINDINGS |
| --- | --- | --- |
| Plain radiographs (x-rays) | Anteroposterior 30 degrees flexion lateral patellofemoral view | Segond fracture<br>Degenerative changes<br>Tibial eminence avulsion fracture (pediatric population) |
| Magnetic resonance imaging (MRI) | Sagittal/oblique sagittal Coronal/oblique coronal | Bone bruise pattern<br>Complete or partially torn ligament |
| Three-dimensional computed tomography (3-D CT) | Medial wall of lateral femoral condyle Tibial plateau | Previous bone tunnel position<br>Lateral intercondylar ridge<br>Lateral bifurcate ridge |

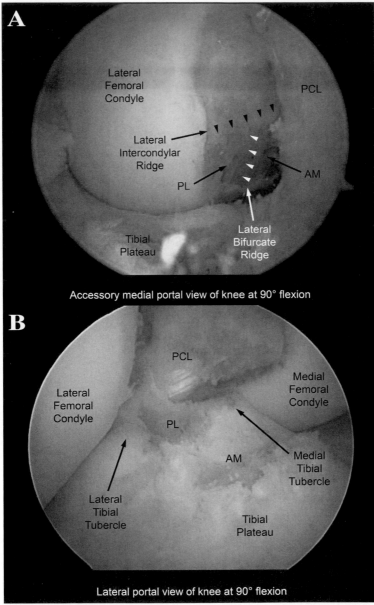

**Figure 12-2.** Arthroscopic images of the right knee at 90 degrees of flexion: (A) the relative position of insertion sites (AM and PL) and bony landmarks/ridges is well-depicted on the femoral side when viewed from the accessory medial portal. (B) The tibial landmarks are best viewed from the high lateral portal.

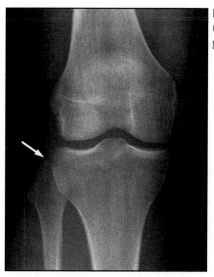

**Figure 12-3.** Segond fracture (arrow) seen on AP plain radiograph of the right knee.

# IMAGING

For any acutely injured knee, plain radiographs should be the first imaging study performed (see Table 12-2). The standard knee series consisting of anteroposterior flexion, 30 degrees lateral, and "Merchant" or "sunrise" views are sufficient in most cases. When appropriate, a longstanding cassette is added to assess lower extremity overall alignment. A Segond fracture, defined as a posterolateral capsular avulsion from the tibia, is considered to be pathognomonic for ACL injury and can be seen on plain x-rays (Figure 12-3).[20,21] Degenerative osteoarthritic changes evident on plain radiographs may indicate chronic ACL deficiency.[22] For pediatric patients, x-rays are important to evaluate for possible tibial eminence avulsion fracture and to assess the status of the physes.

Following plain radiographs, magnetic resonance imaging (MRI) is typically performed when ligamentous knee injury is suspected. MRI has a reported sensitivity of greater than 90% for acute ACL tears.[23] To aid in the visualization of the 2-bundle anatomy and identification of partial or single-bundle tears of the ACL, it is useful to obtain oblique sagittal and

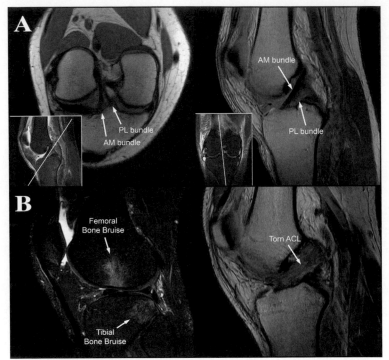

**Figure 12-4.** MRI of the (A) normal ACL with oblique sagittal and oblique coronal cuts, and (B) torn ACL, single sagittal view and typical bone bruise pattern.

oblique coronal MRI cuts that are oriented parallel to the ACL (Figure 12-4A). The MRI also provides other important information. A pathognomonic bone bruise pattern that occurs with acute ACL injury is commonly seen. The bone bruise involves the posterior one-third of the lateral tibial plateau and the middle one-third of the lateral femoral condyle (Figure 12-4B). In addition, associated injury of the PCL, posterolateral corner, collateral ligaments, extensor mechanism, menisci, and articular cartilage can be readily assessed with MRI.

CT scan with 3-D reconstruction of the bony anatomy has recently shown promise as a useful preoperative tool for revision ACL reconstruction cases (Figure 12-5). Accurate assessment of previous bone tunnel position can aid in surgical planning, providing valuable information for revision cases.

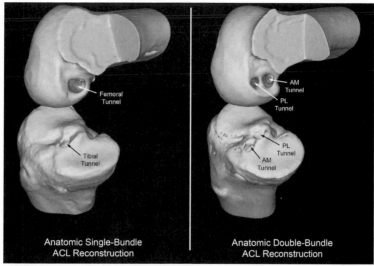

**Figure 12-5.** 3-D CT bone models of anatomic single-bundle and double-bundle ACL reconstructions. Note: Right knee positioned at 90 degrees flexion with the medial femoral condyle subtracted.

Specifically, one can determine whether the previous tunnels can be reused or if they preclude single-stage ACL reconstruction. An ongoing study at the University of Pittsburgh is demonstrating the utility of 3-D CT scan as a tool to assess anatomic bone tunnel position in patients having undergone ACL reconstruction.

# TREATMENT

## Nonoperative Management

Isolated ACL injuries may be treated conservatively depending on several factors, including severity of pain, stability, and the patient's desired activity level. Initial treatment includes assisted weight-bearing and range of motion exercises. Quadriceps and hamstring strengthening exercises are useful to achieve greater stability. If the patient ultimately chooses nonoperative management, then activities involving high-energy cutting motions or other excessive loading of the knee joint must be avoided. It is important to inform patients that there is a high likelihood of recurrent episodes of instability, especially in young, active patients who attempt to return to pre-injury–level sports and activities.[24,25] In addition, each episode of instability risks further damage to the menisci and articular cartilage, and in the unstable knee, the risk of later degenerative changes is high.[26] Thus, surgical management is recommended for patients who wish to maintain active lifestyle levels.

## Operative Management

ACL reconstruction (ACL-R) has evolved from open knee surgery in the 1980s to arthroscopic-assisted surgery starting in the 1990s. Despite variation in technique, several principles remain the same, including appropriate graft selection, graft fixation, graft incorporation/biologic healing, and structured rehabilitation. Most recently, the trend of ACL-R has focused on more accurate anatomic positioning of bone tunnels. Specifically, anatomic ACL reconstruction pays particular attention to the unique anatomy of each individual patient and then attempts to most closely recreate the native anatomy. Though countless surgical techniques for ACL reconstruction have been described, the basic principle should remain constant: the restoration of native anatomy. Regardless of the graft selected or fixation device employed, careful attention must be directed to identification of the native ACL insertion sites and bony landmarks, which will guide anatomic tunnel placement.

### Graft Selection

There are multiple graft options, each with its own set of advantages and disadvantages based on biomechanical properties, healing, donor site morbidity, fixation strength, and time to returning to sports/activities. These factors, in addition to patient age, activity level, and related injuries, must be taken into account when choosing the appropriate graft.

Bone-patellar tendon-bone autografts tend to provide stronger initial fixation due to direct bone-to-bone healing.[27] However, BPTB autograft is contraindicated in patients with patellofemoral chondrosis, extensor mechanism malalignment, or narrow patellar tendon width.[28] Potential complications of patellar tendon harvest include patella fracture,[29] postoperative anterior knee pain, and quadriceps weakness.[30,31] On the other hand, hamstring autografts afford no risk of trauma to the extensor mechanism; however, tendon-to-bone healing is significantly slower, and postoperative protocols should be adjusted accordingly.[32]

Allograft options include bone-patellar tendon-bone, Achilles allograft, and soft tissue allografts, such as tibialis anterior, tibialis posterior, and semitendinosus tendons. The advantage of allograft tissue is the lack of donor site morbidity, smaller incisions, and less postoperative pain.[33,34] Recent studies have shown that allografts require greater time to graft incorporation and have potentially higher revision rates.[35,36] Patients should be counseled regarding the extremely uncommon but potential risk of disease transmission or immune reaction to foreign tissue.[33,37] Also, allograft has higher costs and, in some regions of the world, limited availability. Despite these disadvantages, allograft is often used in revision cases when autograft has been harvested previously, or in cases where autograft will not yield a large enough graft. Other factors such as multi-ligamentous knee injury, patient age older than 30 years, or work conditions/activities requiring kneeling are relative contraindications to the use of autograft tissue.

After ACL reconstruction, the knee is placed in a hinged knee brace for a total of 6 weeks, with the first week locked in full extension. Immediately following surgery, continuous passive motion is started from 0 to 45 degrees of flexion, increasing by 10 degrees each day. Crutches are used for the first postoperative month, and the patient may bear weight as tolerated. At 12 weeks after surgery, patients are typically allowed to begin supervised noncutting and nontwisting activities, such as straight line light running, bicycling, and swimming. Return to full activity and sports is gradually allowed at 7 to 9 months postoperatively.

# CONCLUSION

ACL injury is increasingly common. Anatomical, biological, biomechanical, and kinematic studies have led to improved management of the acutely injured ACL. Still, there remains room for continued improvement in the evaluation, treatment, and assessment of clinical outcomes for the ACL-deficient patient. The principle of anatomy, which forms the basis of orthopedic surgery, drives the treatment of ACL injury. Restoration of knee function and return to full unlimited activity continues to be the ultimate goal for the management of our patients.

# REFERENCES

1. Steckel H, Vadala G, Davis D, Musahl V, Fu FH. 3-T MR imaging of partial ACL tears: a cadaver study. *Knee Surg Sports Traumatol Arthrosc.* 2007;15(9):1066-1071.
2. Dargel J, Schmidt-Wiethoff R, Fischer S, et al. Femoral bone tunnel placement using the transtibial tunnel or the anteromedial portal in ACL reconstruction: a radiographic evaluation. *Knee Surg Sports Traumatol Arthrosc.* 2009;17(3):220-227.
3. Gavriilidis I, Motsis EK, Pakos EE, et al. Transtibial versus anteromedial portal of the femoral tunnel in ACL reconstruction: a cadaveric study. *Knee.* 2008;15(5):364-367.
4. Kaseta MK, DeFrate LE, Charnock BL, Sullivan RT, Garrett WE. Reconstruction technique affects femoral tunnel placement in ACL reconstruction. *Clin Orthop Relat Res.* 2008;466(6):1467-1474.
5. Tashman S, Collon D, Anderson K, Kolowich P, Anderst W. Abnormal rotational knee motion during running after anterior cruciate ligament reconstruction. *Am J Sports Med.* 2004;32(4):975-983.
6. Biau DJ, Tournoux C, Katsahian S, Schranz P, Nizard R. ACL reconstruction: a meta-analysis of functional scores. *Clin Orthop Relat Res.* 2007;458:180-187.
7. Fithian DC, Paxton EW, Stone ML, et al. Prospective trial of a treatment algorithm for the management of the anterior cruciate ligament-injured knee. *Am J Sports Med.* 2005;33(3):335-346.
8. Ishibashi Y, Tsuda E, Fukuda A, Tsukada H, Toh S. Stability evaluation of single-bundle and double-bundle reconstruction during navigated ACL reconstruction. *Sports Med Arthrosc.* 2008;16(2):77-83.
9. Siebold R, Dehler C, Ellert T. Prospective randomized comparison of double-bundle versus single-bundle anterior cruciate ligament reconstruction. *Arthroscopy.* 2008;24(2):137-145.
10. Zantop T, Diermann N, Schumacher T, et al. Anatomical and non-anatomical double-bundle anterior cruciate ligament reconstruction: importance of femoral tunnel location on knee kinematics. *Am J Sports Med.* 2008;36(4):678-685.
11. Musahl V, Plakseychuk A, VanScyoc A, et al. Varying femoral tunnels between the anatomical footprint and isometric positions: effect on kinematics of the anterior cruciate ligament-reconstructed knee. *Am J Sports Med.* 2005;33(5):712-718.

12. Yagi M, Wong EK, Kanamori A, et al. Biomechanical analysis of an anatomic anterior cruciate ligament reconstruction. *Am J Sports Med.* 2002;30(5):660-666.

13. Bach BR, Warren RF, Wickiewicz TL. The pivot shift phenomenon: results and description of a modified clinical test for anterior cruciate ligament insufficiency. *Am J Sports Med.* 1988;16(6):571-576.

14. Hefti F, Müller W, Jakob RP, Stäubli HU. Evaluation of knee ligament injuries with the IKDC form. *Knee Surg Sports Traumatol Arthrosc.* 1993;1(3-4):226-234.

15. Malanga GA, Andrus S, Nadler SF, McLean J. Physical examination of the knee: a review of the original test description and scientific validity of common orthopedic tests. *Arch Phys Med Rehabil.* 2003;84(4):592-603.

16. Harner CD, Irrgang JJ, Paul J, Dearwater S, Fu FH. Loss of motion after anterior cruciate ligament reconstruction. *Am J Sports Med.* 1992;20(5):499-506.

17. Harner CD, Baek GH, Vogrin TM, et al. Quantitative analysis of human cruciate ligament insertions. *Arthroscopy.* 1999;15(7):741-749.

18. Gabriel MT, Wong EK, Woo SL, Yagi M, Debski RE. Distribution of in situ forces in the anterior cruciate ligament in response to rotatory loads. *J Orthop Res.* 2004;22(1):85-89.

19. Fu FH, Jordan SS. The lateral intercondylar ridge—a key to anatomic anterior cruciate ligament reconstruction. *J Bone Joint Surg Am.* 2007;89(10):2103-2104.

20. Stallenberg B, Gevenois PA, Sintzoff SA, et al. Fracture of the posterior aspect of the lateral tibial plateau: radiographic sign of anterior cruciate ligament tear. *Radiology.* 1993;187(3):821-825.

21. Dietz GW, Wilcox DM, Montgomery JB. Segond tibial condyle fracture: lateral capsular ligament avulsion. *Radiology.* 1986;159(2):467-469.

22. Lohmander LS, Englund PM, Dahl LL, Roos EM. The long-term consequence of anterior cruciate ligament and meniscus injuries: osteoarthritis. *Am J Sports Med.* 2007;35(10):1756-1769.

23. Munshi M, Davidson M, MacDonald PB, Froese W, Sutherland K. The efficacy of magnetic resonance imaging in acute knee injuries. *Clin J Sport Med.* 2000;10(1):34-39.

24. Daniel DM, Stone ML, Dobson BE, et al. Fate of the ACL-injured patient. A prospective outcome study. *Am J Sports Med.* 1994;22(5):632-644.

25. Hawkins RJ, Misamore GW, Merritt TR. Followup of the acute non-operated isolated anterior cruciate ligament tear. *Am J Sports Med.* 1986;14(3):205 210.

26. Chaudhari AMW, Briant PL, Bevill SL, Koo S, Andriacchi TP. Knee kinematics, cartilage morphology, and osteoarthritis after ACL injury. *Med Sci Sports Exerc.* 2008;40(2):215-222.

27. Gulotta LV, Rodeo SA. Biology of autograft and allograft healing in anterior cruciate ligament reconstruction. *Clin Sports Med.* 2007;26(4):509-524.

28. Noyes FR, Barber SD, Mangine RE. Bone-patellar ligament-bone and fascia lata allografts for reconstruction of the anterior cruciate ligament. *J Bone Joint Surg Am.* 1990;72(8):1125-1136.

29. Christen B, Jakob RP. Fractures associated with patellar ligament grafts in cruciate ligament surgery. *J Bone Joint Surg Br.* 1992;74(4):617-619.

30. Aglietti P, Buzzi R, D'Andria S, Zaccherotti G. Patellofemoral problems after intraarticular anterior cruciate ligament reconstruction. *Clin Orthop Relat Res.* 1993;(288):195-204.

31. Sachs RA, Daniel DM, Stone ML, Garfein RF. Patellofemoral problems after anterior cruciate ligament reconstruction. *Am J Sports Med.* 1989;17(6):760-765.

32. Uchio Y, Ochi M, Adachi N, Kawasaki K, Kuriwaka M. Determination of time of biologic fixation after anterior cruciate ligament reconstruction with hamstring tendons. *Am J Sports Med.* 2003;31(3):345-352.

33. Rihn JA, Harner CD. The use of musculoskeletal allograft tissue in knee surgery. *Arthroscopy.* 2003;19 Suppl 1:51-66.

34. Pearsall AW, Hollis JM, Russell GV, Scheer Z. A biomechanical comparison of three lower extremity tendons for ligamentous reconstruction about the knee. *Arthroscopy.* 2003;19(10):1091-1096.

35. Prodromos C, Joyce B, Shi K. A meta-analysis of stability of autografts compared to allografts after anterior cruciate ligament reconstruction. *Knee Surg Sports Traumatol Arthrosc.* 2007;15(7):851-856.

36. Malinin TI, Levitt RL, Bashore C, Temple HT, Mnaymneh W. A study of retrieved allografts used to replace anterior cruciate ligaments. *Arthroscopy.* 2002;18(2):163-170.

37. Simonds RJ, Holmberg SD, Hurwitz RL, et al. Transmission of human immunodeficiency virus type 1 from a seronegative organ and tissue donor. *N Engl J Med.* 1992;326(11):726-732.

# 13

# POSTERIOR CRUCIATE LIGAMENT INJURIES

*James R. Romanowski, MD and Christopher D. Harner, MD*

## INTRODUCTION

Posterior cruciate ligament (PCL) injuries remain relatively rare orthopedic events, comprising approximately 3% of all knee ligament injuries.[1] Motor vehicle accidents are responsible for 45% of PCL tears, whereas approximately 40% are attributable to athletic causes.[2] Posterior cruciate tears within the setting of athletics occur most frequently in football (52%); however, they are not unheard of in baseball (17%), skiing (9%), soccer (9%), gymnastics (9%), and basketball (4%).[3]

Low-grade injuries are often treated conservatively. More severe injuries are initially approached conservatively; however, they often have additional soft tissue damage leading

Ranawat A, Kelly BT. *Musculoskeletal Examination of the Hip and Knee: Making the Complex Simple* (pp. 311-332). © 2011 SLACK Incorporated

to functional deficits necessitating surgical intervention. Considerable debate over the management of these injuries remains, as accurate diagnosis is difficult and surgical treatment outcomes have not traditionally been as successful as other ligament reconstructions. Furthermore, evidence-based outcomes concerning knee injuries has been dominated by the attention devoted toward the anterior cruciate ligament (ACL); therefore, there is a paucity of literature available to reliably guide decision-making recommendations related to the PCL.

# HISTORY

Careful evaluation of the injury mechanism can provide critical insight in determining which ligaments and stabilizing structures may be torn. Patients with acute PCL injuries typically describe an anterior to posterior force on the proximal tibia either from a fall or motor vehicle accident—the so-called "dashboard injury." Additional mechanisms are associated with athletic activities such as a posterior tibial force with plantar flexion of the ipsilateral foot, or with more violent forces tearing not only the PCL, but also additional knee ligaments. These injuries may also occur without a posterior tibial force in the scenario of knee hyperextension or hyperflexion.[4]

Patients usually are unaware that a ligamentous injury has occurred in the PCL-deficient knee. This is particularly true with isolated injuries, as the secondary restraints limit the sensation of instability. The low initial morbidity helps explain that more than 50% of patients with PCL disruption wait longer than 1 year before seeking medical treatment.[2] A "popping" sensation is rarely recalled, with the complaints primarily focused on the effusion or pain in the posterior knee. As these injuries become chronic, the discomfort typically shifts to the patellofemoral joint and medial compartments, becoming more noticeable with kneeling or deceleration activities.[5] Furthermore, in the setting of chronic PCL deficiency, patients may describe recurrent joint effusions, instability, and abnormal gait mechanics—particularly varus thrust with more complex posterolateral corner injuries.

# EXAMINATION

A careful physical exam is critical in the evaluation of the PCL-injured knee (Table 13-1). The patient is observed with both extremities exposed to allow for comparison. In the acute setting, both effusion and bruising can direct the exam toward additional pathology. Conversely, a painful, swollen joint can make thorough examination difficult and can require the use of other modalities, such as magnetic resonance imaging (MRI), to help with the diagnosis. Prior surgical incisions should be documented. Limb alignment and gait abnormalities including varus thrust must be carefully evaluated, as these scenarios often require additional or staged surgical procedures.

It is important to recognize the normal relationship of the proximal tibia with the femur. To evaluate *step off*, the patient is supine with the knee flexed to 90 degrees, the hip flexed to 45 degrees, and the ipsilateral foot secured. Palpation of the medial compartment over the anteromedial joint line typically reveals 1 cm of anterior translation of the tibial plateau on the femur. Failure to appreciate this spatial positioning can lead to pseudo-positive testing for ACL tears, as the examiner mistakes the reduction of the PCL-deficient sag for a positive Lachman or anterior drawer test.

The *posterior drawer test* is considered to be the most sensitive physical exam test of PCL dysfunction.[6,7] The maneuver has been shown to detect PCL insufficiency with 90% sensitivity and 99% specificity.[8] With similar positioning as the *step off test*, a posterior force is directed on the proximal tibia with the knee flexed to 90 degrees and the ankle secured. This test assesses the function of the PCL and allows for classification of PCL tears. Injuries are typically categorized into 3 grades. Grade I injuries involve 0 to 5 mm of posterior translation with a medial tibial plateau step off remaining anterior to the femoral condyles. Grade II injuries exhibit 5 to 10 mm of posterior translation, which often correlates to the tibial plateau being flush with the femoral condyles. Grade III injuries represent the most severe type with more than 10 mm of posterior drawer translation. Grade III injuries are often associated with posterolateral corner (PLC) injuries.[9]

**Table 13-1**

## METHODS FOR EXAMINING THE POSTERIOR CRUCIATE LIGAMENT

| Examination | Technique | Illustration | Grading | Significance |
|---|---|---|---|---|
| Posterior drawer | Posterior translation of the tibia at 90 degrees of knee flexion with the foot secured | 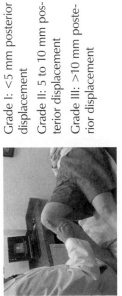 | Grade I: <5 mm posterior displacement<br><br>Grade II: 5 to 10 mm posterior displacement<br><br>Grade III: >10 mm posterior displacement | Flexion at 90 degrees minimizes the secondary restraint of the posterolateral corner<br><br>Increased posterior translation suggests PCL injury when compared to the contralateral knee |
| Step off | Knee is positioned at 90 degrees with the foot secured. Palpate anterior joint line over the medial compartment | | Grade I: <5 mm posterior displacement<br><br>Grade II: 5 to 10 mm posterior displacement<br><br>Grade III: >10 mm posterior displacement | The resting proximal tibia is normally 1 cm anterior to the femur. When the proximal tibia is in plane with the femur, this suggests a Grade II/III PCL tear |

*(continued)*

**Table 13-1 (continued)**

## METHODS FOR EXAMINING THE POSTERIOR CRUCIATE LIGAMENT

| Examination | Technique | Illustration | Grading | Significance |
|---|---|---|---|---|
| Posterior sag (Godfrey) | Assistant elevates bilateral heels with the hips and knees flexed to 90 degrees. Clinician observes from lateral position | 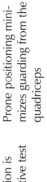 | Posterior subluxation is considered a positive test | Increased posterior sub- luxation suggests injury to the PCL |
| Whipple | Patient is prone with the injured extremity flexed to 70 degrees. Clinician places posterior force on proximal tibia | 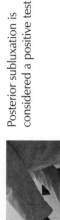 | Posterior subluxation is considered a positive test | Prone positioning mini- mizes guarding from the quadriceps |

*(continued)*

**Table 13-1 (continued)**

## METHODS FOR EXAMINING THE POSTERIOR CRUCIATE LIGAMENT

| Examination | Technique | Illustration | Grading | Significance |
|---|---|---|---|---|
| Quadriceps active test | Knee is positioned at 90 degrees with the foot secured. The quadriceps is then fired | 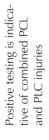 | ≥2 mm of anterior movement of the proximal tibia on the femur is positive[10] | The quadriceps reduces the posteriorly displaced proximal tibia in the PCL-deficient knee |
| Reverse pivot shift | Patient is supine with the knee brought from 90 degrees flexion to extension, with valgus stress, and the foot externally rotated | 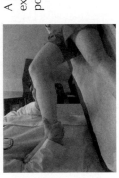 | A palpable shift during extension is considered a positive test | Positive testing is indicative of combined PCL and PLC injuries |

*(continued)*

**Table 13-1 (continued)**

## METHODS FOR EXAMINING THE POSTERIOR CRUCIATE LIGAMENT

| Examination | Technique | Illustration | Grading | Significance |
|---|---|---|---|---|
| External rotation thigh foot angle test (Dial test) | Patient is placed either supine or prone. Both knees are flexed at 30 degrees and 90 degrees. The thigh-foot angles are compared | 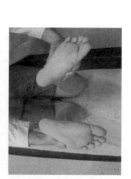 | ≥10 degrees limb to limb external rotation difference is considered a positive test | Increased external rotation at 30 degrees (and not at 90 degrees) suggests an isolated posterolateral corner injury. Increased rotation at both flexion angles suggests disruption of both the PCL and PLC |

*(continued)*

**Table 13-1 (continued)**

## METHODS FOR EXAMINING THE POSTERIOR CRUCIATE LIGAMENT

| Examination | Technique | Illustration | Grading | Significance |
| --- | --- | --- | --- | --- |
| Limb alignment | Weight-bearing visual assessment of lower extremities | 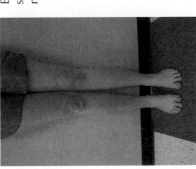 | Excessive varus, valgus, or side-to-side differences are noted | Extreme varus or valgus must be addressed in the reconstructive scenario as these may affect outcome |

(continued)

**Table 13-1 (continued)**

## METHODS FOR EXAMINING THE POSTERIOR CRUCIATE LIGAMENT

| Examination | Technique | Illustration | Grading | Significance |
|---|---|---|---|---|
| Range of motion | Examine at full flexion and full extension | 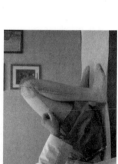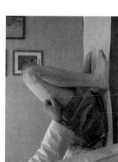 | The range of motion is assessed with a goniometer and documented | Prior to surgical intervention, as well as postoperatively, both limbs should have similar range of motion to maximize function and outcome |

The *posterior sag test,* or *Godfrey test,* may provide additional evidence of a PCL disruption. With the knee and hip flexed to 90 degrees, the heel is supported by the examiner, and the posterior translation is compared between the limbs. The PCL-deficient knee will often exhibit significant posterior translation when compared to the normal leg (Figure 13-1A). The posterior sag may also be assessed by viewing, from the lateral side, the 90 degree flexed knee with foot planted (Figure 13-1B).

The *quadriceps active test* is a dynamic test that will demonstrate reduction of the posteriorly displaced tibia seen with posterior tibial sag. The patient is supine with the foot secured, knee flexed to 90 degrees, and hip positioned at 45 degrees, while actively firing the quadriceps to attempt knee extension. This test viewed laterally shows reduction of the proximal tibia to its native position anterior to the femoral condyles. More than 2 mm of anterior movement of proximal tibia on the femur is considered positive.[10]

The *Whipple test* eliminates the reduction influence of the quadriceps and allows for further assessment of the PCL.[11] The patient is placed prone, and the injured leg is placed in 70 degrees of flexion. The ankle is supported, and a posterior force is placed on the proximal tibia. Increased translation when compared to the contralateral limb is considered a positive test.

Given the association of PLC injuries with PCL tears, it is imperative to assess this region of the knee.[9] The *external rotation thigh foot angle test,* or *dial test,* performed with the knee flexed at 30 and 90 degrees, can provide useful diagnostic information concerning the PLC. The patient may be placed either prone or supine, and both limbs are evaluated at the above angles. Compared to the noninjured limb, increased external rotation of 10 degrees or more at both 30 and 90 degrees suggests disruption of both the PCL and PLC. When the laxity is isolated to the flexed knee at 30 degrees, this is indicative of an isolated PLC injury.[12]

The *reverse pivot shift test* also allows adjunctive assessment of the PLC. With the patient supine, the knee and hip are flexed at 90 degrees with valgus stress, and the foot is externally rotated. The extremity is then brought into extension, observing a "shift" as the lateral plateau reduces from a

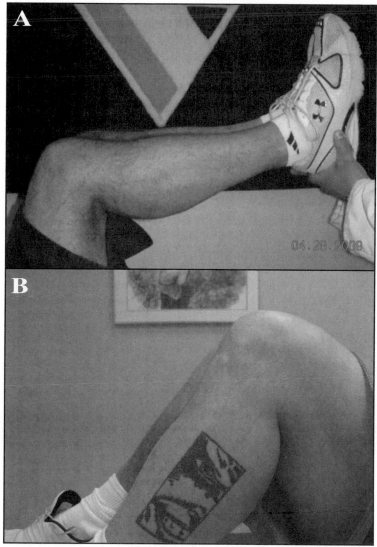

**Figure 13-1.** Posterior sag test (Godfrey test). (A) The examiner flexes the hips and knees to 90 degrees while supporting the heels. The right knee demonstrates posterior tibial translation when compared to the contralateral leg. (B) The knees may also be compared with the feet planted and 90 degrees of knee flexion. The patient illustrates PCL deficiency.

posteriorly subluxed position. This test is considered positive with the pathologic reduction and suggests damage to both the PCL and PLC.[13]

Patients with acute ruptures make the clinical exam challenging, as pain and muscle spasm can interfere with physical findings. Perhaps the most reliable evaluation is an exam under anesthesia (EUA). In the operating room, the injured extremity is tested and compared with the noninjured limb. Fluoroscopy can also provide valuable information as it shows bony position with various stresses placed upon the knee, with additional information obtained by comparison with the opposite leg.

## PATHOANATOMY

Understanding the ligamentous contribution to knee stability and function allows for more accurate correlation of the clinical exam. The PCL is comprised of 2 functional bundles: anterolateral (AL) and posteromedial (PM; Figure 13-2). The AL bundle averages twice the cross-sectional area of the PM bundle.[5] The femoral attachment of the PCL on the lateral surface of the medial femoral condyle is semicircular and averages 32 mm in width, but narrows to 13 mm at its midsection.[14,15] The typical length from its femoral origin to the tibial insertion is approximately 38 mm.[15] The midsubstance cross-sectional area averages 41 mm² — approximately 1.5 times that of the ACL.[16]

Biomechanically, the AL bundle becomes taught in flexion, whereas the PM bundle increases tension with knee extension. The PCL serves as the primary restraint to posterior translation and serves as a secondary stabilizer to external rotation, varus, and valgus stresses.[17,18]

More severe PCL injuries are often associated with damage to the PLC of the knee; therefore, it is imperative to understand these structures' contribution to knee stability. Deficiencies in this region must be recognized, as they influence treatment decisions and have potential deleterious outcome effects if not addressed. This area of the knee may be categorized into static and dynamic stabilizers. Static components include the lateral collateral ligament (LCL), popliteofibular ligament,

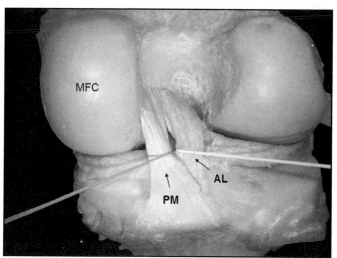

**Figure 13-2.** Anatomic dissection of the posterior cruciate ligament. MFC = medial femoral condyle; AL = anterolateral bundle; PM = posteromedial bundle.

posterior arcuate ligament, condensation of the posterolateral capsule, fabellofibular ligament, and posterior horn of the lateral meniscus. Dynamic stabilizers include the iliotibial band, popliteus muscle complex, and the biceps tendon.[5,19] The PLC primarily serves to resist varus stress and external rotation; however, it contributes secondarily to posterior tibial translation.

Some PCL ligamentous dysfunction grading classification systems are based on posterior translation of the tibia on the femur; therefore, understanding the various contributions to stability helps delineate the degree of damage. Several studies have analyzed the effect of both isolated and combined sectioning of the PCL and PLC. PLC loss alone results in 1.5 to 4.0 mm of posterior translation at all flexion angles (maximum at 30 degrees), but the additional loss of the PCL causes an increased total translation of 10.4 to 13.4 mm.[20] Isolated PLC loss leads to increased external rotation (maximum at 30 degrees) with a minimal increase through the addition of a PCL disruption.

# IMAGING

Radiographs remain a requirement during the evaluation of the PCL-injured knee. The typical knee series includes a weight-bearing AP, lateral (30 degrees flexion), flexion PA (45 degrees), and a long cassette view of the bilateral lower extremities. This modality allows not only for fracture assessment and associated injuries, but special views can provide particular diagnostic insight regarding the PCL. Stress radiographs, or fluoroscopy, looking at the posterior sagittal translation of the tibia on the femur have been shown to be more reliable in the diagnosis of PCL injuries when compared to arthrometer and clinical posterior drawer testing (Figure 13-3).[21]

MRI is an important element in the evaluation of the injured knee. This is particularly true in the acute setting where pain, hemarthrosis, and patient guarding cloud clinical evaluation (Figure 13-4). With this modality, it is important to remember that the majority of PCL injuries are not disruptive tears, but rather elongation injuries. The PCL may be dysfunctional as a continuous structure, even though it is not obviously torn. A particularly helpful criterion for diagnosing acute PCL tears is that the damaged ligament, as seen on sagittal sequences, measures 7 mm or more in anterior-posterior width (94% sensitivity, 92% specificity).[22] For chronic PCL dysfunction, the stretched PCL may appear normal and without edema; therefore, an MRI may be less helpful, and clinical correlation is paramount.[5]

# TREATMENT

Both timing (acute versus chronic) and severity of the injury (isolated versus combined ligamentous deficiency) are important variables to consider during the decision-making process (Table 13-2). For avulsion injuries, early surgical intervention is generally recommended.[23] Acute, isolated injuries additionally allow for immobilization and the potential healing or decrease in severity grade of the PCL disruption. Conservative management of chronic injuries includes physical therapy and activity modifications.

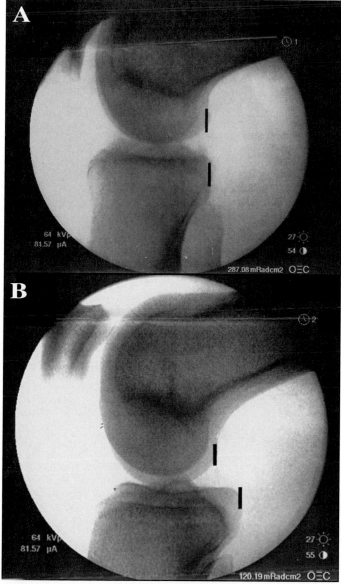

**Figure 13-3.** Fluoroscopic stress radiographs performed during an exam under anesthesia. Black bars represent posterior femoral condylar and tibial plateau surfaces. (A) Lateral view in neutral position. (B) Lateral view with posterior drawer stress.

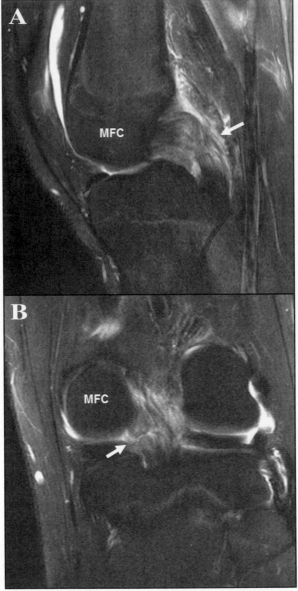

**Figure 13-4.** MRI views of midsubstance PCL rupture. MFC = medial femoral condyle. White arrow represents torn PCL. (A) Sagittal T2 FS. (B) Coronal T2 FS.

**Table 13-2**

## HELPFUL HINTS

- The neurovascular status must be documented and addressed during the initial evaluation of the PCL-injured knee.
- The vast majority of isolated Grade I and Grade II PCL injuries can be treated conservatively.
- Bracing during the acute PCL presentation is more successful and definitive than in patients with chronic PCL deficiency.
- During examination of the PLC, specific testing of the LCL and popliteus complex is necessary as deficiencies affect treatment.
- Stress radiographs combined with clinical exam can accurately predict degree of PCL rupture and damage to associated secondary restraints.
- The clinical exam and exam under anesthesia are critical for determining the extent of ligament reconstruction.
- PCL reconstruction should be performed in medical centers with readily available vascular surgeons.
- Tourniquet use is not necessary for ligament reconstruction of the knee.

Multi-ligamentous injuries involving the PCL (ACL, PLC, and MCL) are typically approached surgically given the complex biomechanical contributions and subsequent dysfunction related to the ligamentous loss. Additional indications for PCL reconstruction are based on patient symptoms—persistent instability, as well as medial compartment and patellofemoral pain. Varus malalignment and an associated varus thrust may be found in a subset of PCL deficient patients. For these individuals, a biplanar osteotomy that corrects both the varus deformity and tibial slope should be performed. Contraindications to surgical intervention include active infection, refusal to follow postoperative rehabilitation guidelines, and severe arthrosis. The complexity and outcomes of surgical PCL reconstruction must be discussed with patients and balanced with their expectations.

Acute Grade I PCL injuries are treated conservatively with 4 weeks of bracing in full extension and a focused quadriceps rehabilitation program with weight-bearing as tolerated. Bracing in full extension limits the posterior translation resulting from hamstring activation during this healing period. Patients are allowed to unlock their brace for structured range of motion exercises—0 to 75 degree motion sets 3 times a day for 1 month. Closed chain exercises are initiated, as well as mini-squats. Within an athletic population, conservative management of isolated PCL injuries has been shown to result in an 84% return-to-sport rate, with 64% returning to the same level of performance.[24] Return to sport usually occurs 1 to 3 months from the time of injury.[5]

Grade II injuries are initially approached conservatively. The natural history of conservatively treated PCL tears after an average of 2.6 years follow-up shows subjective results to be superior to objective results.[4] Subjective scores have been found to be independent of PCL laxity, with nonoperative treatment of isolated PCL tears to be consistently excellent in 40% of patients, consistently good in 10%, and fair in 6%.[25] There is a trend toward medial joint arthrosis, but it is not statistically significant regardless of the degree of PCL laxity.[26] Grade II tears have a portion of the PCL remaining and, if surgery becomes necessary, are usually approached with single-bundle augmentation. The anterolateral bundle is usually reconstructed, as this is the larger of the 2 components.

Isolated Grade III injuries are initially treated nonoperatively, as in Grade I and Grade II injuries. Patients with persistent symptoms are usually approached surgically and often have unrecognized additional ligamentous damage (Figure 13-5). Arthroscopic surgical techniques usually involve single- or double-bundle reconstructions. The modern single-bundle method was originally described by Clancy and colleagues, but more recent focus has been on the theoretical advantages of double-bundle constructs.[27] Given that the native PCL has variable tension within its bundles through the knee's range of motion, recreation of the AL and PM components is an attempt to restore the respective pre-injury kinematic contributions. Randomized comparison studies of the 2 constructs have not been performed; therefore, any advantages are purely observational.[28]

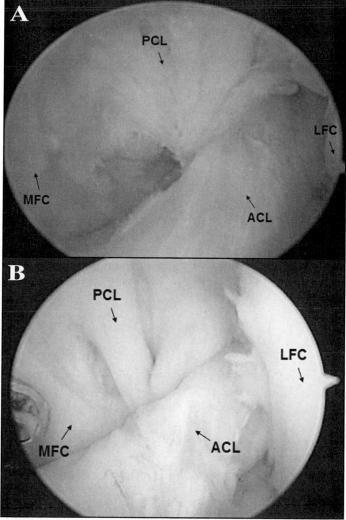

**Figure 13-5.** Arthroscopic view of the knee from the lateral portal. LFC = lateral femoral condyle; MFC = medial femoral condyle; ACL = anterior cruciate ligament; PCL = posterior cruciate ligament. (A) Normal knee. Note the broad, fan shaped insertion of the PCL on the MFC. (B) PCL ruptured knee. The remnant of the PCL is chronically torn and attenuated.

Additional reconstruction techniques have been described and include various tunnel configurations (or a tibial inlay) and a range of fixation devices and graft choices that provide the surgeon with several options when approaching the PCL-deficient knee. The tibial inlay PCL reconstruction method approaches the knee posteriorly and has been shown to decrease graft degradation related to the "killer turn" of anteriorly based soft tissue constructs.[29] Despite all of these surgical methods, it is important to consider a Cochrane analysis that showed no randomized controlled trials have compared techniques or superiority of one particular treatment over another.[28]

## CONCLUSION

PCL injuries represent a complex clinical entity that requires a meticulous evaluation and an appreciation for the natural history and difficulties related to surgical intervention. A thorough clinical exam is critical to recognize and optimize the outcome of these complex injuries. The majority of isolated PCL injuries may be addressed nonoperatively with bracing and rehabilitation. More severe injuries and persistent symptoms after failed rehabilitation often require surgical intervention. Regardless of the severity, patients should be well informed of their injury and the potential for long-term dysfunction. Further research is needed to delineate the clinical results related to the various surgical techniques with the goal being improved patient outcome.

## REFERENCES

1. Harner CD, Höher J. Evaluation and treatment of posterior cruciate ligament injuries. *Am J Sports Med.* 1998;26(3):471-482.
2. Schulz MS, Russe K, Weiler A, Eichhorn HJ, Strobel MJ. Epidemiology of posterior cruciate ligament injuries. *Arch Orthop Trauma Surg.* 2003;123:186-191.
3. Parolie JM, Bergfeld JA. Long-term results of nonoperative treatment of isolated posterior cruciate ligament injuries in the athlete. *Am J Sports Med.* 1986;14(1):35-38.
4. Fowler PJ, Messieh SS. Isolated posterior cruciate ligament injuries in athletes. *Am J Sports Med.* 1987;15:553-557.

5. Margheritini F, Rihn J, Musahl V, Mariani PP, Harner C. Posterior cruciate ligament injuries in the athlete: an anatomical, biomechanical and clinical review. *Sports Med.* 2002;32(6):393-408.

6. Clancy WG Jr, Shelbourne KD, Zoellner GB, Keene JS, Reider B, Rosenberg TD. Treatment of knee joint instability secondary to rupture of the posterior cruciate ligament: report of a new procedure. *J Bone Joint Surg Am.* 1983;65A:310-322.

7. Covey DC, Sapega AA. Injuries to the posterior cruciate ligament. *J Bone Joint Surg Am.* 1993;75A:1376-1386.

8. Ross G, Chapman AW, Newberg AR, Scheller Jr AD. Magnetic resonance imaging for the evaluation of acute posterolateral complex injuries of the knee. *Am J Sports Med.* 1997;25(4):444-448.

9. Sekiya JK, Whiddon DR, Zehms CT, Miller MD. A clinically relevant assessment of posterior cruciate ligament and posterolateral corner injuries. Evaluation of isolated and combined deficiency. *J Bone Joint Surg Am.* 2008;90(8):1621-1627.

10. McAllister DR, Petrigliano FA. Diagnosis and treatment of posterior cruciate ligament injuries. *Curr Sports Med Rep.* 2007;6(5):293-299.

11. Whipple TL, Ellis FD. Posterior cruciate ligament injuries. *Clin Sports Med.* 1991;10(3):515-557.

12. Fanelli GC. The dislocated knee: treatment of combined anterior cruciate ligament-posterior cruciate ligament-lateral side injuries of the knee. *Clin Sports Med.* 2000;19:493-502.

13. Jakob RP, Hassler H, Staeubli HU. Observations on rotatory instability of the lateral compartment of the knee. Experimental studies on the functional anatomy and the pathomechanism of the true and the reversed pivot shift sign. *Acta Orthop Scand Suppl.* 1981;191:1-32.

14. Van Dommelen BA, Fowler PJ. Anatomy of the posterior cruciate ligament. A review. *Am J Sports Med.* 1989;17(1):24-29.

15. Girgis FG, Marshall JL, Al Monajem ARS. The cruciate ligaments of the knee joint: anatomical, functional and experimental analysis. *Clin Orthop.* 1975;106:216-231.

16. Harner CD, Livesay GA, Kashiwaguchi S, Fujie H, Choi NY, Woo SL. Comparative study of the size and shape of human anterior and posterior cruciate ligaments. *J Orthop Res.* 1995;13(3):429-434.

17. Butler DL, Noyes FR, Grood ES. Ligamentous restraints to anterior-posterior drawer in the human knee. A biomechanical study. *J Bone Joint Surg.* 1980;62A:259-270.

18. Gollehon DL, Torzilli PA, Warren RF. The role of the posterolateral and cruciate ligaments in the stability of the human knee. A biomechanical study. *J Bone Joint Surg.* 1987;69A:233-242.

19. Terry GC, LaPrade RF. The posterolateral aspect of the knee: anatomy and surgical approach. *Am J Sports Med.* 1996;24:732-739.

20. Veltri DM, Deng XH, Torzilli PA, Warren RF, Maynard MJ. The role of the cruciate and posterolateral ligaments in stability of the knee: a biomechanical study. *Am J Sports Med.* 1995;23:436-443.

21. Hewett TE, Noyes FR, Lee MD. Diagnosis of complete and partial posterior cruciate ligament ruptures: stress radiography compared with KT-1000 arthrometer and posterior drawer testing. *Am J Sports Med.* 1997;25:648-655.

22. Rodriguez W Jr, Vinson EN, Helms CA, Toth AP. MRI appearance of posterior cruciate ligament tears. *AJR Am J Roentgenol*. 2008;191(4):1031.
23. Richter M, Kiefer H, Hehl G, Kinzl L. Primary repair for posterior cruciate ligament injuries: an eight-year follow up of fifty-three patients. *Am J Sports Med*. 1996;24:298-305.
24. Parolie JM, Bergfeld JA. Long-term results of nonoperative treatment of isolated posterior cruciate ligament injuries in the athlete. *Am J Sports Med*. 1986;14:35-38.
25. Shelbourne KD, Muthukaruppan Y. Subjective results of nonoperatively treated, acute, isolated posterior cruciate ligament injuries. *Arthroscopy*. 2005;21(4):457-461.
26. Shelbourne KD, Davis TJ, Patel DV. The natural history of acute, isolated, nonoperatively treated posterior cruciate ligament injuries. A prospective study. *Am J Sports Med*. 1999;27(3):276-283.
27. Harner CD, Janaushek MA, Kanamori A, et al. Biomechanical analysis of a double-bundle posterior cruciate ligament reconstruction. *Am J Sports Med*. 2000;28:144-151.
28. Peccin MS, Almeida GJ, Amaro J, Cohen M, Soares BG, Atallah AN. Interventions for treating posterior cruciate ligament injuries of the knee in adults. *Cochrane Database Syst Rev*. 2005;2:CD002939.
29. Bergfeld JA, McAllister DR, Parker RD, et al. A biomechanical comparison of posterior cruciate ligament reconstruction techniques. *Am J Sports Med*. 2001;29:129-136.

# MENISCAL INJURIES

*Seth L. Sherman, MD; Bradley S. Raphael, MD;*
*and Scott A. Rodeo, MD*

## INTRODUCTION

Meniscal injuries are common and occur secondary to either athletic activity or activities of daily living. Clinical symptoms of pain, swelling, locking, and motion loss may cause marked physical impairment that requires surgical intervention. Meniscal tears represent approximately 50% of knee injuries that require surgery.[1] Arthroscopic treatment of meniscal injuries has become one of the most common orthopedic surgical procedures in the United States.[2,3] Meniscal tears may occur in isolation or in conjunction with ligamentous injury. The medial meniscus is torn roughly 3 times more often than the lateral meniscus.[1]

Ranawat A, Kelly BT. *Musculoskeletal Examination of the Hip and Knee: Making the Complex Simple* (pp. 333-355).
© 2011 SLACK Incorporated

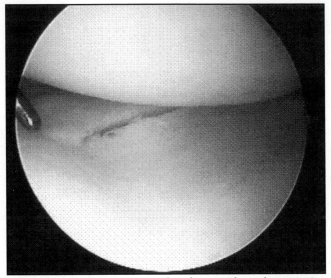

**Figure 14-1.** Arthroscopic peripheral tear with no degenerative changes.

There are 2 types of meniscal tears: traumatic and degenerative. Younger patients are more likely to have acute traumatic sports-related events as the cause of their meniscal pathology. These tears may be peripherally located in a well-vascularized zone, making them more amenable to repair (Figure 14-1). One-third of these tears are associated with an anterior cruciate ligament (ACL) injury.[4] Degenerative tears usually occur in patients in their fourth through sixth decades of life. These may have insidious onset and complex tear patterns (Figure 14-2). Patient age and tear pattern make the majority of these tears unsuitable for meniscal repair.[2]

# HISTORY

Accurate diagnosis of meniscal pathology begins with a careful history. Patient age, onset of symptoms, and mechanism of injury help in the diagnosis of traumatic versus degenerative tears and aid in treatment decisions regarding surgical repair (Table 14-1). Degenerative tears usually occur

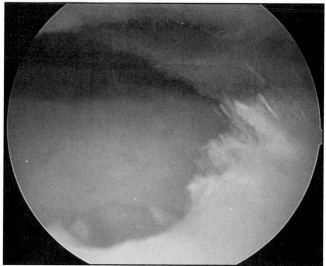

**Figure 14-2.** Arthroscopic degenerative tear with chondral changes.

in older patients with an atraumatic chronic history of joint line pain and swelling. Degenerative tears are often associated with varying degrees of chondral damage. Traumatic tears usually present as a specific sports-related injury to the meniscus, often caused by a twisting injury or an axial load during a hyperflexion event. The patient is typically younger and may present with acute pain and swelling. In contrast to an ACL injury, the swelling in the knee following isolated meniscal injury is usually more gradual in onset.[5] Recurrent or chronic swelling after a twisting event should raise suspicion for meniscal and/or chondral injury. Mechanical symptoms such as locking or clicking may occur with larger tears. Patients may present with a mechanical block to extension due to a displaced bucket handle tear. Smaller tears may produce a clicking or catching sensation without frank locking. Similar complaints may be seen in patients with chondral injury or patellofemoral chondrosis.[2]

A few special situations should raise suspicion for meniscal injury. In the acute ACL tear, lateral meniscal injury is more common secondary to the transient anterior subluxation of the lateral tibial plateau on the lateral femoral condyle during the

**Table 14-1**

# HELPFUL HINTS

## Types of Meniscal Injury

| | AGE | DESCRIPTION/ MECHANISM OF INJURY | TEAR TYPE/ TREATMENT |
|---|---|---|---|
| Traumatic | Males: 21 to 30 Females: 11 to 20 | Sports-related acute event. Twisting or axial load on hyperflexed knee. One-third associated with acute ACL tear | Peripheral (vertical longitudinal or oblique). May be amenable to repair |
| Degenerative | 4th to 6th decade | Atraumatic, insidious onset. Chronic joint line pain and swelling. Varying degree of chondral damage | Complex tear patterns in avascular zone of meniscus. Most are unsuitable for repair and may require meniscectomy |

## Imaging

| IMAGE | PERTINENT VIEWS | FINDINGS |
|---|---|---|
| Plain x-ray | Standard AP, 30 or 45 degrees flexion PA weight-bearing view, true lateral, Merchant, or skyline | Look for joint space narrowing or patellofemoral pathology. Rules out other sources of knee pain |
| MRI | Axial, coronal, sagittal meniscal windows | Accurate for meniscal tears and associated pathology. High intra-meniscal signal and change in meniscus morphology indicate tear (ie, absent bowtie sign, double posterior cruciate ligament [PCL] sign) |

initial event. In the chronic ACL-deficient knee, the posterior horn of the medial meniscus has been shown to function as a secondary constraint to anterior tibial translation. This causes overload of the posterior horn of the medial meniscus and results in an increased incidence of medial meniscus tears in this patient population.[5] Meniscal tears are also frequent in patients with tibial plateau and femoral shaft fractures, with a reported incidence in small series of 47% and 32%, respectively.[5,6]

# EXAMINATION

Physical examination for meniscal injury is similar to other pathologic conditions of the knee. The clinician is required to perform a complete evaluation of the entire lower extremity, with focus on the knee examination including inspection, palpation, range of motion, ligamentous stability testing, and special tests for meniscal injury (Table 14-2). Inspection should focus on the presence or absence of a joint effusion, quadriceps atrophy, and focal joint line swelling or evidence of a meniscal cyst. Palpation of localized joint line tenderness is the most important physical finding in patients with a meniscal tear.[2] Tenderness is likely related to localized synovitis in the adjacent capsule or synovial tissue.[5] Range of motion testing is necessary to rule out a mechanical block to motion and to document any loss of flexion. Ligamentous stability examination is important to evaluate for an acute or chronic ACL tear. In the setting of acute ACL injury, joint line tenderness is not as useful of a clinical indicator in defining meniscal injury preoperatively.[7]

There are numerous special tests for meniscal pathology. The majority of these tests are provocative maneuvers used to trap the meniscus between the femoral and tibial condyles. The McMurray test is performed with the patient supine and the hip and knee flexed to 90 degrees. With one hand on the knee to provide compression, the other hand maneuvers the foot from external rotation to internal rotation. A positive test can trap the meniscus and lead to a palpable pop or click along the joint line that can be felt by the examiner. Pain during this test is also suggestive of meniscal pathology.

**Table 14-2**

## Methods for Examining the Knee With Suspected Meniscal Injury

| Examination | Technique | Illustration | Grading | Significance |
|---|---|---|---|---|
| Inspection | Supine, ambulation from front and back | | | Look for joint effusion, focal swelling, meniscal cyst, quad atrophy. Evaluate standing alignment and gait pattern (ie, antalgic) |
| Palpation | Evaluate joint line | 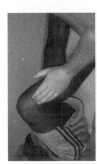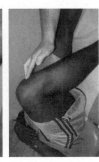 | | Tenderness at joint line most sensitive test for meniscal injury |

(continued)

**Table 14-2 (continued)**

## METHODS FOR EXAMINING THE KNEE WITH SUSPECTED MENISCAL INJURY

| Examination | Technique | Illustration | Grading | Significance |
|---|---|---|---|---|
| Range of motion | Active and passive | 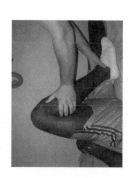 | Degrees | Loss of terminal extension in locked bucket handle tear, loss of motion from degenerative conditions |

(continued)

**Table 14-2 (continued)**

## METHODS FOR EXAMINING THE KNEE WITH SUSPECTED MENISCAL INJURY

| Examination | Technique | Illustration | Grading | Significance |
|---|---|---|---|---|
| Ligamentous stability | ACL, PCL, medial collateral ligament (MCL), lateral collateral ligament (LCL), and posterolateral corner (PLC) exam | | Numeric values based on comparison with the contralateral normal knee | Meniscal tear common with acute ACL tear, medial meniscus tear more likely in chronic ACL deficiency |
| | Lachman | | I: Mild (0-5 mm) | |
| | | | II: Moderate (6-10 mm) | |
| | | | III: Severe (>10 mm) | |
| | | | (A = endpoint, B = no endpoint) | |
| | Pivot shift | | Normal | |
| | | | +: Glide | |
| | | | ++: Clunk | |
| | | | +++: Gross | |

(continued)

**Table 14-2 (continued)**

## METHODS FOR EXAMINING THE KNEE WITH SUSPECTED MENISCAL INJURY

| Examination | Technique | Illustration | Grading | Significance |
|---|---|---|---|---|
| McMurray | Patient supine. Hip and knee flexed to 90 degrees. One hand on joint line, other rotates foot | 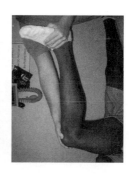 | (+) if pop/click palpated or if pain with exam | Entraps torn meniscus and reproduces patient symptoms |

(continued)

**Table 14-2 (continued)**

## METHODS FOR EXAMINING THE KNEE WITH SUSPECTED MENISCAL INJURY

### SPECIAL TESTS FOR MENISCUS TEAR

| Examination | Technique | Illustration | Grading | Significance |
|---|---|---|---|---|
| Flexion McMurray | Start with knee in maximal flexion and foot either in internal/external rotation. Knee slowly brought into extension | 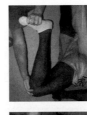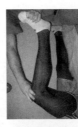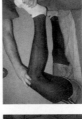 | (+) if patient has pain in either the posteromedial or posterolateral joint line during extension | Internal rotation entraps lateral meniscus, external entraps the medial meniscus |

*(continued)*

**Table 14-2 (continued)**

## METHODS FOR EXAMINING THE KNEE WITH SUSPECTED MENISCAL INJURY

| Examination | Technique | Illustration | Grading | Significance |
|---|---|---|---|---|
| Apley compression | Prone. Knee flexed to 90 degrees. Foot rotated internal/external | 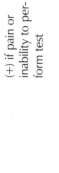 | (+) if patient has pain during rotation of leg | Pain or clicking may indicate meniscal tear |
| Squat test | Repetitive squatting from a standing position, or ask patient to "duck walk" | 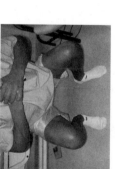 | (+) if pain or inability to perform test | Suggestive of meniscal pathology |

The flexion McMurray test is a variation in which the knee is maximally flexed and the foot is brought to external rotation. Gradual knee extension may produce a positive result if the patient experiences pain over the posteromedial joint line, indicating entrapment of the medial meniscus under the medial femoral condyle. Performing the examination with the foot in full internal rotation attempts to entrap the lateral meniscus under the lateral femoral condyle. The squat test asks a patient to squat repetitively or "duck walk." Symptoms during these maneuvers or inability to perform the test are suggestive of a meniscal tear. The Apley grind test and Steinmann compression test are other adjunct tests that may be useful supplements.[1,2,5]

Joint line tenderness has been shown to be the best clinical test for meniscal tear, with sensitivity of 74% and positive predictive value of 50%. Many of the other clinical tests, in isolation, have poor sensitivity, specificity, and positive predictive values (PPVs). However, the combination of history, physical examination, and plain x-ray to diagnose meniscal tears proved significantly more useful. Using arthroscopic confirmation as a means of definitive diagnosis, this combined evaluation had a sensitivity of 95%, specificity of 72%, and PPV of 85% for medial meniscal tears, and sensitivity of 88%, specificity of 92%, and PPV of 58% for lateral meniscus tears.[8,9]

## PATHOANATOMY

An understanding of the anatomy and biomechanics of these structures is critical in order to diagnose and treat disorders of the meniscus. The menisci are semi-lunar, fibro-cartilaginous wedges positioned between the round femoral condyles and the relatively flat tibial plateau. They have multiple important functions, including load transmission, shock absorption, contributions to joint stability, proprioception, and assistance in lubrication and chondral nutrition of the knee. Loss of meniscal function can be detrimental to the long-term function of the knee. Partial meniscectomy of the inner third of the meniscus and total meniscectomy lead to peak load increases of 65% and 235%, respectively.[5] Clinical

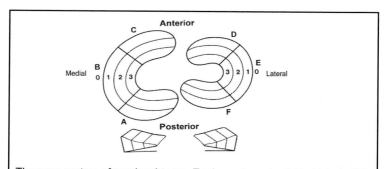

The zone system of meniscal tears. Each meniscus is divided into radial thirds represented by the letter A through F. The meniscus is then subdivided into circumferential thirds represented by 1,2,3. Zone 0 is the meniscosynovial junction.

**Figure 14-3.** Classification of meniscal zones. (Reprinted with permission from *Clin Sports Med*, 10, Cooper D, Arnoczky S, Warren R, Meniscal repair, pp 529-547, Copyright Elsevier 1991.)

findings of radiographic Fairbank's changes (joint space narrowing, osteophyte formation, squaring of the femoral condyles) after partial meniscectomy have been documented in multiple series, with one study demonstrating these findings in 50% of knees only 5 years after partial meniscectomy.[1] As previously discussed, medial meniscectomy in an ACL-deficient knee increases anterior tibial translation of up to 58% at 90 degrees of flexion.[10] Similarly, loss of the posterior horn of the medial meniscus in a patient with an ACL reconstruction places the graft at risk because of increased graft forces in this situation.[11]

Meniscal tears can be classified based on location, orientation, and appearance (Figure 14-3). Cooper and colleagues[12] have divided the location of a tear into 2 different zones: radial and circumferential. The radial zone divides the meniscus into 3 regions: anterior, middle, and posterior. The circumferential zone divides the meniscus into 4 areas (0, 1, 2, or 3). Tears in the 0 or 1 circumferential zone are considered to be peripheral tears, and tears in the 2 or 3 circumferential zone are central.[12] Circumferential zones have implications with regard to the vascularity and healing potential of a tear. These are also described as red-red, red-white, and white-white tears based on circumferential location. Red-red tears are close to

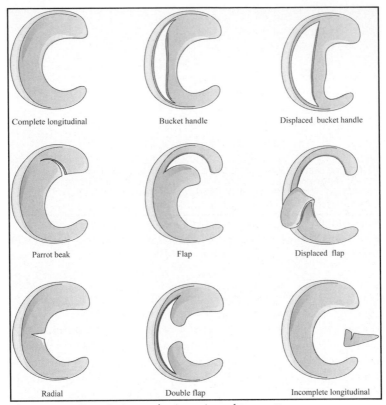

**Figure 14-4.** Description and orientation of tear patterns.

the meniscal capsular junction and have the most favorable healing potential. Red-white tears are in the middle of the meniscus at the junction of the vascular and avascular portions of the tissue. These have intermediate healing potential. White-white tears are in the central portion of the meniscus where there is no blood supply and essentially no healing potential.

Meniscal tears are also classified based on orientation and appearance (Figure 14-4). They are commonly described as vertical longitudinal, oblique, complex (degenerative), transverse (radial), and horizontal. Vertical longitudinal or oblique tears are common and occur in 81% of cases.[13] Vertical longitudinal tears can be complete, as in bucket handle tears, or incomplete. These occur most often in the medial meniscus in young individuals and are often associated with an ACL tear. Oblique tears are often called flap or parrot beak. They occur mainly at the junction of the middle and posterior third of the meniscus. Complex tears occur mostly in the posterior horn and mid-body of older patients, occur in multiple planes, and are often associated with degenerative articular cartilage. Degenerative meniscus tears typically have a horizontal cleavage component. Horizontal tears are the result of shear forces from axial compression. Radial tears occur mainly at the junction of the posterior and middle third of the meniscus or at the posterior attachment of the lateral meniscus. Radial tears also occur at the junction of the anterior horn and mid-body of the lateral meniscus. Complete radial tears result in a loss of load-bearing function. They begin near the inner margin of the meniscus and extend toward the capsule in a plane parallel to the articular surface. They are commonly associated with meniscal cysts, especially with lateral meniscal tears.[2,5]

# IMAGING

The diagnosis of meniscal pathology can be further defined with the use of imaging studies including plain radiograph, arthrography, and magnetic resonance imaging (MRI). With the increased use of MRI, arthrography is infrequently selected for the evaluation of meniscal disease.

Plain radiographs should be the first study ordered for any patient with suspected meniscal injury. Radiograph series includes a standard anteroposterior view in full extension, a 30 or 45 degree flexion posteroanterior weight-bearing view of both knees, a true lateral, and a Merchant or skyline view. While meniscal tears cannot be definitively diagnosed by plain x-ray, these views are important to evaluate for joint space narrowing and patellofemoral pathology. Findings suggestive of traumatic or degenerative chondral or osteochondral injury may be responsible for the painful symptoms, with or without the presence of a meniscal tear. In addition, isolated meniscectomy in the setting of advanced stage arthritis has been shown to be no better than nonoperative treatment or placebo in recent studies.[14,15]

**Figure 14-5.** MRI demonstrating "double PCL sign."

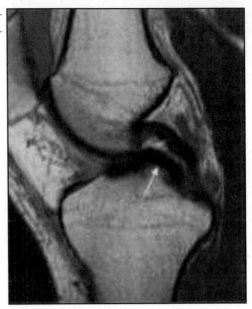

MRI is a highly accurate, noninvasive imaging method, and its advantages include multiplanar imaging of the meniscus, avoidance of ionizing radiation, and ability to evaluate other structures within the knee. The accuracy of MRI in the detection of meniscal tears continues to improve with more powerful magnets and increased experience in reading images. It is now considered to have greater than 95% sensitivity for the detection of a meniscal tear. Diagnosis of meniscal tear by MRI requires evaluation of both intra-meniscal signal and meniscal morphology. The menisci are normally low-signal structures on all pulse sequences with MRI. High intra-meniscal signal that extends to either the femoral or tibial surface of the meniscus is suggestive of a tear. Morphological changes including the "absent bowtie sign" and the "double PCL sign" indicate a displaced bucket handle tear (Figure 14-5).[5]

Treating patients based solely on MRI evidence of meniscal pathology is adamantly discouraged. Clinical judgment and understanding of the entire clinical picture is necessary for proper diagnosis and treatment selection. Studies have shown that 13% of asymptomatic patients younger than 45 years and 36% of asymptomatic patients older than 45 years had positive

MRI findings of meniscus pathology. Another study evaluating asymptomatic 18- to 39-year-old patients with a normal physical examination found a 5.6% rate of meniscal tears on MRI.[16,17] While acknowledgment of these limitations is important, an MRI done in the context of a thorough history and physical examination remains the most powerful imaging tool in the diagnosis of meniscal disease.

# TREATMENT

Treatment options for meniscal injury include conservative treatment, meniscectomy, meniscal repair, and meniscal transplant. The indications for surgical treatment of meniscal pathology include 1) symptoms of meniscal injury that affect activities of daily life, work, and/or sports; 2) positive physical examination findings for meniscal injury (as described previously); 3) failure to respond to nonsurgical management including activity modification, medication, and rehabilitation; and 4) absence of other causes of knee pain identified on plain x-ray or MRI.[2,13] While these criteria are a useful guideline for surgical intervention, operative treatment may still be indicated in the absence of one of more of these criteria. A good example is a locked knee from a displaced meniscal tear. Surgery should be undertaken in an urgent manner in this situation, foregoing attempts at conservative management options. As always, clinical judgment is paramount in deciding the risks and benefits of operative treatment for each individual patient.

# CONSERVATIVE TREATMENT

Some small, stable tears may be asymptomatic and do not require treatment. Meniscal tears that are diagnosed by MRI that do not correlate with history and physical examination findings may also be treated nonoperatively. In the current literature, it is mostly agreed upon that, in a stable knee (or a knee with newly reconstructed ACL), certain tears require no treatment because they heal spontaneously or remain asymptomatic. These include short (<1 cm), stable, vertical longitudinal tears, stable partial thickness tears (<50% depth of meniscus on superior or inferior surface), small (<3 mm) radial tears, or tears displaced only 1 to 2 mm.[1,18]

## Meniscectomy

Due to the well-known association between meniscectomy and late arthritis, total meniscectomy has fallen out of favor (Figure 14-6).[5,19,20] Partial meniscectomy is the treatment of choice for irreparable tears or those not able to spontaneously heal. Surgical management involves removing unstable fragments, thereby eliminating locking and catching, and decreasing pain associated with meniscal instability. Care should be taken to only remove nonfunctional tissue and to preserve as much viable tissue as possible to minimize effects on joint mechanics.[21] Tears most often treated with partial meniscectomy include complex, degenerative tears, horizontal tears, irreparable or deformed bucket handle tears, and centrally located oblique flap and radial tears.[1]

Results have shown more than 95% satisfaction at more than 10 years postoperatively when no degenerative disease is present at the time of surgery. This falls to 62% satisfaction in patients with concomitant degenerative changes.[5] Radiographic deterioration is seen with long-term follow-up of partial meniscectomies. Risk factors for radiographic deterioration were age older than 35 years, presence of medial joint degeneration at arthroscopy, resection of posterior one-third of the meniscus, and meniscal rim resection.

## Meniscal Repair

Attempts to preserve or repair the meniscus should be the main priority for the treating surgeon when possible. Current indications for meniscal repair include 1) complete vertical longitudinal tears longer than 1 cm, 2) tears within the peripheral 10% to 30% of the meniscus or within 3 to 4 mm of the meniscocapsular junction, 3) peripheral tears that can be displaced toward the center of the plateau by probing, 4) absence of secondary degeneration or deformity, 5) a tear in an active patient, and 6) a tear associated with concurrent ligament stabilization or a stable knee (Figure 14-7).[5,22]

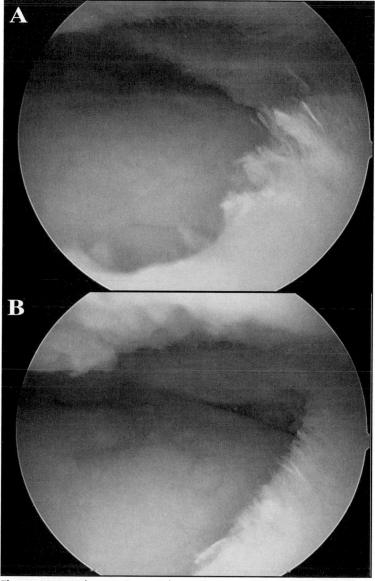

**Figure 14-6.** Arthroscopic partial menisectomy (A) before and (B) after.

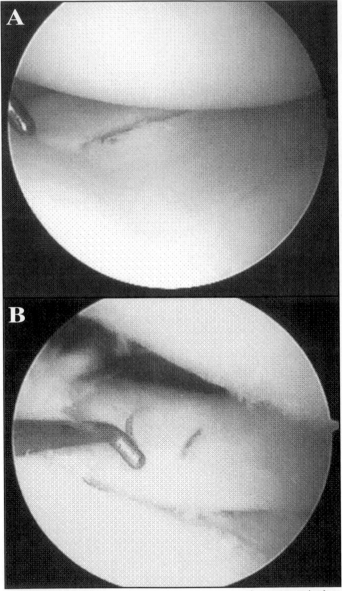

**Figure 14-7.** Arthroscopic or inside-out meniscal repair (A) before and (B) after.

Success of meniscal repair depends on the healing capacity of the tear. In general, better results are seen in patients younger than 40 years old. Tear location (peripheral/red-red more than central/white-white), pattern (vertical longitudinal more than complex or horizontal pattern), chronicity (acute more than chronic), amount of intrasubstance degeneration, and presence of concomitant ligamentous stability also influence healing capacity. Surgical techniques include open meniscal repair, arthroscopic assisted (inside-out repair, outside-in repair), and all-inside arthroscopic repair. While selection of technique is surgeon-dependent, vertical mattress repair with inside-out technique is considered the current "gold standard." All-inside arthroscopic techniques are gaining popularity but lack long-term data on efficacy. Meniscal repairs performed in conjunction with ACL reconstruction tend to heal with more frequency than isolated meniscal repairs. Several authors attribute this to the creation of a favorable healing environment by presence of hemarthrosis following ACL reconstruction. The use of exogenous fibrin clot placed into the repair site of an isolated meniscal tear may augment the healing environment and lead to improved healing rates.

## Meniscal Transplant

Meniscal allograft transplantation has been met with encouraging early success in both animal models and small clinical series.[5,23-25] It is now considered a viable option for the meniscal-deficient patient. The indications for transplant continue to evolve. At present, they include patients who have undergone previous total or near-total meniscectomy, with joint line pain, early chondral changes, and normal (or correctable) anatomic alignment and stability. Osteotomy or ligamentous reconstruction are critical adjunct procedures to correct malalignment and instability in order to normalize joint forces on the graft and prevent early failure. Prophylactic meniscal transplants in young, asymptomatic patients after total or near-total meniscectomy remain controversial. Advanced degenerative tibiofemoral changes are associated with poor outcomes of meniscal transplant, and this procedure is not indicated in these patients. Surgical success requires proper graft selection, graft sizing, and meticulous intraoperative technique. Early short-term results are favorable, but long-term studies are needed to fully evaluate the efficacy of this procedure.[5]

# CONCLUSION

The diagnosis of meniscal injury is based on a focused history, thorough physical examination, and use of appropriate imaging studies. Proper use of all of the tools described in this chapter will allow for rational treatment decisions based on the pertinent pathoanatomy and individualized patient-related factors.

# REFERENCES

1. Miller MD, Cooper DE, Warner JP. *Review of Sports Medicine and Arthroscopy.* 2nd ed. Philadelphia, PA: W.B. Saunders; 2002.
2. Greis PE, Bardana DD, Holmstrom MC, et al. Meniscal injury: I. Basic science and evaluation. *J Am Acad Orthop Surg.* 2002;10(3):168-176.
3. Renstrom P, Johnson RJ. Anatomy and biomechanics of the menisci. *Clin Sports Med.* 1990;9(3):523-538.
4. Poehling GG, Ruch DS, Chabon SJ. The landscape of meniscal injuries. *Clin Sports Med.* 1990;9(3):539-549.
5. Ma CB, Rodeo SA. Meniscal injuries. In: Garrick JG, ed. *Orthopaedic Knowledge Update: Sports Medicine 3.* Rosemont, IL: American Academy of Orthopaedic Surgeons; 2004:199-212.
6. Vangsness CT Jr, Ghaderi B, Hohl M, et al. Arthroscopy of meniscal injuries with tibial plateau fractures. *J Bone Joint Surg Br.* 1994;76(3):488-490.
7. Shelbourne KD, Martini DJ, McCarroll JR, et al. Correlation of joint line tenderness and meniscal lesions in patients with acute anterior cruciate ligament tears. *Am J Sports Med.* 1995;23(2):166-169.
8. Terry GC, Tagert BE, Young MJ. Reliability of the clinical assessment in predicting the cause of internal derangements of the knee. *Arthroscopy.* 1995;11(5):568-576.
9. Weinstabl R, Muellner T, Vecsei V, et al. Economic considerations for the diagnosis and therapy of meniscal lesions: can magnetic resonance imaging help reduce the expense? *World J Surg.* 1997;21(4):363-368.
10. Levy IM, Torzilli PA, Warren RF. The effect of medial meniscectomy on anterior-posterior motion of the knee. *J Bone Joint Surg Am.* 1982;64(6):883-888.
11. Papageorgiou CD, Gil JE, Kanamori A, et al. The biomechanical interdependence between the anterior cruciate ligament replacement graft and the medial meniscus. *Am J Sports Med.* 2001;29(2):226-231.

12. Cooper DE, Arnoczky SP, Warren RF. Arthroscopic meniscal repair. *Clin Sports Med.* 1990;9(3):589-607.
13. Rosenberg TD, Metcalf RW, Gurley WD. Arthroscopic meniscectomy. *Instr Course Lect.* 1988;37:203-208.
14. Moseley JB Jr, Wray NP, Kuykendall D, et al. Arthroscopic treatment of osteoarthritis of the knee: a prospective, randomized, placebo-controlled trial. Results of a pilot study. *Am J Sports Med.* 1996;24(1):28-34.
15. Moseley JB, O'Malley K, Petersen NJ, et al. A controlled trial of arthroscopic surgery for osteoarthritis of the knee. *N Engl J Med.* 2002;347(2):81-88.
16. Boden SD, Davis DO, Dina TS, et al. A prospective and blinded investigation of magnetic resonance imaging of the knee. Abnormal findings in asymptomatic subjects. *Clin Orthop Relat Res.* 1992;282:177-185.
17. LaPrade RF, Burnett QM 2nd, Veenstra MA, et al. The prevalence of abnormal magnetic resonance imaging findings in asymptomatic knees. With correlation of magnetic resonance imaging to arthroscopic findings in symptomatic knees. *Am J Sports Med.* 1994;22(6):739-745.
18. Henning CE, Clark JR, Lynch MA, et al. Arthroscopic meniscus repair with a posterior incision. *Instr Course Lect.* 1988;37:209-221.
19. Jorgensen U, Sonne-Holm S, Lauridsen F, et al. Long-term follow-up of meniscectomy in athletes. A prospective longitudinal study. *J Bone Joint Surg Br.* 1987;69(1):80-83.
20. Wroble RR, Henderson RC, Campion ER, et al. Meniscectomy in children and adolescents. A long-term follow-up study. *Clin Orthop Relat Res.* 1992;279:180-189.
21. Greis PE, Holmstrom MC, Bardana DD, et al. Meniscal injury: II. Management. *J Am Acad Orthop Surg.* 2002;10(3):177-187.
22. Shelbourne KD, Patel DV, Adsit WS, et al. Rehabilitation after meniscal repair. *Clin Sports Med.* 1996;15(3):595-612.
23. Arnoczky SP, Warren RF, McDevitt CA. Meniscal replacement using a cryopreserved allograft. An experimental study in the dog. *Clin Orthop Relat Res.* 1990;252:121-128.
24. Jackson DW, McDevitt CA, Simon TM, et al. Meniscal transplantation using fresh and cryopreserved allografts. An experimental study in goats. *Am J Sports Med.* 1992;20(6):644-656.
25. Milachowski KA, Weismeier K, Wirth CJ. Homologous meniscus transplantation. Experimental and clinical results. *Int Orthop.* 1989;13(1):1-11.

**15**

# CARTILAGE INJURIES

*Volker Musahl, MD; Olufemi R. Ayeni, MD;
and Riley J. Williams III, MD*

## INTRODUCTION

Articular cartilage is avascular and has a limited intrinsic healing capacity. Injuries of articular cartilage will lead to osteoarthritis (OA).[1,2] OA is the leading cause of limitations in activities of daily living and has a significant socioeconomic impact on the health care system.[3] Therefore, simple and effective arthroscopic and open techniques for the treatment of articular cartilage lesions are of great interest.

While chondrocytes make up less than 10% of articular cartilage, they are responsible for maintenance of the glycosaminoglycan-rich matrix.[4] Under normal physiological conditions,

Ranawat A, Kelly BT. *Musculoskeletal Examination of the Hip
and Knee: Making the Complex Simple* (pp. 356-375).
© 2011 SLACK Incorporated

chondrocytes exhibit low metabolic activity, divide infrequently, and are long lasting. In the pathophysiologic condition, however, chondrocytes increase their metabolic activity and may undergo apoptosis.[5] Ultimately, acute treatment of cartilage injury, optimizing survival and recovery of chondrocytes, is desired and may aid in the prevention of OA.

Current surgical approaches are focused on limiting the disease process, providing pain relief, and providing functional recovery. Current techniques rely on either stimulating marrow cells or transplanting tissues that contain viable cells. Minimally invasive techniques include arthroscopic lavage, débridement, abrasion chondroplasty, and microfracture techniques.[6] Reconstructive procedures include osteotomy, meniscal transplantation, osteochondral autograft and allograft transplantation, and autologous chondrocyte transplantation.[7-10]

# HISTORY

Full-thickness articular cartilage defects in the knee are common in patients younger than age 40, and the defects may occur in a variety of clinical settings.[11] A single traumatic event may cause shearing forces of the femur on the tibia, resulting in articular cartilage fracture, laceration, or subchondral shear fracture.[12,13] In contrast, chronic repetitive loading may result in fatigue and failure of articular cartilage. Traumatic events are more common in younger patients, and chronic repetitive events are more common in the middle-aged and older populations. Once the degenerative cascade is initiated, cartilage will undergo softening and fibrillation (Outerbridge Grade I), fissures and cracks in the surface (Grade II), severe fissures and cracks with ulceration (Grade III), and eventually exposure of subchondral bone (Grade IV).[14]

Articular cartilage defects extending to subchondral bone rarely heal without intervention. While some patients may not experience significant problems from acute full-thickness chondral defects, eventual development of degenerative changes is debilitating. Indications for "cartilage procedures" include symptomatic full-thickness chondral defects on the weight-bearing surface of the knee, with a defect size ideally between 1 and 4 cm$^2$, minimal degenerative changes in surrounding tissues and articular cartilage, patient age younger than 50 years, and a compliant patient who has realistic expectations.

Patients with lower activity levels are usually less symptomatic and may respond to minimally invasive techniques, such as chondroplasty and microfracture. Completely asymptomatic articular cartilage lesions should not be treated aggressively and should be followed over time. Location of pain is an important prognostic factor, as is localized pain as opposed to diffuse pain. The best results are reported for isolated femoral condyle lesions, while the worst results are reported for patellar lesions and bipolar lesions. There are limited data with respect to outcome after treatment of tibial lesions.[15] Patients should be evaluated for associated pathology, such as malalignment, meniscal deficiency, ligamentous instability, and generalized OA. Osteotomy, meniscal transplantation, or ligament reconstruction can be performed concomitantly.

## EXAMINATION

Evaluation of a patient with articular cartilage injury should consider age of the patient, activity level, body weight, and overall emotional well-being, as well as addictive behavior patterns. A patient who is not motivated, is unrealistic about expectations or rehabilitation, is a smoker, and is overweight is probably better suited for a different treatment approach.

Physical examination of the knee includes observation of gait, limb alignment, and examination of the ipsilateral hip. The skin should be inspected for the presence of skin incisions, which may affect the intended surgical exposure. Tension in the quadriceps muscle should be inspected and compared to the contralateral side while the patient performs a straight leg raise. With the patient sitting on the side of the examination table, he or she should be asked to straighten the knee from a bend position. This gives the physician an idea about quadriceps function, any contractures, and patella tracking as well. Any amount of quadriceps atrophy is a sign of chronicity of the underlying condition.

After inspection, the knee and surrounding soft tissues should be palpated for any swelling or tenderness. Intra-articular effusion is best determined by squeezing the supra-patellar pouch while simultaneously shifting the patella from medial to lateral. Mild, moderate, or severe effusion is a sign of intra-articular irritation. Knee range of motion should reveal a full flexion-extension arc; any degree of flexion contracture is a poor prognostic indicator. Tightness in hamstring muscles is best determined by the popliteal angle, tightness in the iliotibial band by Ober's test. Tightness in the hip adductors and abductors as well as in the gastrocnemius muscle should also be assessed. Any amount of increased tightness gives the physician an idea about structures to address in a rehabilitation protocol.

Examination of the patella assesses for facet pain, malalignment, or maltracking. The Q-angle is judged by a line drawn from the anterior superior iliac spine to the middle of the patella and then to the middle of the tibial tubercle. Patella maltracking is best assessed by evaluation of the quadriceps angle with the patella in the reduced position with the knee in full extension. The J-sign refers to a lateral deviation (subluxation) of the patella when the knee is brought from flexion to full extension. Ligamentous laxity is assessed with the Lachman test, posterior drawer, and varus and valgus stress tests. Medial and lateral joint lines are examined for meniscal pathology. The neurovascular status of the intended operative limb needs to be assessed and carefully documented (Table 15-1).

## PATHOANATOMY

In 1743, Hunter observed that "ulcerated cartilage is a troublesome thing, once destroyed is not repaired."[16] Because articular cartilage has neither vascular supply nor innervation, articular cartilage has a limited healing potential. A healing response is only then initiated when full-thickness defects also injure the subchondral bone. Resultant fibrocartilaginous repair tissue is histologically dissimilar and biomechanically inferior to normal hyaline cartilage. Fibrocartilage consists predominantly of type I and type III collagen, while hyaline cartilage consists mainly of type II collagen.[17]

**Table 15-1**

## METHODS FOR EXAMINING THE ARTHRITIC KNEE

| Examination | Technique | Illustration | Grading | Significance |
|---|---|---|---|---|
| Alignment | Examine mechanical axis | Varus malalignment 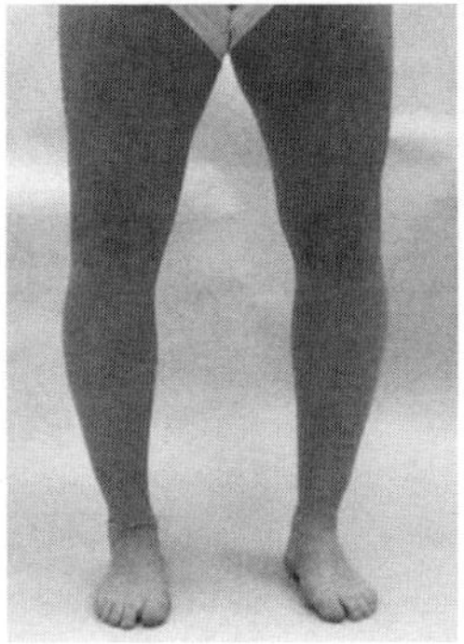 | Varus, neutral, valgus | Malalignment should be corrected prior to cartilage repair, especially when injured compartment overloaded |
| Range of motion | Measure extension and flexion with goniometer | | In degrees | Any flexion contracture is a poor prognostic indicator |

(continued)

**Table 15-1 (continued)**

## METHODS FOR EXAMINING THE ARTHRITIC KNEE

| Examination | Technique | Illustration | Grading | Significance |
|---|---|---|---|---|
| Patella evaluation | A. Facet tenderness<br>B. Lateral lift<br>C. Glide<br>D. Tracking | Lateral patella subluxation<br>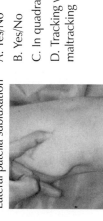 | A. Yes/No<br>B. Yes/No<br>C. In quadrants<br>D. Tracking well versus maltracking | Address appropriate pathology |
| Ligaments | Lachman test<br>Posterior drawer<br>Valgus stress<br>Varus stress | Lachman test<br>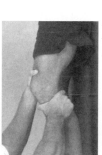 | 1-3 plus endpoint | Concomitant ligament laxity should be addresses prior or simultaneously |

(continued)

**Table 15-1 (continued)**

## METHODS FOR EXAMINING THE ARTHRITIC KNEE

| Examination | Technique | Illustration | Grading | Significance |
|---|---|---|---|---|
| Joint line | A. Palpation<br>B. McMurray test | McMurray test<br>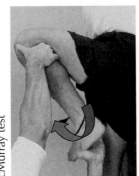 | Postive if click is palpated | Meniscal pathology is different from articular cartilage pathology |

The chondrocyte is the only cell type found in articular cartilage. Chondrocytes are surrounded by their extracellular matrix, and there is no cell-to-cell contact. Mature chondrocytes are spheroidal in shape and synthesize type II collagen, large aggregating proteoglycans, and specific noncollagenous proteins. Chondrocytes sense changes in matrix composition caused by degradation of macromolecules, and degraded matrix components are turned over to maintain the articular surface. To form articular cartilage, chondrocytes organize collagens, proteoglycans, and noncollagenous proteins into a highly ordered structure.[18]

Four zones of articular cartilage are identified: 1) the thin and collagen-rich superficial zone, 2) the transitional zone, 3) the proteoglycan-rich radial zone, and 4) the zone of calcified cartilage. Collagen fibers of the radial zone pass into the tidemark, which corresponds to the boundary between calcified and uncalcified cartilage. The thin zone of calcified cartilage separates the uncalcified cartilage and subchondral bone.

A healing response of articular cartilage can only be found when the injury penetrates the subchondral bone. Optimal healing of articular cartilage would regenerate tissue identical to hyaline cartilage. The repair tissue should fill and seal off the injury with adhesion to subchondral bone and complete integration into surrounding healthy articular cartilage. Repair tissue should be able to resist mechanical wear and should be gradually included in the natural turnover of normal articular cartilage.[18] However, the reality is that no repair tissue and no operative procedure today can restore normal hyaline articular cartilage. Therefore, research is aimed at novel strategies to regenerate and restore tissues affected by cartilage injuries and OA.

# IMAGING

Axial alignment is determined by full-length, hip-to-toe weight-bearing radiographs on a single cassette. Standing anteroposterior, lateral, 45 degrees posteroanterior flexion weight-bearing, and Merchant views are the standard views for every patient (Figures 15-1 through 15-3). These films are

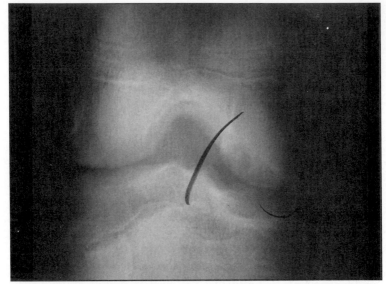

**Figure 15-1.** Posteroanterior flexion weight-bearing radiograph showing medial femoral condyle osteochondral defect.

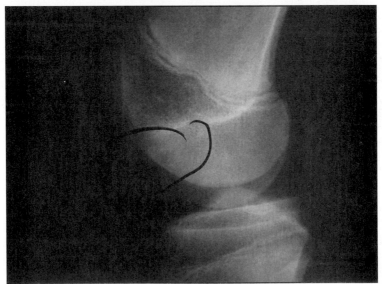

**Figure 15-2.** Corresponding lateral radiograph.

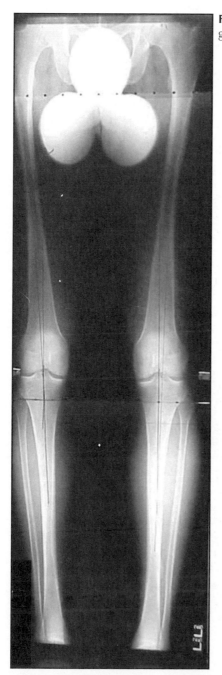

**Figure 15-3.** Alignment radiograph (hip-to-ankle).

useful to assess joint space narrowing, Fairbanks changes, and to rule out bone-on-bone disease, which is a contraindication to cartilage reconstructive procedures. If patella malalignment is suspected, computed tomography (CT) can be used to evaluate the position of the patella in the trochlear groove.

Magnetic resonance imaging (MRI) offers multiplanar tomographic views, eliminating projectional distortion and magnification as well as the problem of superimposing of overlaying structures. Conventional MRI is both sensitive and specific for detecting articular cartilage defects in the knee.[19,20] The volume of articular cartilage can be quantified, and its thickness can be mapped. However, the utilization of MRI should be done cautiously. Studies have shown limited enhanced diagnostic utility over clinical examination, particularly in children.[21]

Cartilage-sensitive pulse sequences consist of T1-weighted 3-dimensional fat-suppressed gradient echo imaging that demonstrates high contrast between low signal-intensity bone and high signal-intensity articular cartilage. Fast spin-echo imaging provides good differential contrast between the intermediate signal intensity of articular cartilage, low signal intensity of fibrocartilage, and high signal intensity of synovial fluid (Figures 15-4 and 15-5). With proper technique, this sequence has the ability to detect partial-thickness chondral lesions and is well-suited to evaluate reconstructed cartilage.[22]

Optical coherence tomography (OCT) is an optical imaging technique that allows for nondestructive high-resolution cross-sectional imaging of articular cartilage and has the potential to be used for early diagnosis of cartilage damage.[23] This technology can be described as similar to ultrasound except that the image generated is an echograph of infrared light instead of ultrasound. OCT has been applied to a wide variety of tissues to obtain high-resolution cross-sectional images comparable to low-power histology and superior to both conventional MRI (150 μm) and ultrasound. When applied to assessment of tissue-engineered cartilage repair, OCT imaging was found to be comparable to low-power histology.[24]

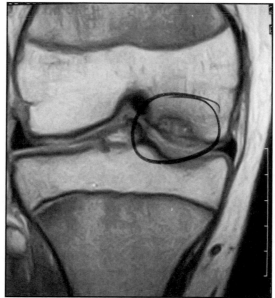

**Figure 15-4.** Coronal fast spin echo MRI showing medial femoral condyle osteochondral defect.

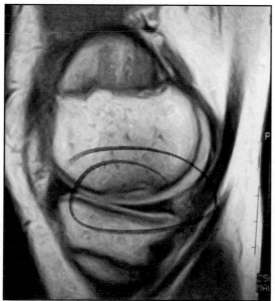

**Figure 15-5.** Corresponding sagittal MRI.

# TREATMENT

Conservative treatment includes physical therapy and activity modification, consisting of range of motion and stretching exercises; strengthening exercises, especially of the quadriceps, hip, and core musculature; as well as aerobic conditioning. Modalities such as hydrotherapy, heat, ultrasound, electrical neuromuscular stimulation, and cryotherapy can be employed. Braces and orthotics have a limited role in cases of malalignment or patella and ligamentous instability. Nonsteroidal anti-inflammatory drugs (NSAIDs) are helpful for short-term treatment. Intra-articular injections of corticosteroids can reduce inflammation and provide temporary relief. Viscosupplementation has become more popular and was shown to have beneficial effects on improvement of pain and function.[25] Glucosamine and chondroitin also have beneficial effects.

Operative strategies for cartilage repair can be classified by the following treatment categories: 1) palliative treatment, 2) enhancement of intrinsic repair, 3) whole-tissue transplantation, 4) cell-based repair, 5) scaffold-based repair, and 6) combined cell- and scaffold-based repair (Table 15-2).[26] Palliative options aim at relieving mechanical symptoms of locking and catching induced by chondral flaps and include débridement, lavage, and chondroplasty. There is no lesion fill with palliative techniques. Strategies that aim at enhancing intrinsic repair rely on accessing marrow-based pluripotent stem cells, such as abrasion arthroplasty, drilling, and microfracture.[6] These stem cells are thought to form a clot and repair tissue at the site of articular cartilage injury. Whole-tissue transplantation includes autologous and allogenous osteochondral transfers, as well as mosaicplasty. Cell-based repair, also known as autologous chondrocyte implantation (ACI), involves local implantation of chondrocytes for the purpose of forming hyaline-like cartilage.[7] Implanted chondrocytes are covered and protected by periosteal patches (ACI) or type I/III collagen patches (collagen-associated chondrocyte implantation).[27] Scaffold-based repairs can be used to treat chondral or osteochondral defects. The TruFit (Smith & Nephew, San Antonio, TX) is a biphasic resorbable synthetic implant that is currently approved for backfill of donor sites when performing mosaicplasty procedures.

**Table 15-2**

# HELPFUL HINTS:
## INDICATIONS FOR CARTILAGE PROCEDURES

## Marrow Stimulating
- Older patient
- Low functional demand
- Grade III-IV unipolar lesion
- Contained lesion
- Size 0.5 to 2 cm$^2$

## Autologous Osteochondrial Transplantation
- Focal, traumatic lesion
- Size 1 to 5 cm$^2$
- Lesion does not need to be contained
- Femur or patella lesions

## Osteochondrial Allograft Transplantation
- Large, uncontained lesion
- Osteochondrial lesion
- Osteochondritis dissecans
- Size 2 to 12 cm$^2$
- Salvage for failed first-line procedure

## Autologous Chondrocyte Implantation
- Younger patient
- High functional demand
- Size 2 to 10 cm$^2$
- Femur, patella, trochlea, tibia lesions
- Uncontained lesion
- Multiple lesions
- Lesion with <6 mm bone loss

Marrow-stimulating techniques are appropriate first-line treatment for grade III or IV lesions of the femur (0.5 to 5 cm$^2$). A stable rim consisting of healthy articular cartilage is prerequisite for blood clot stabilization and successful outcome with this technique. Patients need to be carefully selected. High-demand patients with small lesions (<2 cm$^2$) and low-demand patients with larger lesions (2 cm$^2$ and larger) are appropriate candidates for this approach. Patients with a body mass index (BMI) higher than 30 should not be considered surgical candidates when using this approach. The microfracture technique is a single-stage, cost-effective, first-line approach that results in adequate tissue fill with biomechanically inferior fibrocartilage.[28] The durability of microfracture technique is estimated to be between 2 and 5 years in an athletic population.[29] Compared to ACI, the microfracture technique shows similar satisfactory results in patients 5 years after cartilage repair. However, a third of the patients in the study had early radiographic signs of OA at the time of follow-up.[9]

Autologous osteochondral transplantation (AOT) uses either multiple small osteochondral cylinder plugs (mosaicplasty) or a single large plug (Figures 15-6 through 15-8).[8] AOT is indicated for focal, traumatic lesions 1 to 5 cm$^2$ in size that do not have to be contained. Autogenous tissue is used to recreate hyaline articular cartilage. The donor site is usually the ipsilateral knee, specifically nonweight-bearing portions of the trochlea or notch (see Figure 15-7). Arthrotomy is usually required for a 3-dimensional reconstruction and contouring of articular cartilage. Despite its technical demands, AOT is a good first-line treatment for smaller focal cartilage lesions in high-demand patients. Compared to ACI, mosaicplasty was found to have a faster recovery and a higher degree of hyaline cartilage.[30]

Fresh osteochondral allograft transplantation typically is used as a salvage procedure and for large osteochondral lesions (2 to 12 cm$^2$ or larger). Large uncontained osteochondral lesions, chondral lesions, osteochondritis dissecans lesions, osteonecrotic lesions, and post-traumatic lesions can be treated with this approach.[10,15] Advantages are bony fixation of the press-fit graft and the presence of intact functional hyaline articular cartilage that contains viable chondrocytes. There is no donor site morbidity. However, allografts are limited in supply, can only be stored temporarily, bear the risk of disease transmission, and are costly.

ACI is indicated for large lesions (2 to 10 cm$^2$) in high-demand patients. Chondral lesions of the femur, trochlea, patella, and tibia can be treated with this approach.[7] ACI is a 2-step surgery. Step 1 is harvesting of autologous chondrocytes from a nonweight-bearing area of the knee, usually the notch.

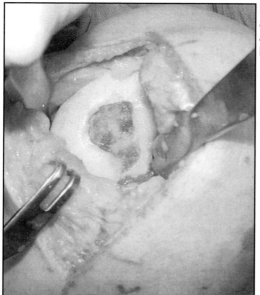

**Figure 15-6.** Intra-operative demonstration of a large osteochondral lesion.

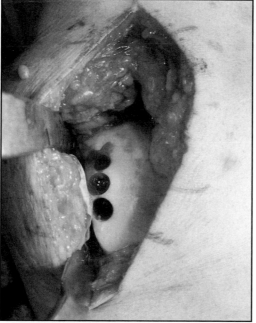

**Figure 15-7.** Harvest of autologous osteochondral plugs from the nonweight-bearing zone of the trochlea.

**Figure 15-8.** Mosaic-plasty.

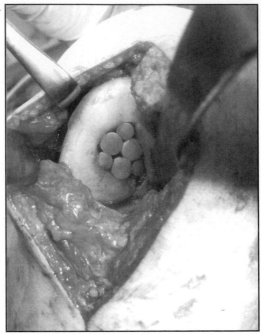

Chondrocytes are expanded and treated in culture for 2 to 3 weeks. Step 2 is an arthrotomy approach with reimplantation of the expanded chondrocytes into the defect under a periosteum or synthetic collagen patch. Good clinical results can be achieved; however, ACI is a technically demanding procedure, patients need to be compliant with staging, there is a high revision rate of 10% to 48%, and the procedure is expensive.[7,31,32]

Cell-based articular cartilage repair with scaffolds are third-generation ACI techniques and include the Hyalograft C chondrocyte seeded implant,[33] the matrix-ACI (MACI),[34] and others. The Hyalograft C implant uses a hyaluronic acid-based patch soaked with autologous chondrocytes. Implantation of the patch can be achieved arthroscopically and requires no suture stabilization or glue. Clinical results are improved at 3 years in 80% of patients, with an arthroscopic appearance of normal articular cartilage in 96% of patients and hyaline-like repair cartilage.[33]

# CONCLUSION

Treatment of articular cartilage lesions presents a difficult clinical challenge. Good clinical outcomes can be achieved when carefully selecting patients. Factors to be considered include patient symptoms, activity level and expectations, previous treatment history, lesion size and quality of surrounding articular cartilage, cruciate ligament status, and limb alignment. Surgeons need to understand the pathophysiology of the cartilage repair method used and its relation to postoperative rehabilitation. Associated pathology, such as malalignment or ligamentous laxity, can be addressed concomitantly or prior to the articular cartilage procedure. Meticulous preoperative planning and proper surgical technique will increase the likelihood of good clinical outcome.

# REFERENCES

1. Caplan AI, Elyaderani M, Mochizuki Y, Wakitani S, Goldberg VM. Principles of cartilage repair and regeneration. *Clin Orthop.* 1997;342:254-269.
2. Hunziker EB. Articular cartilage repair: basic science and clinical progress. A review of the current status and prospects. *Osteoarthritis Cartilage.* 2002;10(6):432-463.
3. Jackson DW, Simon TM, Aberman HM. Symptomatic articular cartilage degeneration: the impact in the new millennium. *Clin Orthop.* 2001;(391 Suppl):S14-S25.
4. Trippel SB, Ehrlich MG, Lippiello L, Mankin HJ. Characterization of chondrocytes from bovine articular cartilage: I. Metabolic and morphological experimental studies. *J Bone Joint Surg Am.* 1980;62(5):816-820.
5. D'Lima DD, Hashimoto S, Chen PC, Colwell CW Jr, Lotz MK. Human chondrocyte apoptosis in response to mechanical injury. *Osteoarthritis Cartilage.* 2001;9(8):712-719.
6. Steadman JR, Rodkey WG, Rodrigo JJ. Microfracture: surgical technique and rehabilitation to treat chondral defects. *Clin Orthop Relat Res.* 2001;(391 Suppl):S362-S369.
7. Brittberg M, Lindahl A, Nilsson A, Ohlsson C, Isaksson O, Peterson L. Treatment of deep cartilage defects in the knee with autologous chondrocyte transplantation. *N Engl J Med.* 1994;331(14):889-895.
8. Hangody L, Rathonyi GK, Duska Z, Vasarhelyi G, Fules P, Modis L. Autologous osteochondral mosaicplasty. Surgical technique. *J Bone Joint Surg Am.* 2004;86-A Suppl 1:65-72.

9. Knutsen G, Drogset JO, Engebretsen L, et al. A randomized trial comparing autologous chondrocyte implantation with microfracture. Findings at five years. *J Bone Joint Surg Am.* 2007;89(10):2105-2012.

10. Williams RJ 3rd, Ranawat AS, Potter HG, Carter T, Warren RF. Fresh stored allografts for the treatment of osteochondral defects of the knee. *J Bone Joint Surg Am.* 2007;89(4):718-726.

11. Curl WW, Krome J, Gordon ES, Rushing J, Smith BP, Poehling GG. Cartilage injuries: a review of 31,516 knee arthroscopies. *Arthroscopy.* 1997;13(4):456-460.

12. Buckwalter JA. Articular cartilage: injuries and potential for healing. *J Orthop Sports Phys Ther.* 1998;28(4):192-202.

13. Mankin HJ. The reaction of articular cartilage to injury and osteoarthritis (first of two parts). *N Engl J Med.* 1974;291(24):1285-1292.

14. Outerbridge RE. The etiology of chondromalacia patellae. *J Bone Joint Surg Br.* 1961;43-B:752-757.

15. Bugbee WD, Convery FR. Osteochondral allograft transplantation. *Clin Sports Med.* 1999;18(1):67-75.

16. Hunter W. Of the structure and diseases of articular cartilages. *Phil Trans.* 1744;42:514-521.

17. Buckwalter JA, Mankin HJ, Grodzinsky AJ. Articular cartilage and osteoarthritis. *Instr Course Lect.* 2005;54:465-480.

18. Buckwalter JA, Mankin HJ. Articular cartilage: degeneration and osteoarthritis, repair, regeneration, and transplantation. *Instr Course Lect.* 1998;47:487-504.

19. Potter HG, Black BR, Chong le R. New techniques in articular cartilage imaging. *Clin Sports Med.* 2009;28(1):77-94.

20. Potter HG, Linklater JM, Allen AA, Hannafin JA, Haas SB. Magnetic resonance imaging of articular cartilage in the knee. An evaluation with use of fast-spin-echo imaging. *J Bone Joint Surg Am.* 1998;80(9):1276-1284.

21. Kocher M, DiCanzio J, Zurakowski D, Micheli L. Diagnostic performance of clinical examination and selective magnetic resonance imaging in the evaluation of intraarticular knee disorders in children and adolescents. *Am J Sports Med.* 2001;29:292-296.

22. Shindle MK, Foo LF, Kelly BT, et al. Magnetic resonance imaging of cartilage in the athlete: current techniques and spectrum of disease. *J Bone Joint Surg Am.* 2006;88 Suppl 4:27-46.

23. Chu CR, Lin D, Geisler JL, Chu CT, Fu FH, Pan Y. Arthroscopic microscopy of articular cartilage using optical coherence tomography. *Am J Sports Med.* 2004;32(3):699-709.

24. Han CW, Chu CR, Adachi N, et al. Analysis of rabbit articular cartilage repair after chondrocyte implantation using optical coherence tomography. *Osteoarthritis Cartilage.* 2003;11(2):111-121.

25. Day R, Brooks P, Conaghan PG, Petersen M. A double blind, randomized, multicenter, parallel group study of the effectiveness and tolerance of intraarticular hyaluronan in osteoarthritis of the knee. *J Rheumatol.* 2004;31(4):775-782.

26. Williams RJ 3rd, Brophy RH. Cartilage repair procedures: clinical approach and decision making. *Instr Course Lect.* 2008;57:553-561.
27. Gooding CR, Bartlett W, Bentley G, Skinner JA, Carrington R, Flanagan A. A prospective, randomised study comparing two techniques of autologous chondrocyte implantation for osteochondral defects in the knee: periosteum covered versus type I/III collagen covered. *Knee.* 2006;13(3):203-210.
28. Minas T, Nehrer S. Current concepts in the treatment of articular cartilage defects. *Orthopedics.* 1997;20(6):525-538.
29. Mithoefer K, Williams RJ 3rd, Warren RF, Wickiewicz TL, Marx RG. High-impact athletics after knee articular cartilage repair: a prospective evaluation of the microfracture technique. *Am J Sports Med.* 2006;34(9):1413-1418.
30. Horas U, Pelinkovic D, Herr G, Aigner T, Schnettler R. Autologous chondrocyte implantation and osteochondral cylinder transplantation in cartilage repair of the knee joint. A prospective, comparative trial. *J Bone Joint Surg Am.* 2003;85-A(2):185-192.
31. Peterson L, Minas T, Brittberg M, Nilsson A, Sjogren-Jansson E, Lindahl A. Two- to 9-year outcome after autologous chondrocyte transplantation of the knee. *Clin Orthop.* 2000;374:212-234.
32. Rosenberger RE, Gomoll AH, Bryant T, Minas T. Repair of large chondral defects of the knee with autologous chondrocyte implantation in patients 45 years or older. *Am J Sports Med.* 2008;36(12):2336-2244.
33. Marcacci M, Berruto M, Brocchetta D, et al. Articular cartilage engineering with Hyalograft C: 3-year clinical results. *Clin Orthop Relat Res.* 2005;435:96-105.
34. Bartlett W, Skinner JA, Gooding CR, et al. Autologous chondrocyte implantation versus matrix-induced autologous chondrocyte implantation for osteochondral defects of the knee: a prospective, randomised study. *J Bone Joint Surg Br.* 2005;87(5):640-645.

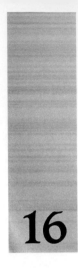

**16**

# POSTEROLATERAL AND POSTEROMEDIAL CORNERS OF THE KNEE

*Keith R. Reinhardt, MD; Mark Drakos, MD; and Russell F. Warren, MD*

## INTRODUCTION

Recent anatomic and biomechanical evidence has renewed interest in the posterolateral corner (PLC) and posteromedial corner (PMC) of the knee through an improved understanding of their contribution to knee stability. Isolated PLC injuries reportedly represent only 1.6% of acute ligamentous knee injuries. However, PLC injuries have been reported to be as high as 43% to 80% with concurrent ligamentous injuries, namely the anterior cruciate ligament (ACL) and posterior cruciate ligaments (PCL).[1,2] Advancements in imaging techniques and increased suspicion by the examining physician has allowed more PLC injuries to be diagnosed that may have

Ranawat A, Kelly BT. *Musculoskeletal Examination of the Hip and Knee: Making the Complex Simple* (pp. 376-402).
© 2011 SLACK Incorporated

been previously unrecognized. Medial-sided knee injuries, on the other hand, are among the most common injuries to the knee.[3] Nevertheless, the anatomy, diagnosis, and treatment of medial collateral ligament (MCL) and PMC injuries can be challenging, and there should be a high index of suspicion for concomitant meniscal and ligamentous injuries.

As with PLC injuries, missed diagnoses on the medial side can lead to significant disability due to persistent instability and articular cartilage degeneration. Additionally, unrecognized PLC and PMC injuries can place the reconstruction of concurrently injured cruciate ligaments at increased risk for failure due to residual knee instability.[4,5] Prompt recognition and proper treatment of these injuries is, therefore, critical to achieving successful outcomes. Given the increasing frequency with which they are diagnosed and the long-term consequences PLC and PMC injuries can have for patients, it is important to gain a comprehensive understanding of the current evaluation and management principles of these injuries.

# HISTORY

Because PLC and PMC injuries can be masked when they occur in combination with other ligamentous injuries, close attention to a patient's history (in particular, the mechanism of injury and the presenting symptoms) is critical for early detection of these injuries. Symptoms can be variable depending on the severity of injury, amount of instability, and presence of associated injuries. Patients with acute PLC injuries often present complaining of pain in the posterolateral aspect of the knee, with up to 16% experiencing neurological symptoms from peroneal nerve injury.[6-8] During the subacute phase when pain and swelling have subsided, patients may note symptoms of instability, specifically buckling into hyperextension or a varus thrust during the stance phase of gait.[9] Chronic posterolateral injuries can present with medial joint-line pain, lateral joint-line pain, and/or posterolateral pain, as well as complaints of instability with activities such as ascending and descending stairs or slopes and with pivoting or cutting maneuvers.[10] Patients with MCL and PMC injuries will present complaining of medial and posteromedial knee pain and a subjective feeling of instability.[11]

Sports-related trauma, motor vehicle accidents, and falls are the most common causes of PLC and PMC injuries.[2,7,12] Isolated PLC injuries can result from a posterolaterally directed blow to the anteromedial tibia with the knee at or near full extension, resulting in hyperextension and a varus force.[2,8] More commonly, PLC injuries occur in combination with other ligamentous injuries and can be the result of both contact and noncontact hyperextension with external rotation of the tibia, a direct blow to the flexed knee, or high-energy trauma.[6,8,13,14] Injuries to the MCL and PMC are caused most often by a valgus stress to a flexed knee with a planted foot, but can also result from an external rotation pivoting injury or a direct blow to the anterolateral knee. Concomitant meniscal or ligamentous injuries associated with PMC and MCL injuries occur frequently, with some reports as high as 80% in higher-grade MCL sprains.[15] Isolated MCL injuries will rarely injure the medial meniscus but can be associated with lateral compartment chondral injuries. Combined injuries of either the PLC or the PMC and associated structures about the knee may also occur from a complete knee dislocation, in which case a thorough neurovascular assessment is advised, including ankle brachial indices and possible arteriography, to assess potential vascular injury of the limb.[16] Furthermore, a medial knee dislocation with rupture of the MCL may result in a locked dislocation.

# EXAMINATION

Initially, a general examination of the knee including inspection for swelling and ecchymossis, careful palpation for localization of tenderness, and range of motion testing should be conducted. Isolated collateral ligament tears will produce localized swelling with no or minimal effusion. If associated with intra-articular pathology such as an ACL tear or meniscal injury, one would expect an effusion to be present, but if there is capsular disruption from a capsular ligament tear, the hemarthrosis may extravasate and an effusion may not be appreciated.[17] A complete neurovascular assessment of the extremity is essential, especially after higher energy mechanisms of injury or suspected knee dislocation. Additionally, you may discover a peroneal nerve palsy in a patient who suffered a varus injury to the knee. It is also important to assess the patient's gait and limb alignment as injuries to the PLC can cause a standing varus malalignment or varus thrust, whereby the knee buckles into varus during the stance phase of gait.[9,13] Likewise, an MCL or posteromedial corner injury may produce a valgus standing malalignment, and the patient may exhibit a vaulting-type gait secondary to the attempt of the quadriceps to stabilize the knee joint.

From the initial assessment and localization of the injury, as well as the patient's history and symptoms, a more focused physical exam involving specific ligamentous tests for stability should then be performed (Table 16-1). The contralateral uninjured knee is always examined first, providing a basis for comparison for the examiner as well as to give the patient some expectation for the exam on the injured knee. The most commonly used exam to assess the integrity of the lateral collateral ligament (LCL) is the varus stress test (see Table 16-1). During this exam, a varus force is applied to the knee at 30 degrees of flexion and at full extension, with the thigh stabilized against the examining table. Lateral joint line opening at 30 degrees of flexion suggests LCL injury, while opening of the lateral joint line at full extension usually indicates a more severe injury that often includes a complete tear of the LCL as well as injury to the various structures of the PLC.[6] Generally speaking, a 3- to 4-mm opening laterally of the joint line suggests LCL injury alone, whereas a larger opening is seen when additional PLC structures are injured, specifically the popliteus. The most commonly utilized exam to assess asymmetry in tibial external rotation in suspected PLC injuries is the Dial test (see Table 16-1). With the patient prone or supine, the lower legs are synchronously externally rotated at both 30 and 90 degrees of knee flexion and compared. A significant PLC injury is suggested by an increase in tibial external rotation by 10 degrees compared to the uninjured side. The prone position may allow easier measurement of the difference in rotation using the thigh-foot angle (Figure 16-1).[14] An increase in external rotation at 30 degrees that is lessened at 90 degrees suggests an isolated PLC injury, whereas increased external rotation at both 30 and 90 degrees indicates a combined PLC/PCL injury.[18]

**Table 16-1**

## METHODS FOR EXAMINING THE POSTEROLATERAL AND POSTEROMEDIAL CORNERS OF THE KNEE

### LCL and Posterolateral Corner

| EXAMINATION | TECHNIQUE | ILLUSTRATION | GRADING | SIGNIFICANCE |
|---|---|---|---|---|
| Varus stress test | Phase I: Varus force applied to the flexed knee at 30 degrees of flexion<br><br>Phase II: Varus force applied to the knee in full extension | 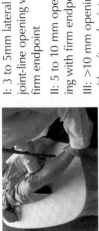 | I: 3 to 5mm lateral joint-line opening with firm endpoint<br><br>II: 5 to 10 mm opening with firm endpoint<br><br>III: >10 mm opening with soft endpoint | Lateral joint-line opening at 30 degrees compared to uninjured knee suggests LCL injury<br><br>Lateral joint opening in full extension suggests combined LCL/PLC injury |
| Tibial external rotation (Dial) test | Simultaneous external rotation of bilateral tibia at 30 and 90 degrees of knee flexion (patient prone or supine) | | + test = Injured side external rotation (ER) 10 degrees greater than uninjured side | Increased ER at 30 degrees compared to uninjured side suggests PLC injury; if lessened at 90 degrees, PLC injury is isolated. If greater ER at 90 degrees than 30 degrees, suggests combined PCL/PLC injury      *(continued)* |

**Table 16-1 (continued)**

## METHODS FOR EXAMINING THE POSTEROLATERAL AND POSTEROMEDIAL CORNERS OF THE KNEE

| EXAMINATION | TECHNIQUE | ILLUSTRATION | GRADING | SIGNIFICANCE |
| --- | --- | --- | --- | --- |
| Posterolateral drawer test | Posterior force on proximal tibia at 90 degrees of knee flexion and 15 degrees of ER | 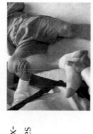 | + test = Posterior and external rotation of lateral tibial plateau compared to medial plateau | + test suggests an incompetent PLC (popliteal tendon and/or popliteofibular ligament) |
| External rotation recurvatum test | Legs in full extension are lifted from the great toes, using gravity as the posteriorly directed force | 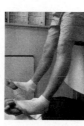 | + test = Injured leg falls into relative hyperextension and varus from tibial external rotation compared to normal side | + test suggests PLC injury |
| Reverse pivot-shift | Passive extension of flexed knee in external rotation with simultaneous valgus force | 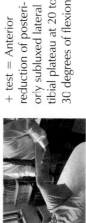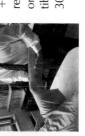 | + test = Anterior reduction of posteriorly subluxed lateral tibial plateau at 20 to 30 degrees of flexion | + test suggests PLC injury. Compare to normal side—can see + test in normal knees |

(continued)

**Table 16-1 (continued)**

## Methods for Examining the Posterolateral and Posteromedial Corners of the Knee

### MCL and Posteromedial Corner

| Examination | Technique | Illustration | Grading | Significance |
|---|---|---|---|---|
| Valgus stress test in external rotation | Phase I: Valgus force applied to the knee flexed at 30 degrees and externally rotated<br><br>Phase II: Valgus force applied to the knee in full extension and externally rotated | | I: 3 to 5 mm medial joint-line opening with firm endpoint<br><br>II: 5 to 10 mm opening with firm endpoint<br><br>III: >10 mm opening with soft endpoint | Medial joint-line opening compared to uninjured knee suggests MCL injury. AMRI suggests PMC injury<br><br>Medial joint opening in full extension suggests combined Grade III MCL and PMC damage |
| External rotation anterior drawer test | Anterior translation of the tibia at 80 degrees of knee flexion and 15 degrees of external rotation | | + test = Greater anterior translation of the medial tibial plateau on injured side compared to uninjured side | Increased anterior translation (AMRI) suggests disruption of meniscotibial ligaments of the PMC |

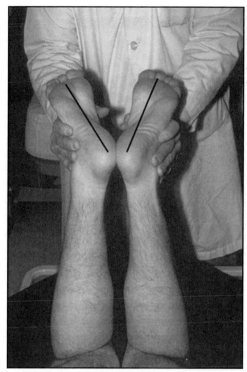

**Figure 16-1.** Photo demonstrating the prone position and proper positioning for the Dial test. Note the ease of measuring the thigh-foot angles.

Rotational stability can also be assessed using the posterolateral drawer test and the external rotation recurvatum test,[19] where the former is performed with the knee in flexion and the latter with the knee in extension (see Table 16-1). When performing the posterolateral drawer test, the knee is flexed to 90 degrees with the foot externally rotated 15 degrees, and a posterior force is applied to the proximal tibia. In the external rotation recurvatum test, both legs are lifted by the examiner grasping the great toes and are observed for relative hyperextension and external rotation of the injured extremity (Figure 16-2). Positive findings in either of these exams denotes likely PLC injury. The reverse pivot shift test[20] (see Table 16-1), a dynamic form of the posterolateral drawer test, is performed by bringing the knee from flexion into extension with the foot in external rotation while applying a valgus force to the knee. A positive test is noted when the posteriorly subluxed lateral

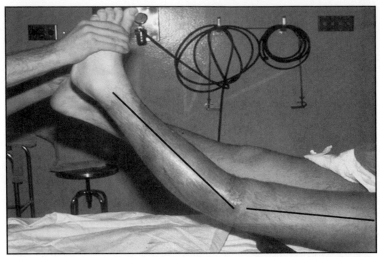

**Figure 16-2.** Photo depicting a left knee PLC injury evident during this positive external rotation recurvatum test. Note the significant recurvatum highlighted by the black lines.

tibial plateau reduces anteriorly at 20 to 30 degrees of flexion as the force vector on the iliotibial band changes from flexion to extension.

The cornerstone of diagnosing and grading injuries to the MCL and PMC is valgus stress testing at 0 degrees and 30 degrees of knee flexion (see Table 16-1). With concomitant PCL or ACL tears, MCL tears are unstable at both 0 degrees and 30 degrees, but with an intact PCL, MCL injuries are stable at 0 degrees but unstable at 30 degrees of knee flexion.[14] Grading of MCL injuries is based on the amount of medial joint line opening. For this exam, the patient lies supine with the hip slightly abducted and flexed and the leg cradled between the examiner's waist and elbow. Alternatively, the patient's leg can be allowed to drop off the side of the examining table with the thigh resting on the table while the exam is performed. A valgus force is applied first with the knee at 30 degrees of flexion to isolate the MCL, with the opposite hand used to palpate the medial joint line to assess the amount of joint opening. In addition to grading, the specific degree of MCL injury may also be elucidated by experienced examiners. A first-degree sprain of the MCL will have tenderness over the

MCL without instability. Second-degree sprains are characterized by increased valgus laxity but maintain a firm endpoint,
while a third-degree sprain will have no definitive endpoint.
Valgus stress testing is then performed with the knee in full
extension. Medial joint line opening in full extension is indicative of a more significant injury, usually a complete Grade III
MCL tear associated with PMC damage as well as ACL and/or
PCL injuries. During these maneuvers, the examiner can also
place a hand over the plantar surface of the foot to provide an
external rotation force and observe for any anteromedial rotation of the medial tibial plateau on the medial femoral condyle. Anteromedial rotatory instability (AMRI) with anterior
subluxation of the medial tibial plateau suggests PMC injury.
In addition to valgus stressing, PMC injuries can be evaluated
using the external rotation anterior drawer test (see Table 16-1).
During this maneuver, an anterior force is applied to the tibia
with the knee flexed to 80 degrees and in 15 degrees of external rotation. Increased anterior translation of the medial tibial
plateau compared to the uninjured side is indicative of disruption of the medial meniscotibial ligaments.[14]

# PATHOANATOMY

Knowledge of the anatomy and biomechanical functions
of the individual structures of the PLC and PMC of the knee
is essential to recognizing, diagnosing, and treating injuries
to these areas. Ongoing efforts to more clearly define the
complex anatomy of these regions has improved the understanding of the roles of the PLC and PMC in maintaining knee
stability. First described more than 25 years ago, the posterolateral aspect of the knee consists of 3 distinct anatomic layers
(Table 16-2 and Figure 16-3).[21] Layer I, the most superficial,
consists of the iliotibial tract and the superficial portion of the
biceps tendon. The common peroneal nerve lies deep to Layer
I on the posterior aspect of the long head of the biceps. Layer II
contains the patellar retinaculum anteriorly and patellofemoral ligaments posteriorly. The deepest layer, Layer III, is
divided into a superficial lamina, which encompasses the LCL
and ends at the fabellofibular ligament, and a deep lamina,
which forms the coronary ligament and popliteal hiatus,

## Table 16-2

### HELPFUL HINTS IN EVALUATING POSTEROLATERAL AND POSTEROMEDIAL CORNER INJURIES

#### Anatomy of the Knee

| | LAYER | ANATOMICAL STRUCTURES |
|---|---|---|
| Lateral side of the knee | I | Iliotibial tract, superficial biceps tendon |
| | II | Patellar retinaculum, lateral patellofemoral ligament |
| | III | LCL, fabellofibular ligament, coronary ligament, arcuate ligament, popliteofibular ligament, popliteus tendon, lateral joint capsule |
| Medial side of the knee | I | Deep crural fascia, sartorius muscle |
| | II | Superficial MCL (POL), medial patellofemoral ligament, and ligaments of the gracilis/semitendinosus/ semimembranosus |
| | III | Deep MCL, true medial joint capsule |

#### Imaging of the Knee in Suspected PLC/PMC Injuries

| MODALITY | FINDING | SIGNIFICANCE |
|---|---|---|
| Standard radiographs (x-rays) | Arcuate sign | Fibula styloid fracture associated with PLC injury |
| | Segond fracture (seen with associated ACL injury) | Joint capsule avulsion fracture off proximal tibia |
| | Pellegrini-Stieda Lesion | MCL calcification associated with chronic MCL injury |
| T2-weighted magnetic resonance imaging (MRI) | High signal superficial to MCL/LCL fibers, fibers intact | Grade I LCL or MCL injury |
| | High signal throughout MCL/LCL fibers, fibers partially intact | Grade II LCL or MCL injury |
| | Complete disruption of MCL/LCL fibers | Grade III LCL or MCL injury |

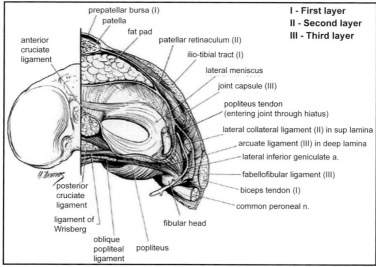

prepatellar bursa (I)
patella
fat pad
anterior cruciate ligament
patellar retinaculum (II)
ilio-tibial tract (I)
lateral meniscus
joint capsule (III)
popliteus tendon (entering joint through hiatus)
lateral collateral ligament (II) in sup lamina
arcuate ligament (III) in deep lamina
lateral inferior geniculate a.
fabellofibular ligament (III)
biceps tendon (I)
common peroneal n.
posterior cruciate ligament
ligament of Wrisberg
fibular head
oblique popliteal ligament
popliteus

I - First layer
II - Second layer
III - Third layer

**Figure 16-3.** Anatomic layers and structures of the lateral side of the knee. (Reprinted with permission from *J Bone Joint Surg Am*, Seebacher JR, Inglis AE, Marshall JL, Warren RF. The structure of the posterolateral aspect of the knee. 1982;64(4):536-541.)

terminating at the arcuate ligament. The popliteofibular ligament and lateral joint capsule are other components of Layer III.

The LCL is the primary static stabilizer to varus instability of the knee, especially during the first 30 degrees of flexion,[6] but receives secondary dynamic stabilization from the iliotibial band. The lateral capsular ligament is also thought to provide stability under varus stress. The popliteus muscle and tendon complex, including the popliteomeniscal fascicles and popliteofibular ligament, serve as the primary dynamic restraints to external tibial rotation.

Like the lateral side, the medial side of the knee has been described anatomically as consisting of 3 distinct layers (Figure 16-4; see Table 16-2).[22] Layer I, the most superficial layer, is comprised of the deep crural fascia investing the sartorius muscle. The superficial MCL; medial patellofemoral ligament; and ligaments of the gracilis, semitendinosus, and semimembranosus all constitute Layer II. The posterior oblique fibers of the superficial MCL has been described as

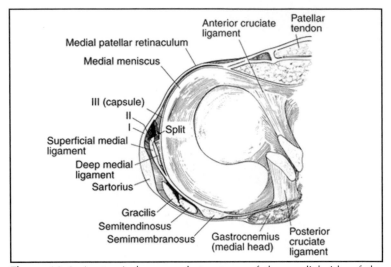

**Figure 16-4.** Anatomic layers and structures of the medial side of the knee. (Reprinted with permission from *J Bone Joint Surg Am,* Warren LF, Marshall JL. The supporting structures and layers on the medial side of the knee: an anatomical analysis. 1979;61(1):56-62.)

a separate anatomic structure—the posterior oblique ligament (POL).[23] The deepest layer, Layer III, consists of the true capsule of the knee joint, which thickens beneath the MCL to form the deep MCL or medial capsular ligament. The deep MCL can be divided into 2 parts via its attachment to the medial meniscus: the meniscotibial (coronary) ligament and meniscofemoral ligament, which attach to the tibia and femur, respectively. At the posteromedial corner of the knee, Layers II and III coalesce to form the posteromedial capsule, which is supported by the fibers of the tendon and sheath of the semimembranosus. The constituents of the "posteromedial corner" include the meniscotibial ligaments, the posterior oblique ligament (POL), the oblique popliteal ligament (OPL), the semimembranosus expansions, and the posterior horn of the medial meniscus.

Although the PMC contributes to knee stability under valgus forces, the superficial MCL, composed of parallel and oblique fibers, is the primary restraint to valgus stress in the knee.[24] The anterior parallel fibers of the superficial MCL are tensioned in knee flexion. In extension, the POL is

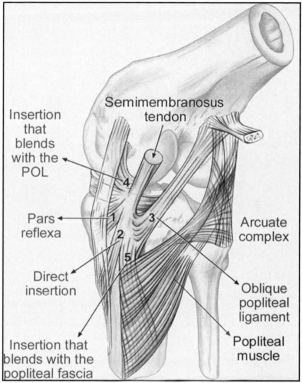

**Figure 16-5.** Illustration of the insertional extensions of the superficial MCL. (From Sims WF, Jacobson KE, *Am J Sports Med*, 32(2), pp. 337-345, copyright © 2004. Reprinted by permission of SAGE publications.)

under tension, while the anterior parallel fibers relax. Similar to the POL, the deep MCL relaxes in flexion and is tight in extension. Additionally, the deep MCL, superficial MCL, and POLs all serve as dynamic restraints to anteromedial rotatory instability of the knee, although the structure providing the primary restraint remains controversial. Finally, through its attachment to the POL and tibia, the semimembranosus contributes to the dynamic stabilization of the PMC. Five expansions of the semimembranosus have been described: (1) pars reflexa, passing anteriorly to insert on the tibia beneath the MCL; (2) direct posteromedial tibial insertion; (3) the OPL insertion; (4) the extension to the POL; and (5) the popliteus aponeurosis expansion (Figure 16-5).[25]

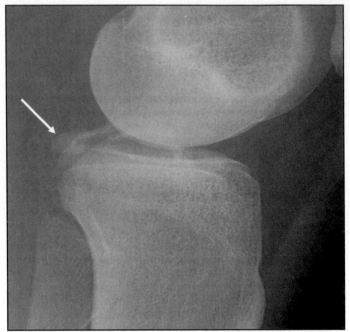

**Figure 16-6.** Lateral radiograph demonstrating the "arcuate sign," or a fracture of the fibula styloid (fragment indicated by arrow), that may be associated with a posterolateral corner injury. In this particular case, the patient also had a posterior cruciate ligament injury.

# IMAGING

For patients with suspected posterolateral or posteromedial corner injuries, a complete series of knee radiographs including standing AP, tunnel (45 degrees flexion), Merchant, and lateral views should be obtained. Findings on knee radiographs suggestive of a PLC injury include abnormal widening of the lateral joint space, an "arcuate" sign (fibula styloid fracture) (Figure 16-6), a Gerdy tubercle avulsion, or a Segond fracture if associated with an ACL injury (avulsion fracture of lateral capsule).[1,2] Similarly, acute MCL and PMC injuries may reveal a widened medial joint space on AP radiographs. In skeletally immature patients, one should always rule out physeal injury to the proximal tibia or distal femur, as these

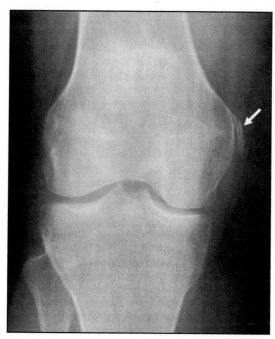

**Figure 16-7.** AP radiograph demonstrating a Pellegrini-Stieda lesion (indicated by arrow), or calcification of the medial collateral ligament associated with chronic injury to the MCL.

are more likely to be injured than the relatively stronger ligaments. Chronic MCL injuries can demonstrate calcification within the substance of the ligament that may be seen on radiographs, known as a Pellegrini-Stieda lesion (Figure 16-7). Stress radiography for PMC or PLC injuries may provide diagnostic assistance in the operating room, but is used infrequently outside the OR given its questionable clinical use and the availability of magnetic resonance imaging (MRI) as a diagnostic modality.

MRI is the primary imaging tool used for assessment of the soft tissues that comprise the posterolateral and posteromedial corners of the knee, although some structures remain difficult to visualize. The normal LCL and MCL appear as taut black structures on T1-weighted, T2-weighted, and proton density MRI images in the coronal plane (Figure 16-8). Injury to the MCL often appears as increased signal intensity on T2-weighted images or disruption of the continuity of the fibers on T1-weighted and proton density images (Figure 16-9).

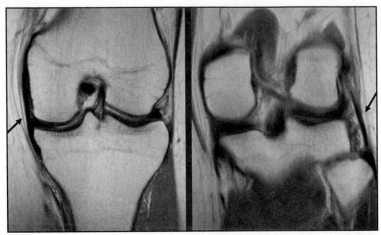

**Figure 16-8.** Coronal proton density MRI images demonstrating the normal taut black appearance of the MCL and LCL (arrows). Note that one should not be able to visualize the entire LCL on a single coronal cut because it has an oblique course. Visualization of the entire LCL on a single coronal cut implies an injury to the ACL.

**Figure 16-9.** Coronal proton density MRI image demonstrating a complete disruption of the fibers of the MCL (indicated by the arrow).

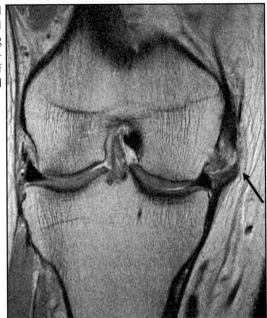

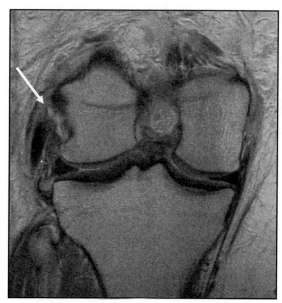

**Figure 16-10.** Coronal proton density MRI image showing a complete tear of the LCL (indicated by the arrow).

Grade I LCL sprains will exhibit high T2 signal superficial to the fibers but the fibers of the ligament remain intact. Grade II LCL sprains will show edema or high T2 signal throughout the ligament fibers, and Grade III demonstrates complete disruption of the ligament without any intact fibers[26] (Figure 16-10). These injuries can be proximal, mid-substance, or distal avulsions. Although MRI can accurately diagnose collateral ligament injuries, the ability to visualize the posteromedial corner, specifically the posteromedial capsule, even in uninjured knees, remains difficult. Like the posteromedial corner, the structures of the posterolateral corner are not consistently visualized on traditional MR sequences. To best visualize the arcuate ligament, fabellofibular ligament, and popliteofibular ligament in their oblique course, it is recommended to add a thin-cut coronal oblique T2-weighted series to the MR imaging protocol.[27] With this addition, the ability to identify these ligaments on MR has been reported at 48%, 46%, and 53%, respectively.[28]

# TREATMENT

## Posterolateral Corner

### Nonoperative Treatment

The treatment of LCL and PLC injuries is guided by the severity (Grading) of injury. Grade I and mild-moderate Grade II LCL injuries can be managed nonoperatively with good outcomes.[7] The nonoperative treatment regimen consists of an initial period of immobilization in a hinged knee brace with the knee locked in extension and protected weight-bearing for 3 to 4 weeks, followed by early mobilization with progressive range of motion exercises and weight-bearing. Return to normal activities is typically permitted by 4 to 6 weeks after injury, but this is patient- and activity-specific and depends on the severity of the injury. Conversely, residual ligamentous laxity and poor functional outcomes have been encountered with nonoperative management of severe Grade II and all Grade III injuries.[7] For this reason, it is recommended that severe Grade II and all Grade III injuries to the LCL/PLC be treated by surgical means, but again the level of activity of the patient, whether he or she is an athlete, and the presence of other injuries all play a role in the treatment decision.

### Operative Treatment

Surgical treatment of LCL/PLC injuries, in particular avulsion injuries, depends heavily on the timing of the injury and the presence of other associated injuries. Ideally, these injuries are addressed in the acute setting (less than 3 weeks from injury)[29] before soft tissue scarring obscures the precise anatomy of the PLC. The options for these injuries are direct primary repair, with or without augmentation, or primary reconstruction, both of which have demonstrated good outcomes when performed acutely.[7,29,30] Associated ACL and PCL injuries are usually addressed first and repaired or reconstructed, followed by the PLC.[29] It is very important to address PLC and MCL injuries when reconstructing the ACL or PCL because missed injuries can place the reconstruction at risk of failure due to increased loads (Figure 16-11). In performing the PLC surgical repair or reconstruction, each anatomic structure of the PLC should be identified and addressed individually to maximize restoration

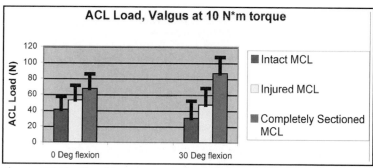

**Figure 16-11.** Graphic representation of the relative increase in load seen by the ACL with injuries to or sectioning of the MCL in cadavers (Reprinted with permission from Dr. Russel F. Warren.).

of native anatomy and biomechanics. Choice of repair, augmentation, or reconstruction will depend on the quality of the tissue and the location of the injury (at osseous insertion or midsubstance). Avulsion injuries should be repaired with rigid internal fixation or sutures. Avulsions from the proximal fibula can readily be reattached en mass in the acute setting. Finally, the peroneal nerve should always be identified and may need to be released to prevent injury during surgery.

In chronic PLC injuries (more than 3 to 4 weeks after injury), scar tissue makes it difficult to identify and anatomically restore the individual structures of the PLC. As such, reconstruction is recommended with attention paid to the LCL, popliteal attachment to the tibia, and the popliteofibular ligament, which are believed to be the most important posterolateral static stabilizers.[29] Limb alignment in the patient with chronic posterolateral instability should be assessed and corrected if necessary using a high tibial osteotomy, prior to PLC reconstructions, because limb malalignment or a varus thrust can lead to failure of the PLC reconstruction from excessive forces during gait.[31] Reconstruction procedures of the PLC are generally divided into fibula-based (nonanatomic) and combined tibia-fibula-based (anatomic) techniques. Fibula-based reconstructions focus on restoration of static varus stability to the knee rather than recreating normal anatomic relationships. Nonanatomic procedures can reconstruct the LCL and popliteofibular ligament[29] and achieve good clinical outcomes with a less technically demanding technique compared to tibia-fibula–based reconstructions.[32] The "anatomic" PLC reconstructions, also known as the tibia-fibula–based techniques, are so-called because they attempt to restore the anatomy of the popliteus in addition to the LCL and popliteofibular ligament. A number of "anatomic" reconstruction techniques have been described, and overall recent short-term results of these procedures in chronic posterolateral instability of the knee appear encouraging (Table 16-3).[33,34]

# Posteromedial Corner

## Nonoperative Treatment

Like the posterolateral corner, Grade I and II injuries to the posteromedial corner are amenable to nonoperative management with good clinical outcomes.[35] A hinged knee brace allows early range of motion while protecting against valgus stresses, and progressive weight-bearing is allowed once pain has subsided. Return to normal activities is permitted by 1 to 2 weeks in Grade I injuries, 3 to 4 weeks in Grade II, and 6 to 8 weeks in Grade III injuries.

## Operative Treatment

The treatment of Grade III injuries to the MCL and posteromedial corner is more controversial than for the lateral side of the knee. Traditionally, Grade III MCL injuries have had good outcomes with conservative therapy, but some patients experienced persistent valgus laxity and poor functional outcomes, which may be the result of underappreciated PMC injuries in those knees.[11] While some authors recommend acute operative treatment of MCL injuries,[36] most authors recommend a trial period of nonoperative treatment for 4 to 6 weeks, with repair or reconstruction reserved for persistent valgus laxity or rotatory instability despite brace therapy.[11,15,37] In patients with combined ACL and MCL/PMC injuries, it is advised to allow the MCL to heal prior to repairing/reconstructing the ACL because MCL injuries can increase loads on the anterior cruciate and jeopardize the reconstruction.[5] The goal of operative repair/reconstruction of the MCL and PMC is to restore the kinematics of the medial side of the knee. This requires anatomic restoration of the posteromedial corner (medial meniscus, POL, and expansions of the semimembranosus) in addition to the superficial MCL.

## Table 16-3

# TECHNIQUES FOR RECONSTRUCTION OF THE LATERAL COLLATERAL LIGAMENT AND POSTEROLATERAL CORNER

## Nonanatomic

| TECHNIQUE | DESCRIPTION | ILLUSTRATION |
|---|---|---|
| Posterolateral complex advancement[10] | Intact but stretched posterolateral complex is advanced en bloc in line with LCL to the lateral femoral epicondyle to restore tension | 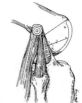 |
| Posterolateral corner sling procedure[38] | Reconstruction of the popliteus using iliotibial band allograft (or other graft) through tibial transosseous tunnel | 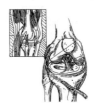 |
| Biceps tenodesis[29] | Central slip of biceps tendon is transferred anteriorly to the lateral femoral epicondyle, recreating LCL and restoring tension to PLC | 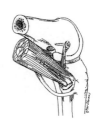 |
| Larson technique[39] | Reconstruction of LCL and PFL with semitendinosus autograft through fibular tunnel | 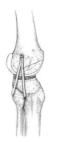 |

*(continued)*

## Table 16-3 (continued)

### TECHNIQUES FOR RECONSTRUCTION OF THE LATERAL COLLATERAL LIGAMENT AND POSTEROLATERAL CORNER

#### Anatomic

| TECHNIQUE | DESCRIPTION | ILLUSTRATION |
| --- | --- | --- |
| 2-graft reconstruction[34] | Two separate grafts (Achilles tendon) passed through tibial and fibular tunnels to reconstruct the LCL, popliteus, and PFL |   |
| Bone-patella tendon-bone (B-PT-B) reconstruction[31] | Combined popliteus muscle-tendon-ligament unit (PMTL) and LCL graft reconstruction with B-PT-B. PMTL is sutured to restore the PFL | 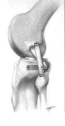 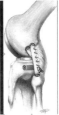 |

Figure 1 is reprinted with permission from *J Bone Joint Surg Am,* Hughston JC, Jacobson KE. Chronic posterolateral rotatory instability of the knee. 1985;67(3):351-359.

Figure 2 is reprinted with permission from Albright JP, Brown AW. Management of chronic posterolateral rotatory instability of the knee: surgical technique for the posterolateral corner sling procedure, in Cannon WD Jr, ed: *Instructional Course Lectures,* volume 47. Rosemont, IL, American Academy of Orthopaedic Surgeons, 1998.

Figure 3 is reprinted with permission from *Clin Sports Med,* 13(3), Veltri DM, Warren RF, Operative treatment of posterolateral instability of the knee, pp 615-627. Copyright Elsevier 1994.

Figure 4 is reprinted with permission from Larson R, Tingstad E. Lateral and posterior instabilities of the knee in the adult. In: DeLee JC, Drez D, eds. *DeLee and Drez's Orthopaedic Sports Medicine: Principles and Practice.* 2nd ed. Philadelphia, PA: Saunders; 2003:1968-1993. Copyright Elsevier 2003.

Figure 5 is from LaPrade RF, Johansen S, Wentorf FA, Engebretsen L, Esterberg JL, Tso A, *Am J Sports Med,* 32(6), pp. 1405-1414, copyright © 2004. Reprinted by permission of SAGE Publications.

Figure 6 is from Noyes FR, Barber-Westin SD, Albright JC, *Am J Sports Med,* 34(9), pp. 1419-1430, copyright © 2006. Reprinted by permission of SAGE Publications.

## Table 16-4

### TECHNIQUES FOR RECONSTRUCTION OF THE MEDIAL COLLATERAL LIGAMENT AND POSTERIOR OBLIQUE LIGAMENT

| Technique | Description | Illustration |
|---|---|---|
| Autogenous hamstring reconstruction of the MCL[40] | Semitendinosus and gracilis autograft is looped through a medial femoral epicondyle drill hole and passed through a transtibial tunnel to reconstruct the anterior fibers of the MCL. | 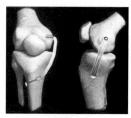 |
| Semitendinosus autograft reconstruction of MCL and POL[41] | Ipsilateral semitendinosus autograft, with pes insertion left intact, is looped into a medial femoral epicondyle drill hole and then passed through a posterior to anterior tibial tunnel to reconstruct the MCL and POL anatomically. | 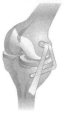 |

Figure 1 is from Yoshiya S, Kuroda R, Mizuno K, Yamamoto T, Kurosaka M, *Am J Sports Med*, 33(9), pp. 1380-1385, copyright © 2005. Reprinted by permission of SAGE Publications.

Figure 2 is from Lind M, Jakobsen BW, Lund B, Hansen MS, Abdallah O, Christiansen SE, *Am J Sports Med*, 37(6), pp. 1116-1122, copyright © 2009. Reprinted by permission of SAGE Publications.

Primary repair of the structures of the posteromedial corner and distal MCL injuries can usually be accomplished. More proximal MCL tears or injuries with poor quality tissue may be better treated with semitendinosus augmentation. However, the superficial MCL may require reconstruction using one of a number of described techniques (Table 16-4).[40,42] Newer techniques aim to reconstruct both the MCL and the POL anatomically in patients with chronic posteromedial instability (see Table 16-4).[41]

# Conclusion

Physicians with high clinical suspicions can reliably diagnose posterolateral and posteromedial corner injuries via a thorough patient history and physical examination employing the provocative maneuvers described in this chapter. Advancements in MRI imaging have further increased the ability to correctly diagnose these injuries. Clinical and surgical management of LCL/posterolateral and MCL/posteromedial corner injuries can be challenging, especially in the multiligamentously injured knee. Techniques for reconstructing these structures have most recently turned toward anatomic approaches to maximizing restoration of knee stability, with promising early results.

# References

1. Covey DC. Injuries of the posterolateral corner of the knee. *J Bone Joint Surg Am*. 2001;83-A(1):106-118.
2. DeLee JC, Riley MB, Rockwood CA Jr. Acute posterolateral rotatory instability of the knee. *Am J Sports Med*. 1983;11(4):199-207.
3. Miyasaka KC, Daniel DM, Stone ML, Hirshman P. The incidence of knee ligament injuries in the general population. *Am J Knee Surg*. 1991;4:3-8.
4. O'Brien SJ, Warren RF, Pavlov H, Panariello R, Wickiewicz TL. Reconstruction of the chronically insufficient anterior cruciate ligament with the central third of the patellar ligament. *J Bone Joint Surg Am*. 1991;73(2):278-286.
5. Battaglia MJ 2nd, Lenhoff MW, Ehteshami JR, et al. Medial collateral ligament injuries and subsequent load on the anterior cruciate ligament: a biomechanical evaluation in a cadaveric model. *Am J Sports Med*. 2009;37(2):305-311.
6. LaPrade RF, Terry GC. Injuries to the posterolateral aspect of the knee: association of anatomic injury patterns with clinical instability. *Am J Sports Med*. 1997;25(4):433-438.
7. Krukhaug Y, Molster A, Rodt A, Strand T. Lateral ligament injuries of the knee. *Knee Surg Sports Traumatol Arthrosc*. 1998;6(1):21-25.
8. Baker CL Jr, Norwood LA, Hughston JC. Acute posterolateral rotatory instability of the knee. *J Bone Joint Surg Am*. 1983;65(5):614-618.
9. Veltri DM, Warren RF. Anatomy, biomechanics, and physical findings in posterolateral knee instability. *Clin Sports Med*. 1994;13(3):599-614.
10. Hughston JC, Jacobson KE. Chronic posterolateral rotatory instability of the knee. *J Bone Joint Surg Am*. 1985;67(3):351-359.
11. Sims WF, Jacobson KE. The posteromedial corner of the knee: medial-sided injury patterns revisited. *Am J Sports Med*. 2004;32(2):337-345.

12. Fleming RE Jr, Blatz DJ, McCarroll JR. Posterior problems in the knee: posterior cruciate insufficiency and posterolateral rotatory insufficiency. *Am J Sports Med.* 1981;9(2):107-113.

13. Hughston JC, Andrews JR, Cross MJ, Moschi A. Classification of knee ligament instabilities. Part II: the lateral compartment. *J Bone Joint Surg Am.* 1976;58(2):173-179.

14. Hughston JC, Andrews JR, Cross MJ, Moschi A. Classification of knee ligament instabilities. Part I: the medial compartment and cruciate ligaments. *J Bone Joint Surg Am.* 1976;58(2):159-172.

15. Fetto JF, Marshall JL. Medial collateral ligament injuries of the knee: a rationale for treatment. *Clin Orthop Relat Res.* 1978;132(132):206-218.

16. Ranawat A, Baker CL 3rd, Henry S, Harner CD. Posterolateral corner injury of the knee: evaluation and management. *J Am Acad Orthop Surg.* 2008;16(9):506-518.

17. Kurzweil PR, Kelley ST. Physical examination and imaging of the medial collateral ligament and posteromedial corner of the knee. *Sports Med Arthrosc.* 2006;14(2):67-73.

18. Veltri DM, Deng XH, Torzilli PA, Warren RF, Maynard MJ. The role of the cruciate and posterolateral ligaments in stability of the knee. A biomechanical study. *Am J Sports Med.* 1995;23(4):436-443.

19. Hughston JC, Norwood LA Jr. The posterolateral drawer test and external rotational recurvatum test for posterolateral rotatory instability of the knee. *Clin Orthop Relat Res.* 1980;147(147):82-87.

20. Jakob RP, Hassler H, Staeubli HU. Observations on rotatory instability of the lateral compartment of the knee. Experimental studies on the functional anatomy and the pathomechanism of the true and the reversed pivot shift sign. *Acta Orthop Scand Suppl.* 1981;191:1-32.

21. Seebacher JR, Inglis AE, Marshall JL, Warren RF. The structure of the posterolateral aspect of the knee. *J Bone Joint Surg Am.* 1982;64(4):536-541.

22. Warren LF, Marshall JL. The supporting structures and layers on the medial side of the knee: an anatomical analysis. *J Bone Joint Surg Am.* 1979;61(1):56-62.

23. Hughston JC, Eilers AF. The role of the posterior oblique ligament in repairs of acute medial (collateral) ligament tears of the knee. *J Bone Joint Surg Am.* 1973;55(5):923-940.

24. Wymenga AB, Kats JJ, Kooloos J, Hillen B. Surgical anatomy of the medial collateral ligament and the posteromedial capsule of the knee. *Knee Surg Sports Traumatol Arthrosc.* 2006;14(3):229-234.

25. Muller W. *The Knee: Form, Function and Ligament Reconstruction.* Berlin, Germany: Springer-Verlag; 1983.

26. Sanders TG, Miller MD. A systematic approach to magnetic resonance imaging interpretation of sports medicine injuries of the knee. *Am J Sports Med.* 2005;33(1):131-148.

27. LaPrade RF, Gilbert TJ, Bollom TS, Wentorf F, Chaljub G. The magnetic resonance imaging appearance of individual structures of the posterolateral knee. A prospective study of normal knees and knees with surgically verified grade III injuries. *Am J Sports Med.* 2000;28(2):191-199.

28. Yu JS, Salonen DC, Hodler J, Haghighi P, Trudell D, Resnick D. Posterolateral aspect of the knee: improved MR imaging with a coronal oblique technique. *Radiology*. 1996;198(1):199-204.

29. Veltri DM, Warren RF. Operative treatment of posterolateral instability of the knee. *Clin Sports Med*. 1994;13(3):615-627.

30. Stannard JP, Brown SL, Farris RC, McGwin G Jr, Volgas DA. The posterolateral corner of the knee: repair versus reconstruction. *Am J Sports Med*. 2005;33(6):881-888.

31. Noyes FR, Barber-Westin SD, Albright JC. An analysis of the causes of failure in 57 consecutive posterolateral operative procedures. *Am J Sports Med*. 2006;34(9):1419-1430.

32. Khanduja V, Somayaji HS, Harnett P, Utukuri M, Dowd GS. Combined reconstruction of chronic posterior cruciate ligament and posterolateral corner deficiency. A two- to nine-year follow-up study. *J Bone Joint Surg Br*. 2006;88(9):1169-1172.

33. Yoon KH, Bae DK, Ha JH, Park SW. Anatomic reconstructive surgery for posterolateral instability of the knee. *Arthroscopy*. 2006;22(2):159-165.

34. LaPrade RF, Johansen S, Wentorf FA, Engebretsen L, Esterberg JL, Tso A. An analysis of an anatomical posterolateral knee reconstruction: an in vitro biomechanical study and development of a surgical technique. *Am J Sports Med*. 2004;32(6):1405-1414.

35. Lundberg M, Messner K. Long-term prognosis of isolated partial medial collateral ligament ruptures. A ten-year clinical and radiographic evaluation of a prospectively observed group of patients. *Am J Sports Med*. 1996;24(2):160-163.

36. Frolke JP, Oskam J, Vierhout PA. Primary reconstruction of the medial collateral ligament in combined injury of the medial collateral and anterior cruciate ligaments. short-term results. *Knee Surg Sports Traumatol Arthrosc*. 1998;6(2):103-106.

37. Jacobson KE, Chi FS. Evaluation and treatment of medial collateral ligament and medial-sided injuries of the knee. *Sports Med Arthrosc*. 2006;14(2):58-66.

38. Albright JP, Brown AW. Management of chronic posterolateral rotatory instability of the knee: surgical technique for the posterolateral corner sling procedure. *Instr Course Lect*. 1998;47:369-378.

39. Larson R, Tingstad E. Lateral and posterior instabilities of the knee in the adult. In: DeLee JC, Drez D, eds. *DeLee and Drez's Orthopaedic Sports Medicine: Principles and Practice*. 2nd ed. Philadelphia, PA: Saunders; 2003:1968-1993.

40. Yoshiya S, Kuroda R, Mizuno K, Yamamoto T, Kurosaka M. Medial collateral ligament reconstruction using autogenous hamstring tendons: technique and results in initial cases. *Am J Sports Med*. 2005;33(9):1380-1385.

41. Lind M, Jakobsen BW, Lund B, Hansen MS, Abdallah O, Christiansen SE. Anatomical reconstruction of the medial collateral ligament and posteromedial corner of the knee in patients with chronic medial collateral ligament instability. *Am J Sports Med*. 2009;37(6):1116-1122.

42. Fenton RL. Surgical repair of a torn tibial collateral ligament of the knee by means of the semitendinosus tendon (bosworth procedure); report of twenty-eight cases. *J Bone Joint Surg Am*. 1957;39-A(2):304-308.

**17**

# KNEE MALALIGNMENT AND HIGH TIBIAL OSTEOTOMY

*Volker Musahl, MD and Thomas L. Wickiewicz, MD*

## INTRODUCTION

The rationale for realignment osteotomies about the knee is to transfer weight-bearing forces from an overloaded compartment of the knee to a relatively healthy compartment of the knee.[1] Although other surgical options for treatment of the arthritic knee confined to a single compartment show good clinical outcome, osteotomy about the knee remains a valuable option.[2,3] This is particularly true in knees with concomitant ligament, meniscus, or articular cartilage injury.[2,4,5]

Osteotomy of the knee was first reported by Jackson in 1958.[6] In 1964, Garpiepy described a closing wedge technique that was later further modified and popularized by Coventry.[1,7]

Ranawat A, Kelly BT. *Musculoskeletal Examination of the Hip and Knee: Making the Complex Simple* (pp. 403-420).
© 2011 SLACK Incorporated

Modifications of the lateral closing wedge or Coventry osteotomy continue to be in use today. Several modifications to the classic technique described by Coventry in 1965 have been described.[8-10] The technology of locked plating has improved both union rates and the ability of early accelerated rehabilitation.[11] Computer navigation systems have been used to increase the accuracy of osteotomy procedures and prevent surgical errors.[12]

There are several disadvantages to the lateral closing wedge osteotomy. Tibial slope is more difficult to control and is often inadvertently decreased. This may alter tension in the posterior cruciate ligament (PCL) and adversely affect knee kinematics in PCL-deficient patients.[13] Lateral closing wedge osteotomies require 2 cuts to be made, and intraoperative adjustments are more difficult. The proximal tibiofibular joint is violated, and there is an increased risk to the peroneal nerve. Furthermore, and most importantly, lateral closing wedge osteotomy alters the shape of the proximal tibia with bone loss and changes in patella height, complicating subsequent total knee arthroplasty (TKA) procedures. However, clinical outcomes for TKA following osteotomy were shown to be similar to patients with primary TKA.[14,15]

The medial opening wedge osteotomy was developed as an alternative to the lateral closing wedge osteotomy to avoid the above-mentioned disadvantages.[16] Opening wedge osteotomies may be technically easier to perform than closing wedge osteotomies because they require only one bone cut. Multiplanar correction can be obtained, and opening wedge osteotomies can be used to treat varus malalignment and lesser degrees of valgus malalignment. Instead of removing bone, and effectively shortening the extremity, opening wedge osteotomies add bone to the diseased and collapsed side.[17] In addition, disruption of the proximal tibiofibular joint or osteotomy of the fibula is not required as it is with closing wedge osteotomy.[8] There are also disadvantages with the medial opening wedge osteotomy. There is a potential need for bone grafting materials. Autogenous bone graft has the disadvantage of harvest site morbidity, and allogenic bone graft has the disadvantage of increased risk for delayed union or nonunion and risk for disease transmission. In addition, the postoperative rehabilitation protocol needs to be adjusted with a longer period of nonweight-bearing. Bleeding complications are more common because the medullary canal is opened instead of closed.

The key to successful osteotomy procedures is careful patient selection. Absolute contraindications to osteotomy are 1) diffuse, nonspecific pain, 2) primary patellofemoral pain, 3) meniscectomy in the contralateral compartment, 4) osteoarthritis (OA) in the contralateral compartment, and 5) inflammatory arthritis. Relative contraindications are 1) older than age 60, 2) range of motion arc less than 90 degrees, 3) obesity, 4) severe OA, 5) tibiofemoral subluxation, and 6) uncorrected moderate or severe ligamentous laxity (Table 17-1).

# HISTORY

The ideal patient for osteotomy is a thin, active patient in the fifth or sixth decade of life, with localized, activity-related pain confined to one compartment of the knee, without patellofemoral symptoms, a stable knee, full range of motion, and realistic expectations with respect to clinical outcomes. Emphasis on the quality and location of pain as well as the desired activity level postsurgery is important. Although symptoms related to ligamentous laxity, if untreated, present a contraindication to osteotomy, combined osteotomy and ligament reconstruction become increasingly more common.

Patients with a history of inflammatory arthritis should not be treated with osteotomy.[18] Post-traumatic arthritis, osteochondritis dissecans, or unilateral meniscectomy have not been shown to adversely affect patient outcomes. Combined medial and lateral meniscectomies, however, present a contraindication.[19] In most patients older than 60 years, arthroplasty provides more complete pain relief and shorter rehabilitation and is more reliable than osteotomy.[20] Uni-compartmental arthroplasty as a temporizing procedure is becoming more popular; however, long-term results are inferior to those of TKA as are results of revision arthroplasty. Tibial osteotomy remains the procedure of choice in younger, active patients with uni-compartmental arthritis, and TKA is preferred in older, lower-demand patients.[21]

**Table 17-1**

## *HELPFUL HINTS:*
## *CONTRAINDICATIONS TO OSTEOTOMY*

### Absolute
- Diffuse knee pain
- Primary patellofemoral pain
- Meniscectomy in contralateral compartment
- OA in contralateral compartment
- Inflammatory arthritis

### Relative
- Older than age 60
- Obesity
- Range of motion arc less than 90 degrees
- Severe OA
- Tibiofemoral subluxation
- Uncorrected ligamentous laxity

# EXAMINATION

Physical examination starts with inspection of gait. Observations should be made regarding antalgic gait, favoring one side, Trendelenburg gait (should lead to assessment of hip function), thrust (ligamentous incompetence), foot arch (hyperpronating individuals tend to overload the patellofemoral joint), and limb alignment. Next, the ipsilateral hip, ankle joint, and lower back should be examined. Decreased range of motion in any of the above-mentioned joints should be further evaluated for the presence of OA or other pathologies. Particularly, hip joint pathology can present with referred pain down the adductors and the knee. Inspection of the limb in the supine position should confirm the presence of malalignment (Table 17-2). The skin should be inspected for the presence of skin incisions, which may affect the intended surgical exposure.

**Table 17-2**

## METHODS FOR EXAMINING THE MALALIGNED KNEE

| Examination | Technique | Illustration | Grading | Significance |
|---|---|---|---|---|
| Gait | Examine hip, knee, ankle, foot | Varus thrust 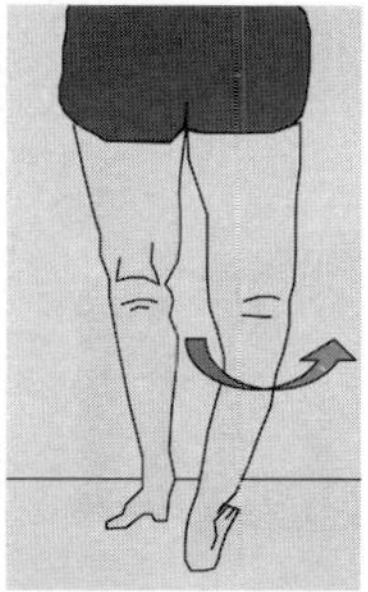 | Presence, Yes/No | Trendelenburg gait may be related to hip. Thrust is related to ligament incompetence. High arch may be related to neuromuscular conditions |
| Range of motion | Measure extension and flexion with goniometer | Flexion contracture 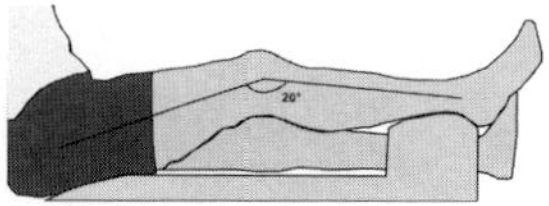 | In degrees | Fixed flexion contractures greater than 10 degrees represent contraindication |

*(continued)*

**Table 17-2 (continued)**

### METHODS FOR EXAMINING THE MALALIGNED KNEE

| Examination | Technique | Illustration | Grading | Significance |
|---|---|---|---|---|
| Alignment | Examine mechanical axis of limb | Bilateral, R>L tibial varus 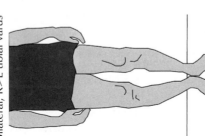 | >1 degree varus = varus<br><1 degree varus = valgus | Severe varus (>20 degrees) may be treated with dome osteotomy. Severe valgus (>12 degrees) may be treated with femoral osteotomy |

Knee range of motion should reveal a full flexion-extension arc with less than 10 degrees of fixed flexion contracture. Examination of the patella should not reveal any significant pain, malalignment, or maltracking. Medial and lateral joint lines should be free of any significant meniscal pathology. The McMurray test is best applied in deep flexion with the examiner's finger on the joint line and the other hand exerting varying degrees of internal-external rotation and varus-valgus torques. The neurovascular status of the intended operative limb needs to be assessed and carefully documented. Obesity is associated with lower success rates and needs to be openly discussed with the patient. Alternative procedures and nutritional advice should be discussed.

## Pathoanatomy

OA is a result of loss of balance between biological resistance of the joint and the stresses acting on it. Excessive pressure has a deleterious effect on articular cartilage, and higher levels of deformity increase the magnitude of contact pressure in the compartment toward the load axis.[22,23] Maquet's biomechanical theory of joint stability states that, in a normal knee, there exists equilibrium between 2 forces. The resulting force creates compressive stresses across the knee and must act perpendicular to the weight-bearing surface.[24] Altered forces in cases of malalignment, therefore, lead to increased bone mineral density of the affected femoral and tibial condyles.[25] These increased densities decrease significantly at 1 year following adequate realignment osteotomy.[26]

The goal of osteotomy procedures is to correct coronal plane alignment, relieve pain, improve function, and maintain normal knee kinematics otherwise precluded by arthroplasty procedures. However, with traditional osteotomy procedures, changes in sagittal plane alignment can occur. These changes can adversely affect postsurgical outcomes in patients with concomitant ligamentous laxity. Increasing tibial slope can adversely affect outcomes for patients with anterior cruciate ligament (ACL) deficiency while decreasing tibial slope can adversely affect outcomes for patients with PCL deficiency.[27] Traditional osteotomies have also been shown to alter the

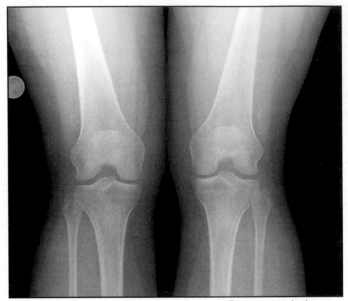

**Figure 17-1.** Posteroanterior 45 degrees flexion weight-bearing radiograph.

anatomical relationship between the patella and tibial tubercle. Patella infera can occur after both opening and closing wedge osteotomies.[28]

# IMAGING

Standing anteroposterior, 45 degrees posteroanterior flexion weight-bearing (Figure 17-1), lateral (Figure 17-2), and Merchant views (Figure 17-3) are the standard views to evaluate for severity of OA (Figure 17-4). Careful inspection of the contralateral tibiofemoral compartment for marginal osteophytes or condylar flattening is warranted to assess the presence of diffuse, multi-compartmental OA. A full-length, hip-to-toe weight-bearing radiograph is used to determine the mechanical axis of the limb. Long cassette films of the femur and tibia are helpful to determine deformities in the femur and tibia that may have an effect on overall limb alignment.

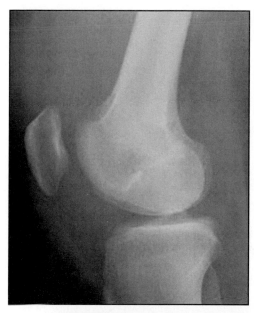

**Figure    17-2.**    Lateral radiograph.

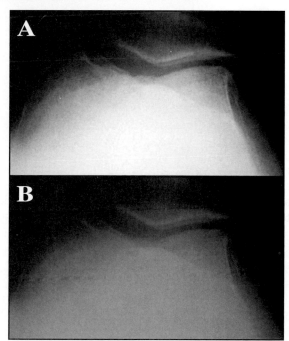

**Figure 17-3.** Merchant view.

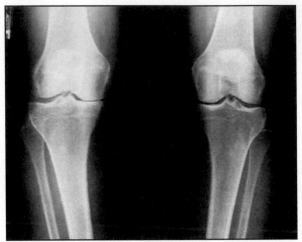

**Figure 17-4.** AP radiograph demonstrating bilateral tibial varus and medial joint space narrowing, right > left.

Preoperative planning is essential when performing osteotomies. Location (femur, tibia, obliquity, defects, laxity), direction (sagittal, coronal, rotational), and magnitude of malalignment must be assessed. Undercorrection or overcorrection are reasons for premature failure and may be secondary to poor preoperative planning or surgical technique. The anatomic axis, or femoral-tibial axis, is measured from standing radiographs and normally measures 5 to 7 degrees of valgus. The height of a tibial osteotomy wedge is estimated by the rule of thumb that each millimeter cut provides 1 degree of angular correction. However, these measurements are only accurate for tibiae that are 56 mm in width. Knowing that the mean tibial width is 80 mm in men and 70 mm in women, this method invariably leads to undercorrection of the deformity.

The mechanical axis is based on a line connecting the center of the femoral head and center of the ankle mortise and normally measures 1.2 degrees of varus. This axis is more accurate, particularly when femoral and tibial deformities are present. The measurement for the medial edge of the proximal tibia to this line divided by the entire width of the tibia determines the weight-bearing axis. The appropriate coordinate for the mechanical axis is at 62% from medial to lateral (Figure 17-5).[29]

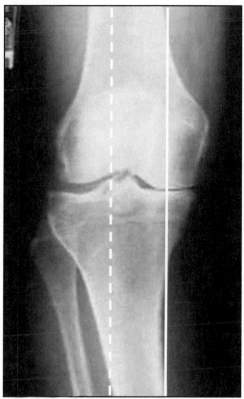

**Figure 17-5.** Mechanical axis shifted into the medial compartment (solid line). Desired mechanical axis in the noninvolved compartment (dashed line).

# TREATMENT

Conservative treatment options include patient education with respect to body weight, nutrition, and activity modification. Rehabilitation is aimed at improving muscle control, core strength, and proprioception. A short course of nonsteroidal anti-inflammatory drugs (NSAIDs) may be beneficial for acute flare-ups. Glucosamine and chondroitin have been shown to have beneficial effects in some patients. As a diagnostic and therapeutic tool, one can use unloader braces or shoe wedges. The role of arthroscopy is limited to patients with mechanical symptoms and should be carefully indicated.[30]

The authors' preferred osteotomy is the coronal plane high tibial osteotomy.[31] Regional anesthesia is preferred. A radiolucent operating table is required, and the patient is supine

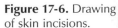
**Figure 17-6.** Drawing of skin incisions.

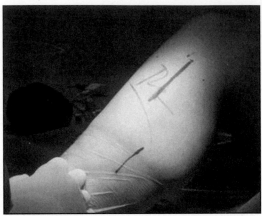

with a tourniquet over the proximal thigh elevated to 250 mm Hg. Fluoroscopic assistance during surgery is essential, and an EKG lead may be used over the center of the femoral head for intraoperative determination of the mechanical axis. The affected extremity is draped free. Arthroscopy is carried out in case of loose bodies, meniscus tears, or articular cartilage flap tears that warrant débridement.

A 2 cm straight lateral incision is taken down through skin and subcutaneous tissue approximately 4 to 7 cm distal to the fibular head (Figure 17-6). After division of the periosteum overlying the fibula, 2 mini-Hohman retractors are placed around the fibula. An oblique (superolateral to inferomedial) osteotomy is completed with a sagittal mini-oscillating saw.

An incision is carried out laterally midway between tubercle and fibula starting at the level of the inferior pole of the patella and continuing 8 cm distally. The anterior compartment fascia is incised longitudinally, and the tibialis anterior muscle is elevated off the tibia with a periosteal elevator (Figure 17-7). A Bennet retractor was placed posteriorly, protecting the anterior compartment musculature and deep neurovascular structures. The laterally based oblique osteotomy consists of one cut extending inferoposteriorly from the tibial tubercle (Figure 17-8). Prior to completion of the osteotomy, 2 drill holes are created in the distal aspect of the osteotomy with a 4.5 mm AO drill bit.

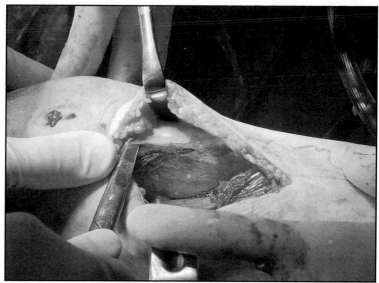

**Figure 17-7.** Elevation of the tibialis anterior muscle off the tibia.

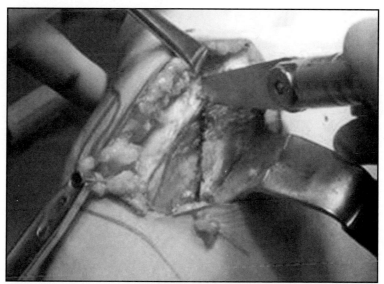

**Figure 17-8.** Laterally based oblique osteotomy extending inferoposteriorly from the tibial tubercle.

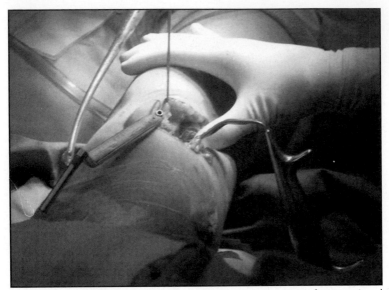

**Figure 17-9.** Steinmann pin in place across osteotomy for rotational control and to prevent shortening. Angular correction is performed manually.

The direction of the drill holes should be perpendicular to the osteotomy and aimed at the posterior tibial diaphysis. The osteotomy is completed with a sagittal saw and 1 inch osteotomes. A smooth Steinmann pin is placed across the osteotomy prior to completion to provide rotational control and prevent shortening. Angular correction is performed under fluoroscopy control, shifting the mechanical axis 62% into the uninvolved compartment using the electrocautery cord (Figures 17-9 and 17-10). The coronal plane osteotomy can be used for both varus and valgus deformities. While stabilizing the osteotomy with bone-holding forceps, two 4.5-mm cortical screws are used as lag screws. It is preferred to use 6.5-mm cancellous screws if screw purchase is poor secondary to extension of the drill hole into the soft posterior tibial metaphysis. A laterally based neutralization plate is then used on the tibia to provide initial stability to the osteotomy site; locked plate techniques have been shown to be beneficial for increased union rates and early weight-bearing (Figure 17-11).[11]

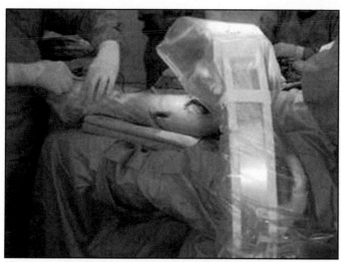

**Figure 17-10.** Angular correction is performed under fluoroscopy control.

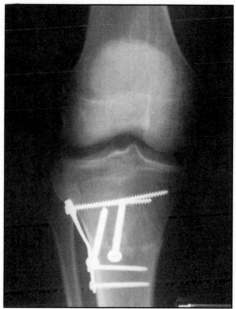

**Figure 17-11.** Postoperative AP radiograph.

Irrigation of wounds is performed, and fascia and skin are closed over a drain in standard fashion. A soft, sterile dressing is applied, after which the leg is placed in a hinged knee brace locked in extension. Patients are usually admitted for one night to monitor bleeding, neurovascular status, and compartment checks. Postoperatively, patients remain nonweight-bearing for 6 to 8 weeks until there is both radiographic and clinical evidence of healing. Range of motion exercises are initiated on the day of surgery using a continuous passive motion (CPM) machine. After the healing phase, patients are progressed to active and active-assisted range of motion exercises with the physical therapist. Patients are then gradually progressed to closed-chain strengthening exercises. More strenuous exercises are allowed after 5 to 6 months postoperatively.

## CONCLUSION

The coronal plane high tibial osteotomy is a technique that can be used for treatment of varus or valgus malalignment. When using TKA as an endpoint, 5-year clinical follow-up results show 84% survival of varus-malaligned knees and 60% survival of valgus-malaligned knees. In contrast to closing wedge osteotomy and opening wedge osteotomy, the coronal plane osteotomy results in no significant change in Insall-Salvati ratio and proximal tibial slope.[31] Osteotomy about the knee presents a good treatment alternative for carefully selected patients. Although current indications for osteotomy are narrow, the long-term results linked with careful preoperative planning, accurate surgical technique, and appropriate postoperative alignment are good, and a 10-year survival of 50% to 75% of realigned knees can be expected.[32,33] Osteotomy remains an important treatment alternative to arthroplasty in the active, middle-aged patient.

## REFERENCES

1. Coventry MB. Osteotomy of the upper portion of the tibia for degenerative arthritis of the knee: a preliminary report. *J Bone Joint Surg Am.* 1965;47:984-990.

2. Mont MA, Stuchin SA, Paley D, et al. Different surgical options for monocompartmental osteoarthritis of the knee: high tibial osteotomy versus unicompartmental knee arthroplasty versus total knee arthroplasty: indications, techniques, results, and controversies. *Instr Course Lect.* 2004;53:265-283.

3. Swienckowski JJ, Pennington DW. Unicompartmental knee arthroplasty in patients sixty years of age or younger. *J Bone Joint Surg Am.* 2004;86-A Suppl 1(Pt 2):131-142.

4. McGuire DA, Carter TR, Shelton WR. Complex knee reconstruction: osteotomies, ligament reconstruction, transplants, and cartilage treatment options. *Arthroscopy.* 2002;18(9 Suppl 2):90-103.

5. Sterett WI, Steadman JR. Chondral resurfacing and high tibial osteotomy in the varus knee. *Am J Sports Med.* 2004;32(5):1243-1249.

6. Jackson J. Osteotomy for osteoarthritis of the knee. In: Proceedings of the Sheffield Regional Orthopaedic Club. *J Bone Joint Surg Br.* 1958;40B:826.

7. Gariepy G. Genu varum treated by high tibial osteotomy. In: Proceedings of the Joint Meeting of Orthopaedic Associations. *J Bone Joint Surg Br.* 1964;46B:783-784.

8. Amendola A, Fowler PJ, Litchfield R, Kirkley S, Clatworthy M. Opening wedge high tibial osteotomy using a novel technique: early results and complications. *J Knee Surg.* 2004;17(3):164-169.

9. Koshino T, Murase T, Saito T. Medial opening-wedge high tibial osteotomy with use of porous hydroxyapatite to treat medial compartment osteoarthritis of the knee. *J Bone Joint Surg Am.* 2003;85-A(1):78-85.

10. Lobenhoffer P, Agneskirchner JD. Improvements in surgical technique of valgus high tibial osteotomy. *Knee Surg Sports Traumatol Arthrosc.* 2003;11(3):132-138.

11. Staubli AE, De Simoni C, Babst R, and Lobenhoffer P. TomoFix: a new LCP-concept for open wedge osteotomy of the medial proximal tibia—early results in 92 cases. *Injury.* 2003;34 Suppl 2:B55-B62.

12. Pearle AD, Goleski P, Musahl V, and Kendoff D. Reliability of image-free navigation to monitor lower-limb alignment. *J Bone Joint Surg Am.* 2009;91 Suppl 1:90-94.

13. Giffin JR, Vogrin TM, Zantop T, Woo SL, Harner CD. Effects of increasing tibial slope on the biomechanics of the knee. *Am J Sports Med.* 2004;32(2):376-382.

14. Meding JB, Keating EM, Ritter MA, Faris PM. Total knee arthroplasty after high tibial osteotomy. A comparison study in patients who had bilateral total knee replacement. *J Bone Joint Surg Am.* 2000;82(9):1252-1259.

15. Parvizi J, Hanssen AD, Spangehl MJ. Total knee arthroplasty following proximal tibial osteotomy: risk factors for failure. *J Bone Joint Surg Am.* 2004;86-A(3):474-479.

16. Marti RK, Verhagen RA, Kerkhoffs GM, Moojen TM. Proximal tibial varus osteotomy. Indications, technique, and five to twenty-one-year results. *J Bone Joint Surg Am.* 2001;83-A(2):164-170.

17. Amendola A. Unicompartmental osteoarthritis in the active patient: the role of high tibial osteotomy. *Arthroscopy.* 2003;19 Suppl 1:109-116.

18. Coventry MB. Upper tibial osteotomy. *Clin Orthop Relat Res.* 1984;182:46-52.
19. Morrey BF. Upper tibial osteotomy for secondary osteoarthritis of the knee. *J Bone Joint Surg Br.* 1989;71(4):554-559.
20. Insall JN, Joseph DM, Msika C. High tibial osteotomy for varus gonarthrosis. A long-term follow-up study. *J Bone Joint Surg Am.* 1984;66(7):1040-1048.
21. Sculco TP. Orthopaedic crossfire—can we justify unicondylar arthroplasty as a temporizing procedure? In opposition. *J Arthroplasty.* 2002;17(4 Suppl 1):56-58.
22. McKellop HA, Sigholm G, Redfern FC, Doyle B, Sarmiento A, Luck JV Sr. The effect of simulated fracture-angulations of the tibia on cartilage pressures in the knee joint. *J Bone Joint Surg Am.* 1991;73(9):1382-1391.
23. Ogata K, Whiteside LA, Lesker PA, Simmons DJ. The effect of varus stress on the moving rabbit knee joint. *Clin Orthop Relat Res.* 1977;129:313-318.
24. Maquet P. Valgus osteotomy for osteoarthritis of the knee. *Clin Orthop Relat Res.* 1976;120:143-148.
25. Akamatsu Y, Koshino T, Saito T, Wada, J. Changes in osteosclerosis of the osteoarthritic knee after high tibial osteotomy. *Clin Orthop Relat Res.* 1997;334:207-214.
26. Koshino T, Ranawat NS. Healing process of osteoarthritis in the knee after high tibial osteotomy. Through observation of strontium-85 scintimetry. *Clin Orthop Relat Res.* 1972;82:149-156.
27. Giffin JR, Stabile KJ, Zantop T, Vogrin TM, Woo SL, Harner CD. Importance of tibial slope for stability of the posterior cruciate ligament deficient knee. *Am J Sports Med.* 2007;35(9):1443-1449.
28. Scuderi GR, Windsor RE, Insall JN. Observations on patellar height after proximal tibial osteotomy. *J Bone Joint Surg Am.* 1989;71(2):245-248.
29. Dugdale TW, Noyes FR, Styer D. Preoperative planning for high tibial osteotomy. The effect of lateral tibiofemoral separation and tibiofemoral length. *Clin Orthop Relat Res.* 1992;274:248-264.
30. Kirkley A, Birmingham TB, Litchfield RB, et al. A randomized trial of arthroscopic surgery for osteoarthritis of the knee. *N Engl J Med.* 2008;359(11):1097-1107.
31. Baumgarten KM, Fealy S, Lyman S, Wickiewicz TL. The coronal plane high tibial osteotomy. Part 1: a clinical and radiographic analysis of intermediate term outcomes. *Hss J.* 2007;3(2):147-154.
32. Billings A, Scott DF, Camargo MP, Hofmann AA. High tibial osteotomy with a calibrated osteotomy guide, rigid internal fixation, and early motion. Long-term follow-up. *J Bone Joint Surg Am.* 2000;82(1):70-79.
33. Sprenger TR, Doerzbacher JF. Tibial osteotomy for the treatment of varus gonarthrosis. Survival and failure analysis to twenty-two years. *J Bone Joint Surg Am.* 2003;85-A(3):469-474.

**18**

# PATELLOFEMORAL INSTABILITY

*James P. Bradley, MD*

## INTRODUCTION

Acute patellar dislocation is the second most common cause of traumatic knee hemarthrosis[1] and can be the cause of persistent pain and disability. While the incidence of primary patellofemoral dislocation in the general population is 5.8 per 100,000, it is significantly increased (29 per 100,000) in the 10- to 17-year-old age group.[2,3] Pain and instability from primary dislocation is common, with up to 55% of patients failing to return to their previous level of sports activity.[4] While nonoperative treatment is largely considered successful, recurrence rates with this method of treatment are not insignificant and have been reported between 15% and 44%.[3]

Ranawat A, Kelly BT. *Musculoskeletal Examination of the Hip and Knee: Making the Complex Simple* (pp. 421-439).
© 2011 SLACK Incorporated

Furthermore, those who have at least one subsequent dislocation have a 50% chance of having recurrent instability.[2]

While defining patellofemoral instability may be relatively
simple, treatment requires an understanding of the many factors involved and their relationship with one another. These
factors include limb alignment, bony architecture, soft tissue
constraints, and the surrounding musculature.[5]

# HISTORY

A thorough history should evaluate the onset and duration of symptoms, mechanism of injury, prior patellofemoral
symptoms, and any prior treatment.[6] If a complete dislocation
occurred, the examiner should ask if the patella had to be
manually reduced or if it spontaneously reduced. Finally, the
location and quality of any current pain should be discussed
as well as any aggravating or alleviating factors (Table 18-1).

# EXAMINATION

The physical examination of the knee for patellofemoral
instability follows the same principles for evaluating other
conditions. These principles include visual inspection, palpation, range of motion, strength testing, instability tests, and
gait analysis. In addition, there are several specific tests used
for establishing the diagnosis of patellofemoral instability.

It is important to first perform a visual inspection of the
knee and entire lower extremity with the patient standing and supine. Specifically, with the patient standing, the
examiner should evaluate for excessive femoral anteversion,
genu valgum, external tibial torsion, and foot pronation. The
Q-angle should be measured and recorded with the patient's
knee both in the slightly flexed (Figure 18-1) and 90 degree
flexed (seated) position (Figure 18-2). This angle is created
by the formation of 2 lines on the lower extremity. The first
line connects the anterior superior iliac spine to the center
of the patella, and the second connects the center of the
patella to the center of the tibial tubercle. The average Q-
angle is 10 degrees in males and 15 degrees in females, and
it should not be more than 8 degrees at 90 degrees of flexion.

## Table 18-1

# HELPFUL HINTS

## Risk Factor

| PATHOANATOMY | PHYSICAL EXAM/ RADIOGRAPHIC FINDINGS | EFFECT ON PATELLOFEMORAL JOINT |
|---|---|---|
| Excessive femoral antetorsion | Greater hip internal rotation than external rotation | Intoeing gate/genu valgum/ increased Q-angle |
| Genu valgum | Increased valgus angle at knee | Increased Q-angle |
| Pes planus | Hindfoot valgus, forefoot supination, and abduction | Increased genu valgum/Q-angle |
| Patellar dysplasia | Abnormal morphology seen on axial x-ray or CT scan | Decreased bony restraint to lateral subluxation/dislocation |
| Trochlear dysplasia | Shallow trochlea groove seen on axial x-ray or CT scan | Decreased bony restraint to lateral subluxation/dislocation |
| Patella alta | Insall-Salvati ratio >1.2 or Blackburne-Peel ratio >1.0 on weight-bearing lateral x-ray | Decreased bony contact in extension/decreased resistance to lateral subluxation |
| Vastus medialis obliquus atrophy | Wasting of vastus medialis obliquus | Decreased dynamic control of patella |
| Ligamentous laxity | Increased pliability of soft tissues, hyperextension of joints | Increased pliability of medial soft tissues |
| Medial patellofemoral ligament injury | Tenderness at medial epicondyle, increase lateral patellar glide | Loss of main soft tissue restraint to lateral translation |

## Imaging

| IMAGE | PERTINENT IMAGE VIEWS | FINDINGS |
|---|---|---|
| Plain radiographs (x-rays) | Weight-bearing 30 degrees flexed PA bilateral knees, weight-bearing 30 degrees flexed lateral, Merchant view | Assess for patellar tilt, patellar subluxation, trochlear dysplasia, and patellar height |
| Computed tomography (CT) | Axial | Evaluate for patellar or trochlear dysplasia |
| Magnetic resonance imaging (MRI) | Axial | Evaluate for medial patellofemoral ligament injury, hemarthrosis, osteochondral injuries of the medial patellar facet, and lateral femoral condyle |

**Figure 18-1.** Supine Q-angle.

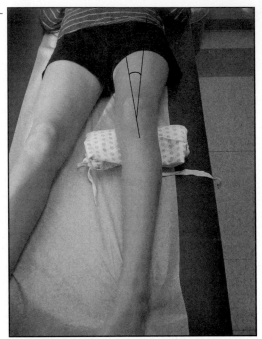

**Figure 18-2.** 90 degree (seated) Q-angle.

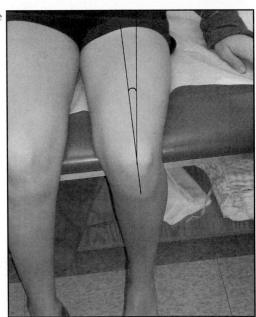

In patients with lateral subluxation of the patella, the Q-angle can be falsely low if the angle is measured with the knee in full extension.

Palpation of the entire patella (including patellar facets) and parapatellar structures should be performed to assess for an effusion or any areas of tenderness. Specifically, tenderness at the medial epicondyle could be indicative of an injury to the medial patellofemoral ligament in acute or recurrent instability (Bassett's sign):

- Joint range of motion as well as muscle strength and tightness should be evaluated. As this is performed, the patellofemoral joint should be palpated for signs of crepitus. Range of motion is followed by ligament testing including Lachman exam, anterior/posterior drawer, pivot shift test, rotatory instability tests, and stability to varus and valgus stresses. Because ligament injury can occur in the setting of acute patellofemoral dislocation, these must be assessed.

The remainder of the physical exam focuses on the patellofemoral joint and begins with assessing patellar tilt. The examiner raises the lateral facet of the patella off of the lateral trochlea. The inability to raise the lateral facet to the horizontal position suggests tightness of the lateral retinacular tissues.

Determining the patellar glide assesses patella mobility and is done by applying a medially and then laterally directed force to the patella. The number of quadrants the patella can be displaced is recorded and compared to the contralateral side. Typically, the patella cannot be translated more than half its width medially or laterally. This test is performed in the extended position and repeated with the knee in 30 to 45 degrees of flexion. As a lateral pressure is applied, the examiner observes the patient for signs of discomfort or reflex quadriceps activation. If this lateral pressure recreates the patient's subluxation symptoms, it is a positive apprehension test. If the patient is unable to relax the quadriceps, this test is difficult to perform and may also be done in the prone position with the knee off the table.[6]

Next, the examiner assesses patellar tracking as the knee is brought from flexion to extension. Typically, the patella follows a straight line while centered in the trochlea as the knee is brought from flexion to extension. In cases with lateral subluxation, there will be lateral movement of the patella as the knee reaches terminal extension, termed the "J" sign (Table 18-2).

## PATHOANATOMY

There are several anatomic locations that need to be addressed when evaluating for patellofemoral joint instability. The bony alignment of the lower limb must be evaluated, including the presence of increased femoral antetorsion, genu valgum, and pes planus. These pathologic processes effectively increase the Q-angle and, therefore, may be a predisposing factor to lateral subluxation/dislocation.

Pathologies specific to the patellofemoral joint include patellar dysplasia, trochlear dysplasia, and the presence of patella alta. These 3 conditions reduce the contact area of the patellofemoral joint and, therefore, decrease the force necessary for patella dislocation.

Soft tissue abnormalities, including vastus medialis obliquus atrophy, may also contribute to patellofemoral instability. Decreased strength of the vastus medialis obliquus leads to an unbalanced vastus lateralis and, therefore, a tendency toward lateral translation of the patella. Additionally, patients with general ligamentous laxity may be susceptible to patellofemoral subluxation secondary to the structural abnormality of the collagen within their tissues.

In cases of acute primary dislocation, there is often damage to the medial patellofemoral ligament, the primary soft tissue stabilizer to lateral translation of the patella. Other areas of potential injury include the medial patellar facet and lateral femoral condyle, as these 2 areas often contact each other in acute patellofemoral dislocations.

## IMAGING

Standard radiographs include posteroanterior weight-bearing views of both knees in 45 degrees of flexion, lateral views, and Merchant views. The Merchant view, in particular, is used to assess for patellar tilt, subluxation, and trochlear dysplasia.

**Table 18-2**

## METHODS FOR EXAMINING THE UNSTABLE KNEE

| Examination | Technique | Illustration | Grading | Significance |
|---|---|---|---|---|
| Range of motion | Examine passive and active | 1. Flexion<br>2. Extension | | Hamstring tightness and flexion contractures can contribute to anterior knee pain |
| Strength testing | Manual strength testing: flexion and extension | | Grade 5 = Full strength<br>Grade 4 = <Full strength<br>Grade 3 = Movement against gravity<br>Grade 2 = Movement with gravity eliminated<br>Grade 1 = Visible contraction | |
| Patellar tilt | Lift lateral facet away from lateral femoral trochlea | 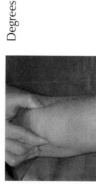 | Degrees | Inability to lift lateral facet to horizontal signifies lateral retinacular tightness |

*(continued)*

**Table 18-2 (continued)**

## METHODS FOR EXAMINING THE UNSTABLE KNEE

| Examination | Technique | Illustration | Grading | Significance |
|---|---|---|---|---|
| Patellar glide | Apply medial and lateral force to patella; Repeat at 30 to 45 degrees of flexion | 1. Medial 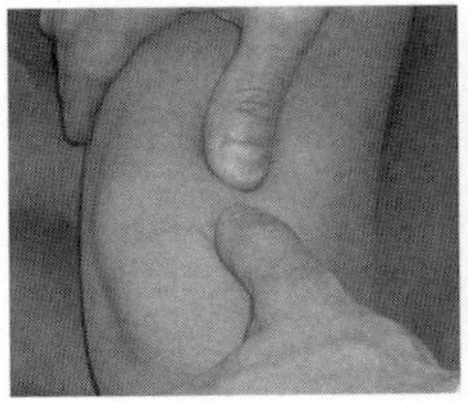    2. Lateral 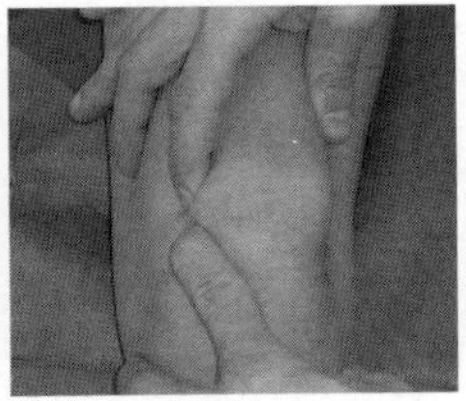 | Quadrants | Glide greater than 2 quadrants may signify patellofemoral instability |
| Bassett's sign | Palpate the medial epicondyle | | Positive = Tenderness | Indicates potential injury to the medial patellofemoral ligament |

(continued)

**Table 18-2 (continued)**

## METHODS FOR EXAMINING THE UNSTABLE KNEE

| Examination | Technique | Illustration | Grading | Significance |
|---|---|---|---|---|
| Apprehension sign | Apply lateral pressure to patella testing lateral mobility | 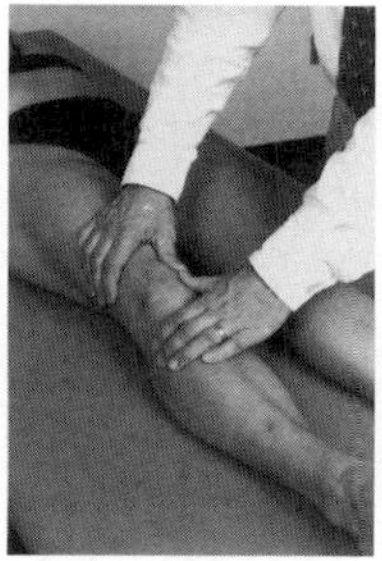 Reprinted with permission from Konin JG, Wiksten DL, Isear Jr JA, Brader H. Special Tests for Orthopedic Examination. 3rd ed. Thorofare, NJ: SLACK Incorporated; 2006. | Positive = Reproduction of instability symptoms or reflex quadriceps activation | Indicates lateral patella instability |

*Patellofemoral Instability MRI Findings*

| STRUCTURE | MRI FINDING |
|---|---|
| Medial patellofemoral ligament | Tearing, attenuation, edema (midsubstance, patellar attachment, medial epicondyle attachment) |
| Medial patella facet | Bone edema, osteochondral defect |
| Lateral femora condyle | Bone edema, osteochondral defect |
| Patella | ± Dysplasia |
| Trochlea | ± Dysplasia |
| Joint | ± Hemarthrosis |

*(continued)*

**Table 18-2 (continued)**

## METHODS FOR EXAMINING THE UNSTABLE KNEE

*Pertinent Anatomy in Patellofemoral Instability*

| STRUCTURE(S) | FUNCTION | IMPORTANCE |
|---|---|---|
| Trochlear groove | Provides bony restraint to lateral translation of the patella at extension and early flexion | A shallow trochlear groove allows increased lateral translation of the patella |
| Quadriceps and patellar tendons | Provides posterior force during flexion, providing increased patellar stability | A relatively long patellar tendon (patella alta) is associated with decreased patellar contact areas and increased patellar instability |
| Iliotibial band | Attaches to the patella and quadriceps tendon and provides resistance to medial translation of the patella | Tightness causes lateral tracking of the patella |
| Lateral patellofemoral band | Provides resistance to medial translation of the patella | Tightness causes lateral tracking of the patella |
| Medial patellofemoral ligament | Primary passive soft-tissue restraint to lateral displacement of the patella | Injury allows increased lateral translation of the patella |
| Vastus Medialis obliquus | Provides dynamic restraint to lateral translation of the patella | First quadriceps muscle to weaken with decreased function; allows increased lateral translation |

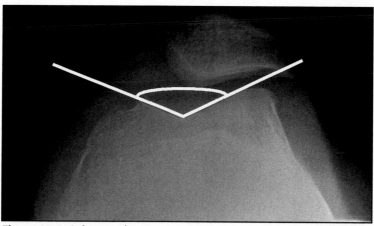

**Figure 18-3.** Sulcus angle.

On the Merchant view taken at 45 degrees of flexion, the sulcus angle can be measured as the angle created by the highest points on the medial and lateral condyles and the lowest point in the intercondylar sulcus[7] (Figure 18-3). The average sulcus angle is 138 degrees (±6 degrees),[8] and an angle greater than 145 degrees is consistent with trochlear hypoplasia.[9]

The congruence angle is used to measure the relationship of the patella to the trochlear groove and is determined by first drawing a line bisecting the sulcus angle to establish a zero reference line. A line is also drawn from the lowest point in the intercondylar sulcus to the lowest point on the patellar articular ridge. The angle between this line and the zero reference line is the congruence angle (Figure 18-4). The average congruence angle is 6 degrees medial, and an angle greater than 16 degrees lateral is abnormal at the 95th percentile.[8]

The lateral patellofemoral angle is taken at 20 degrees of flexion and is used to measure the patellar tilt. This angle is calculated by drawing 2 lines, one connecting the highest points on the medial and lateral femoral condyles and another line joining the limits of the lateral patellar facet. The angle between these 2 lines is the lateral patellofemoral angle and is typically open laterally in normal individuals. Parallel lines or an angle that opens medially is worrisome for patellar instability and subluxation.[10]

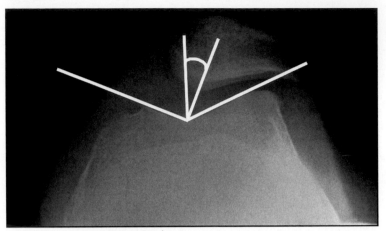

**Figure 18-4.** Congruence angle.

Several measurements have been used to determine patellar height. Classically, the Insall-Salvati ratio is defined as the distance from the inferior pole of the patella to the tibial tubercle (patellar tendon length) divided by the greatest diagonal length of the patella. A ratio greater than 1.2 signifies patella alta, while a ratio less than 0.8 signifies patella baja.[11] The Blackburne-Peel ratio has been shown to have better interobserver reliability[12,13] and is defined as the patellar articular surface length (AL) divided by the perpendicular length (PL) from the lower pole of the articular surface of the patella to the tibial plateau line (Figure 18-5).[14] A ratio greater than 1.0 signifies patella alta, while a ratio less than 0.5 indicates patella baja.

Computed tomography is useful in defining the bony anatomy of the femoral trochlea and tibial tubercle and can be used to determine the tibial tuberosity-to-trochlear groove distance by superimposing axial images of the tibial tubercle and trochlear groove with the knee in full extension. The distance is then measured on this superimposed image and is normally 10 to 15 mm (Figure 18-6).[15]

Magnetic resonance imaging (MRI) is most useful for evaluating soft tissue structures, including injury to the medial patellofemoral ligament.[16] Additional MRI findings in acute patellofemoral dislocations include bony edema, osteochondral damage to the medial patellar facet and the lateral femoral condyle, and the presence of a hemarthrosis (Figure 18-7).[17]

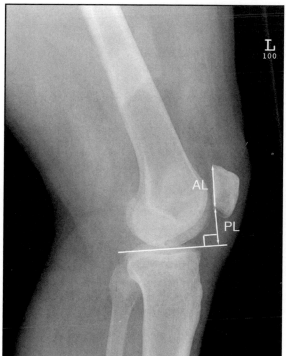

**Figure    18-5.**
Blackburne-Peel ratio.

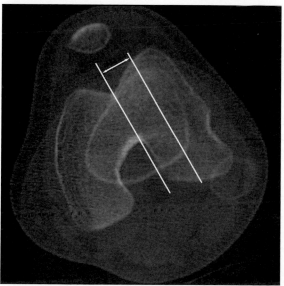

**Figure    18-6.**
Tibial tuberosity to trochlear groove distance.

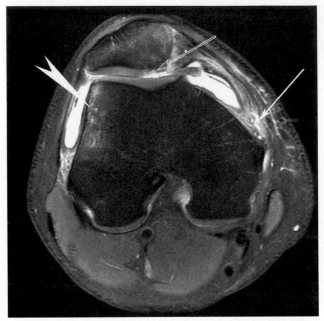

**Figure 18-7.** Axial MRI image after a patellar dislocation showing injury to the MPFL (solid arrow), medial patellar facet (arrow), and lateral femoral condyle (arrowhead).

# MANAGEMENT

## Conservative

Initial treatment after a patellar dislocation focuses on reducing swelling, promoting quadriceps activity, and restoring range of motion. Several studies have explored the outcomes of various nonoperative treatment protocols ranging from patellar taping and braces to immobilization in cylinder casts.[18,19] In general, primary nonoperative treatment for acute patellar dislocations should consist of a brief period of immobilization followed by functional rehabilitation.[19] Patellar bracing during this rehabilitation phase may be beneficial in improving patellofemoral contact area and alignment.[20]

In patients with chronic patellar instability, nonoperative treatment should focus on physical therapy to regain motion, proprioception, and strength of the quadriceps and gluteal muscles.[5] Additional methods, such as patellar taping, may be beneficial in activating the vastus medialis obliquus and decreasing patellar instability.[21]

# Operative

There are more than 100 operative techniques described in the literature for the treatment of patellar instability with no clear advantage of any one technique. These procedures can be broadly classified into soft tissue, bony procedures, or both. Ultimately, the performed surgical procedure should address the underlying pathology and often consists of a combination of procedures from both categories.

## Soft Tissue Procedures

Soft tissue procedures include lateral release, medial repair, medial imbrication, and medial patellofemoral ligament reconstruction. Lateral release of tight retinacular structures can be performed either arthroscopically or open, but is associated with a high recurrence rate when performed alone for patellofemoral instability.[22] It is, however, often used in combination with other soft tissue or bony procedures.

Acute primary repair and medial imbrication procedures can also be performed arthroscopically or open, but have largely fallen out of favor. While acute repair after a primary patellar dislocation seems tempting, several studies have shown no benefit when compared to conservative treatment.[23,24] Medial imbrication has been criticized as a nonanatomic repair and potentially over-tightens the medial soft tissues, creating abnormal patellofemoral motion.[25] Additionally, this procedure fails to address the pathology of the patellofemoral ligament.[5,26]

Several methods of medial patellofemoral ligament reconstruction have been described with various graft choices and methods of fixation. While results are relatively preliminary, they are promising, with several authors reporting success in preventing future subluxations or dislocations.[27-29] One cadaveric study has suggested that medial patellofemoral ligament reconstruction provides more stability against a lateral subluxation force than does a medial tibial tubercle transfer.[26] Ligament reconstruction has been advocated in cases with

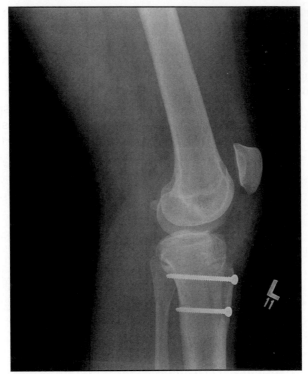

**Figure 18-8.** Postoperative x-ray after a tibial tubercle osteotomy.

recurrent instability, normal patellar height, normal tibial tuberosity to trochlear groove distance,[5] and in cases with trochlea dysplasia.[30]

## Bone Procedures

The tibial tubercle osteotomy and transfer has been used for the treatment of patellofemoral instability for several decades, particularly in situations where the tibial tuberosity to trochlear groove distance is increased.[5] Several different variations of tubercle osteotomies have been described, including the medial transfer (Elmslie-Trillat procedure)[31] and the antero-medial transfer (Fulkerson osteotomy)[32] (Figure 18-8). Good results have been reported with both procedures[33,34] for the treatment of instability; however, thorough preoperative evaluation should be performed to ensure that there is no evidence of patellofemoral articular cartilage damage. Some authors have advised against performing a transfer in cases where there is proximal, medial, or diffuse patellar chondral damage.[35]

Trochleoplasty is another bony procedure designed to treat patellar instability in cases with trochlear dysplasia. Trochleoplasty has been used in Europe with variable results.[36] However, concerns regarding its effectiveness and articular cartilage viability has limited its use in the United States.[5]

## CONCLUSION

The diagnosis and treatment of patellofemoral instability requires a thorough understanding of the physical exam and radiographic findings. While nonoperative treatment is often successful in cases of acute primary dislocation, surgical intervention is often required for the treatment of recurrent instability. The correct surgical procedure addresses the areas of pathology as outlined in this chapter.

## REFERENCES

1. Harilainen A, Myllynen P, Antila H, Seitsalo S. The significance of arthroscopy and examination under anaesthesia in the diagnosis of fresh injury haemarthrosis of the knee joint. *Injury.* 1988;19(1):21-24.
2. Fithian DC, Paxton EW, Stone ML, et al. Epidemiology and natural history of acute patellar dislocation. *Am J Sports Med.* 2004;32(5):1114-1121.
3. Hawkins RJ, Bell RH, Anisette G. Acute patellar dislocations. The natural history. *Am J Sports Med.* 1986;14(2):117-120.
4. Atkin DM, Fithian DC, Marangi KS, Stone ML, Dobson BE, Mendelsohn C. Characteristics of patients with primary acute lateral patellar dislocation and their recovery within the first 6 months of injury. *Am J Sports Med.* 2000;28(4):472-479.
5. Colvin AC, West RV. Patellar instability. *J Bone Joint Surg Am.* 2008;90(12):2751-2762.
6. Boden BP, Pearsall AW, Garrett WE Jr, Feagin JA Jr. Patellofemoral instability: evaluation and management. *J Am Acad Orthop Surg.* 1997;5(1):47-57.
7. Brattstroem H. Shape of the intercondylar groove normally and in recurrent dislocation of patella. A clinical and x-ray-anatomical investigation. *Acta Orthop Scand Suppl.* 1964;68(SUPPL 68):61-148.

8. Merchant AC, Mercer RL, Jacobsen RH, Cool CR. Roentgenographic analysis of patellofemoral congruence. *J Bone Joint Surg Am.* 1974;56(7):1391-1396.

9. Dejour H, Walch G, Nove-Josserand L, Guier C. Factors of patellar instability: an anatomic radiographic study. *Knee Surg Sports Traumatol Arthrosc.* 1994;2(1):19-26.

10. Laurin CA, Dussault R, Levesque HP. The tangential x-ray investigation of the patellofemoral joint: x-ray technique, diagnostic criteria and their interpretation. *Clin Orthop Relat Res.* 1979;(144):16-26.

11. Insall J, Salvati E. Patella position in the normal knee joint. *Radiology.* 1971;101(1):101-104.

12. Seil R, Muller B, Georg T, Kohn D, Rupp S. Reliability and interobserver variability in radiological patellar height ratios. *Knee Surg Sports Traumatol Arthrosc.* 2000;8(4):231-236.

13. Berg EE, Mason SL, Lucas MJ. Patellar height ratios. A comparison of four measurement methods. *Am J Sports Med.* 1996;24(2):218-221.

14. Blackburne JS, Peel TE. A new method of measuring patellar height. *J Bone Joint Surg Br.* 1977;59(2):241-242.

15. Dejour D, Le Coultre B. Osteotomies in patello-femoral instabilities. *Sports Med Arthrosc.* 2007;15(1):39-46.

16. Sanders TG, Morrison WB, Singleton BA, Miller MD, Cornum KG. Medial patellofemoral ligament injury following acute transient dislocation of the patella: MR findings with surgical correlation in 14 patients. *J Comput Assist Tomogr.* 2001;25(6):957-962.

17. Kirsch MD, Fitzgerald SW, Friedman H, Rogers LF. Transient lateral patellar dislocation: diagnosis with MR imaging. *AJR Am J Roentgenol.* 1993;161(1):109-113.

18. Maenpaa H, Lehto MU. Patellar dislocation. The long-term results of nonoperative management in 100 patients. *Am J Sports Med.* 1997;25(2):213-217.

19. Stefancin JJ, Parker RD. First-time traumatic patellar dislocation: a systematic review. *Clin Orthop Relat Res.* 2007;455:93-101.

20. Powers CM, Ward SR, Chan LD, Chen YJ, Terk MR. The effect of bracing on patella alignment and patellofemoral joint contact area. *Med Sci Sports Exerc.* 2004;36(7):1226-1232.

21. Cowan SM, Bennell KL, Hodges PW. Therapeutic patellar taping changes the timing of vasti muscle activation in people with patellofemoral pain syndrome. *Clin J Sport Med.* 2002;12(6):339-347.

22. Kolowich PA, Paulos LE, Rosenberg TD, Farnsworth S. Lateral release of the patella: indications and contraindications. *Am J Sports Med.* 1990;18(4):359-365.

23. Christiansen SE, Jakobsen BW, Lund B, Lind M. Isolated repair of the medial patellofemoral ligament in primary dislocation of the patella: a prospective randomized study. *Arthroscopy.* 2008;24(8):881-887.

24. Sillanpaa PJ, Maenpaa HM, Mattila VM, Visuri T, Pihlajamaki H. Arthroscopic surgery for primary traumatic patellar dislocation: a prospective, nonrandomized study comparing patients treated with and without acute arthroscopic stabilization with a median 7-year follow-up. *Am J Sports Med.* 2008;36(12):2301-2309.

25. Ostermeier S, Holst M, Hurschler C, Windhagen H, Stukenborg-Colsman C. Dynamic measurement of patellofemoral kinematics and contact pressure after lateral retinacular release: an in vitro study. *Knee Surg Sports Traumatol Arthrosc.* 2007;15(5):547-554.

26. Ostermeier S, Stukenborg-Colsman C, Hurschler C, Wirth CJ. In vitro investigation of the effect of medial patellofemoral ligament reconstruction and medial tibial tuberosity transfer on lateral patellar stability. *Arthroscopy.* 2006;22(3):308-319.

27. Panagopoulos A, van Niekerk L, Triantafillopoulos IK. MPFL reconstruction for recurrent patella dislocation: a new surgical technique and review of the literature. *Int J Sports Med.* 2008;29(5):359-365.

28. Mikashima Y, Kimura M, Kobayashi Y, Miyawaki M, Tomatsu T. Clinical results of isolated reconstruction of the medial patellofemoral ligament for recurrent dislocation and subluxation of the patella. *Acta Orthop Belg.* 2006;72(1):65-71.

29. Nomura E, Inoue M. Hybrid medial patellofemoral ligament reconstruction using the semitendinous tendon for recurrent patellar dislocation: minimum 3 years' follow-up. *Arthroscopy.* 2006;22(7):787-793.

30. Steiner TM, Torga-Spak R, Teitge RA. Medial patellofemoral ligament reconstruction in patients with lateral patellar instability and trochlear dysplasia. *Am J Sports Med.* 2006;34(8):1254-1261.

31. Trillat A, Dejour H, Couette A. Diagnosis and treatment of recurrent dislocations of the patella. *Rev Chir Orthop Reparatrice Appar Mot.* 1964;50:813-824.

32. Fulkerson JP, Becker GJ, Meaney JA, Miranda M, Folcik MA. Anteromedial tibial tubercle transfer without bone graft. *Am J Sports Med.* 1990;18(5):490-496; discussion 496-497.

33. Barber FA, McGarry JE. Elmslie-Trillat procedure for the treatment of recurrent patellar instability. *Arthroscopy.* 2008;24(1):77-81.

34. Pritsch T, Haim A, Arbel R, Snir N, Shasha N, Dekel S. Tailored tibial tubercle transfer for patellofemoral malalignment: analysis of clinical outcomes. *Knee Surg Sports Traumatol Arthrosc.* 2007;15(8):994-1002.

35. Pidoriano AJ, Weinstein RN, Buuck DA, Fulkerson JP. Correlation of patellar articular lesions with results from anteromedial tibial tubercle transfer. *Am J Sports Med.* 1997;25(4):533-537.

36. Verdonk R, Jansegers E, Stuyts B. Trochleoplasty in dysplastic knee trochlea. *Knee Surg Sports Traumatol Arthrosc.* 2005;13(7):529-533.

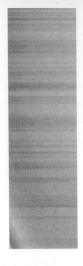

# FINANCIAL DISCLOSURES

*Dr. Olufemi R. Ayeni* has no financial or proprietary interest in the materials presented herein.

*Dr. Martin Beck* has no financial or proprietary interest in the materials presented herein.

*Dr. Asheesh Bedi* has not disclosed any relevant financial relationships.

*Dr. James P. Bradley* receives royalties and research grants from Arthrex.

*Dr. Robert L. Buly* is a stock holder for Pivot Medical.

*Dr. Sunny Cheung* has no financial or proprietary interest in the materials presented herein.

*Dr. Mark Drakos* has no financial or proprietary interest in the materials presented herein.

*Dr. Freddie H. Fu* receives research and educational funding from Smith & Nephew.

*Dr. Reinhold Ganz* is a consultant for Pivot Medical.

*Dr. Christopher D. Harner* receives research funding from DePuy Mitek and Smith & Nephew.

*Dr. Victor M. Ilizaliturri Jr* is a consultant and paid speaker for and receives research support and royalties from Smith & Nephew Endoscopy. He is also a paid speaker and consultant for Buimet Orthopaedics.

*Dr. Michael S. H. Kain* has no financial or proprietary interest in the materials presented herein.

*Dr. Bryan T. Kelly* is a consultant for Pivot Medical and A-2 Surgical and an educational advisor for Smith & Nephew.

*Dr. Eric J. Kropf* has no financial or proprietary interest in the materials presented herein.

*Dr. Michael Leunig* has no financial or proprietary interest in the materials presented herein.

*Dr. C. Benjamin Ma* receives research support from Wyeth Histogenics.

*Dr. Hal David Martin* is a consultant for Smith & Nephew and Pivot Medical

*Dr. RobRoy L. Martin* has not disclosed any relevant financial relationships.

*Dr. Douglas N. Mintz* has no financial or proprietary interest in the materials presented herein.

*Dr. Ryan G. Miyamoto* has no financial or proprietary interest in the materials presented herein.

*Dr. Nicola Mondanelli* has no financial or proprietary interest in the materials presented herein.

*Dr. Volker Musahl* has no financial or proprietary interest in the materials presented herein.

*Dr. Michael H. Ngo* has not disclosed any relevant financial relationships.

Dr. *Andrew D. Pearle* has no financial or proprietary interest in the materials presented herein.

Dr. *Marc J. Philippon* receives a grant or research support from Smith & Nephew Endoscopy, Ossur, Arthrex, Savcony, OrthoRehab, Opedix, and Siemens. He receives royalties from Smith & Nephew, Arthrosurface, Bledsoe, and DonJoy. He receives publishing support from SLACK Incorporated. He is a consultant and stock holder for Smith & Nephew and also holds stock in Arthrosurface.

Dr. *Anil Ranawat* is a consultant and owns stock in Conformis. He is also a consultant for Mako.

Dr. *Bradley S. Raphael* has no financial or proprietary interest in the materials presented herein.

Dr. *Keith R. Reinhardt* has no financial or proprietary interest in the materials presented herein.

Dr. *Scott A. Rodeo* has no financial or proprietary interest in the materials presented herein.

Dr. *James R. Romanowski* has no financial or proprietary interest in the materials presented herein.

Dr. *Jon K. Sekiya* is a consultant, receives royalties, and is a stock holder for OrthoDynamix, LLC.

Dr. *Seth L. Sherman* has no financial or proprietary interest in the materials presented herein.

Dr. *Matthew V. Smith* has no financial or proprietary interest in the materials presented herein.

Dr. *Russell F. Warren* has no financial or proprietary interest in the materials presented herein.

Dr. *Thomas L. Wickiewicz* receives royalties from Mako Surgical.

Dr. *Riley J. Williams III* has not disclosed any relevant financial relationships.

Dr. *Andrew K. Wong* has no financial or proprietary interest in the materials presented herein.

# INDEX

# Wait...There's More!

Throughout the *Musculoskeletal Examination Series*, you will find a thorough review of the most common pathologic conditions, techniques for diagnosis, and appropriate treatment methods. These pocket-sized books include very clear photographic demonstrations, tables, and charts, taking complex subjects and bringing them to a level that will be welcomed by all.

**Series Editor: Steven B. Cohen, MD**

## Musculoskeletal Examination of the Foot and Ankle: Making the Complex Simple

Shepard R. Hurwitz, MD; Selene Parekh, MD

275 pp., Soft Cover, 2011, ISBN 13 978-1-55642-919-4, Order #19193, **$44.95**

## Musculoskeletal Examination of the Hip and Knee: Making the Complex Simple

Anil Ranawat, MD; Bryan T. Kelly, MD

480 pp., Soft Cover, 2011, ISBN 13 978-1-55642-920-0, Order #19207, **$48.95**

## Musculoskeletal Examination of the Shoulder: Making the Complex Simple

Steven B. Cohen, MD

240 pp., Soft Cover, 2011, ISBN 13 978-1-55642-912-5, Order #19126, **$44.95**

## Musculoskeletal Examination of the Spine: Making the Complex Simple

Jeffrey A. Rihn, MD; Eric B. Harris, MD

275 pp., Soft Cover, 2011, ISBN 13 978-1-55642-996-5, Order #19965, **$44.95**

## Musculoskeletal Examination of the Elbow, Wrist, and Hand: Making the Complex Simple

Randall Culp, MD

275 pp., Soft Cover, 2011, ISBN 13 978-1-55642-918-7, Order #19185, **$44.95**

---

Please visit **www.slackbooks.com** to order any of the above title

*24 Hours a Day...7 Days a Week!*

# Attention Industry Partners!

Whether you are interested in buying multiple copies of a book, chapter reprints, or looking for something new and different — we are able to accommodate your needs.

## MULTIPLE COPIES

At attractive discounts starting for purchases as low as 25 copies for a single title, SLACK Incorporated will be able to meet all your of your needs.

## CHAPTER REPRINTS

SLACK Incorporated is able to offer the chapters you want in a format that will lead to success. Bound with an attractive cover, use the chapters that are a fit specifically for your company. Available for quantities of 100 or more.

## CUSTOMIZE

SLACK Incorporated is able to create a specialized custom version of any of our products specifically for your company.

*Please contact the Marketing Communications Director for further details on multiple copy purchases, chapter reprints, or custom printing at 1-800-257-8290 or 1-856-848-1000.*

*\*Please note all conditions are subject to change.*

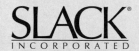